Ophthalmic Pathology and Intraocular Tumors

Section 4
2007–2008

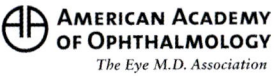

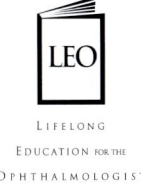

LIFELONG
EDUCATION FOR THE
OPHTHALMOLOGIST

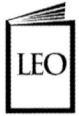 The Basic and Clinical Science Course is one component of the Lifelong Education for the Ophthalmologist (LEO) framework, which assists members in planning their continuing medical education. LEO includes an array of clinical education products that members may select to form individualized, self-directed learning plans for updating their clinical knowledge. Active members or fellows who use LEO components may accumulate sufficient CME credits to earn the LEO Award. Contact the Academy's Clinical Education Division for further information on LEO.

> The American Academy of Ophthalmology is accredited by the Accreditation Council for Continuing Medical Education to provide continuing medical education for physicians.
>
> The American Academy of Ophthalmology designates this educational activity for a maximum of 30 *AMA PRA Category 1 Credits*™. Physicians should only claim credit commensurate with the extent of their participation in the activity.

The Academy provides this material for educational purposes only. It is not intended to represent the only or best method or procedure in every case, nor to replace a physician's own judgment or give specific advice for case management. Including all indications, contraindications, side effects, and alternative agents for each drug or treatment is beyond the scope of this material. All information and recommendations should be verified, prior to use, with current information included in the manufacturers' package inserts or other independent sources, and considered in light of the patient's condition and history. Reference to certain drugs, instruments, and other products in this course is made for illustrative purposes only and is not intended to constitute an endorsement of such. Some material may include information on applications that are not considered community standard, that reflect indications not included in approved FDA labeling, or that are approved for use only in restricted research settings. The FDA has stated that it is the responsibility of the physician to determine the FDA status of each drug or device he or she wishes to use, and to use them with appropriate patient consent in compliance with applicable law. The Academy specifically disclaims any and all liability for injury or other damages of any kind, from negligence or otherwise, for any and all claims that may arise from the use of any recommendations or other information contained herein.

Copyright © 2007
American Academy of Ophthalmology
All rights reserved
Printed in Singapore

Basic and Clinical Science Course

Thomas J. Liesegang, MD, Jacksonville, Florida, *Senior Secretary for Clinical Education*
Gregory L. Skuta, MD, Oklahoma City, Oklahoma, *Secretary for Ophthalmic Knowledge*
Louis B. Cantor, MD, Indianapolis, Indiana, *BCSC Course Chair*

Section 4

Faculty Responsible for This Edition

Debra J. Shetlar, MD, *Chair,* Houston, Texas
Patricia Chévez-Barrios, MD, Houston, Texas
Sander Dubovy, MD, Miami, Florida
Robert H. Rosa, Jr, MD, Temple, Texas
Nasreen Syed, MD, Iowa City, Iowa
Matthew W. Wilson, MD, Memphis, Tennessee
Ron W. Pelton, MD, PhD, Colorado Springs, Colorado
 Practicing Ophthalmologists Advisory Committee for Education

Jacob Pe'er, MD, *Consultant*, Jerusalem, Israel

Dr Rosa has received grant support from Eli Lilly & Company; (OSI) Eyetech, Inc; Genentech, Inc; and the National Eye Institute.

The other authors state that they have no significant financial interest or other relationship with the manufacturer of any commercial product discussed in the chapters that they contributed to this course or with the manufacturer of any competing commercial product.

Recent Past Faculty

Harry H. Brown, MD
Ben J. Glasgow, MD
Hans E. Grossniklaus, MD
Timothy G. Murray, MD
David J. Wilson, MD

In addition, the Academy gratefully acknowledges the contributions of numerous past faculty and advisory committee members who have played an important role in the development of previous editions of the Basic and Clinical Science Course.

American Academy of Ophthalmology Staff

Richard A. Zorab, *Vice President, Ophthalmic Knowledge*
Hal Straus, *Director, Publications Department*
Carol L. Dondrea, *Publications Manager*
Christine Arturo, *Acquisitions Manager*
Nicole DuCharme, *Production Manager*
Stephanie Tanaka, *Medical Editor*
Steven Huebner, *Administrative Coordinator*

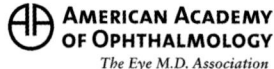

655 Beach Street
Box 7424
San Francisco, CA 94120-7424

Contents

General Introduction xiii

Objectives. 1
Introduction 3
Historical Introduction—The History of Ophthalmic Pathology 5

PART I Ophthalmic Pathology 9

1 Introduction to Part I 11
Organization 11
   Topography 12
   Disease Process 12
   General Diagnosis 18
   Differential Diagnosis 18

2 Wound Repair 21
General Aspects of Wound Repair 21
Healing in Specific Ocular Tissues 21
   Cornea 21
   Sclera 24
   Limbus 24
   Uvea 24
   Lens 26
   Retina 26
   Vitreous 26
   Eyelid, Orbit, and Lacrimal Tissues 26
Histologic Sequelae of Ocular Trauma 27

3 Specimen Handling 33
Communication 33
Orientation 34
Transillumination 35
Gross Dissection 35
Processing and Staining 37
   Fixatives 37
   Tissue Processing 37
   Tissue Staining 38

4 Special Procedures ... 41
Immunohistochemistry ... 41
Flow Cytometry, Molecular Pathology, and Diagnostic Electron
   Microscopy ... 44
      Flow Cytometry ... 44
      Molecular Pathology ... 46
      Diagnostic Electron Microscopy ... 47
Special Techniques ... 47
      Fine-Needle Aspiration Biopsy ... 47
      Frozen Section ... 50

5 Conjunctiva ... 53
Topography ... 53
Congenital Anomalies ... 53
      Choristomas ... 53
      Hamartomas ... 54
Inflammations ... 55
      Papillary versus Follicular Conjunctivitis ... 56
      Infectious Conjunctivitis ... 57
      Noninfectious Conjunctivitis ... 58
Degenerations ... 60
      Pinguecula and Pterygium ... 60
      Amyloid Deposits ... 61
Neoplasia ... 62
      Epithelial Lesions ... 62
      Subepithelial Lesions ... 66
      Melanocytic Lesions ... 68

6 Cornea ... 73
Topography ... 73
Congenital Anomalies ... 74
      Congenital Hereditary Endothelial Dystrophy ... 74
      Dermoid ... 75
      Posterior Keratoconus ... 76
      Sclerocornea ... 76
      Congenital Corneal Staphyloma ... 77
Inflammations ... 77
      Infectious ... 77
      Noninfectious ... 80
Degenerations and Dystrophies ... 80
      Degenerations ... 80
      Dystrophies ... 83
Pigment Deposits ... 88
Neoplasia ... 89

7 Anterior Chamber and Trabecular Meshwork ... 91
Topography ... 91
      Trabecular Beams and Endothelium ... 91

	Congenital Anomalies. 91
	Degenerations 94
		Iridocorneal Endothelial Syndrome 94
		Secondary Glaucoma With Material in the Trabecular Meshwork . . . 95
	Neoplasia 100

8 Sclera. 101
	Topography 101
		Episclera 101
		Stroma 101
		Lamina Fusca 102
	Congenital Anomalies. 102
		Choristoma 102
		Nanophthalmos 103
	Inflammations 103
		Episcleritis 103
		Scleritis 103
	Degenerations 105
	Neoplasia 106

9 Lens 109
	Topography 109
		Capsule 109
		Epithelium 109
		Cortex and Nucleus 109
		Zonular Fibers 109
	Congenital Anomalies. 110
		Ectopia Lentis 110
		Congenital Cataract 111
	Inflammations 112
		Phacoantigenic Endophthalmitis 112
		Phacolytic Glaucoma 113
		Propionibacterium acnes Endophthalmitis 113
	Degenerations 113
		Cataract and Other Abnormalities 113
	Neoplasia and Associations With Systemic Disorders 118
	Pathology of Intraocular Lenses 119
		Decentration 119
		Inflammation 120
		Corneal Complications 121
		Retinal Complications 121

10 Vitreous 123
	Topography 123
	Congenital Anomalies. 124
		Persistent Fetal Vasculature 124
		Bergmeister Papilla 125
		Mittendorf Dot 125

viii • Contents

```
        Peripapillary Vascular Loops . . . . . . . . . . . . . . 125
        Vitreous Cysts . . . . . . . . . . . . . . . . . . . . . 125
    Inflammations . . . . . . . . . . . . . . . . . . . . . . . 125
    Degenerations . . . . . . . . . . . . . . . . . . . . . . . 126
        Syneresis and Aging . . . . . . . . . . . . . . . . . . 126
        Hemorrhage . . . . . . . . . . . . . . . . . . . . . . 126
        Asteroid Hyalosis . . . . . . . . . . . . . . . . . . . 128
        Vitreous Amyloidosis . . . . . . . . . . . . . . . . . 128
        Posterior Vitreous Detachment . . . . . . . . . . . . 129
        Rhegmatogenous Retinal Detachment and
            Proliferative Vitreoretinopathy . . . . . . . . . . 130
        Macular Holes . . . . . . . . . . . . . . . . . . . . . 132
    Neoplasia . . . . . . . . . . . . . . . . . . . . . . . . . 133
        Intraocular Lymphoma . . . . . . . . . . . . . . . . 133
```

11 Retina and Retinal Pigment Epithelium 137

```
    Topography . . . . . . . . . . . . . . . . . . . . . . . . 137
        Retina . . . . . . . . . . . . . . . . . . . . . . . . . 137
        Retinal Pigment Epithelium . . . . . . . . . . . . . . 139
    Congenital Anomalies . . . . . . . . . . . . . . . . . . . 139
        Albinism . . . . . . . . . . . . . . . . . . . . . . . . 139
        Myelinated (Medullated) Nerve Fibers . . . . . . . . 142
        Vascular Anomalies . . . . . . . . . . . . . . . . . . 142
        Congenital Hypertrophy of the RPE . . . . . . . . . 142
    Inflammations . . . . . . . . . . . . . . . . . . . . . . . 144
        Infectious . . . . . . . . . . . . . . . . . . . . . . . 144
        Noninfectious . . . . . . . . . . . . . . . . . . . . . 146
    Degenerations . . . . . . . . . . . . . . . . . . . . . . . 147
        Typical and Reticular Peripheral Cystoid Degeneration . . . . . . 147
        Typical and Reticular Degenerative Retinoschisis . . . . . . . . . 147
        Lattice Degeneration . . . . . . . . . . . . . . . . . 148
        Paving-Stone Degeneration . . . . . . . . . . . . . . 149
        Ischemia . . . . . . . . . . . . . . . . . . . . . . . . 149
        Specific Ischemic Retinal Disorders . . . . . . . . . 156
        Diabetic Retinopathy . . . . . . . . . . . . . . . . . 159
        Retinopathy of Prematurity . . . . . . . . . . . . . 160
        Age-Related Macular Degeneration . . . . . . . . . 161
        Polypoidal Choroidal Vasculopathy . . . . . . . . . 165
        Macular Dystrophies . . . . . . . . . . . . . . . . . 167
        Generalized Chorioretinal Degeneration . . . . . . 171
    Neoplasia . . . . . . . . . . . . . . . . . . . . . . . . . 171
        Retinoblastoma . . . . . . . . . . . . . . . . . . . . 171
        Medulloepithelioma . . . . . . . . . . . . . . . . . . 176
        Fuchs Adenoma . . . . . . . . . . . . . . . . . . . . 177
        Combined Hamartoma of the Retina and RPE . . . 177
        Other Retinal Tumors . . . . . . . . . . . . . . . . 178
        Adenomas and Adenocarcinomas of the RPE . . . 178
```

12 Uveal Tract **179**
- Topography 179
  - Iris 179
  - Ciliary Body 180
  - Choroid 181
- Congenital Anomalies. 181
  - Aniridia 181
  - Coloboma 182
- Inflammations 182
  - Infectious 183
  - Noninfectious 183
- Degenerations 186
  - Rubeosis Iridis 186
  - Hyalinization of the Ciliary Body 187
  - Choroidal Neovascularization 187
- Neoplasia 187
  - Iris 187
  - Choroid and Ciliary Body 189
  - Metastatic Tumors 194
  - Other Uveal Tumors 195
- Trauma 197

13 Eyelids **199**
- Topography 199
- Congenital Anomalies. 201
  - Distichiasis 202
  - Phakomatous Choristoma 202
  - Dermoid Cyst 202
- Inflammations 202
  - Infectious 202
  - Noninfectious 203
- Degenerations 205
  - Xanthelasma 205
  - Amyloid 205
- Neoplasia 207
  - Epidermal Neoplasms 207
  - Dermal Neoplasms 213
  - Appendage Neoplasms 213
  - Melanocytic Neoplasms 215

14 Orbit **219**
- Topography 219
  - Bony Orbit and Soft Tissues 219
- Congenital Anomalies. 220
  - Dermoid and Other Epithelial Cysts 220

Inflammations 221
    Infectious 221
    Noninfectious 222
Degenerations 225
    Amyloid 225
Neoplasia 226
    Lacrimal Gland Neoplasia 226
    Lymphoproliferative Lesions 228
    Vascular Tumors 230
    Tumors With Muscle Differentiation 231
    Tumors With Fibrous Differentiation 234
    Bony Lesions of the Orbit 234
    Nerve Sheath Tumors 235
    Adipose Tumors 236
    Metastatic Tumors 236

15 Optic Nerve 237
Topography 237
Congenital Anomalies 239
    Pits 239
    Colobomas 239
Inflammations 239
    Infectious 239
    Noninfectious 240
Degenerations 241
    Optic Atrophy 241
    Drusen 242
Neoplasia 243
    Melanocytoma 243
    Glioma 243
    Meningioma 244

PART II Intraocular Tumors: Clinical Aspects 247

16 Introduction to Part II 249

17 Melanocytic Tumors 251
Iris Nevus 251
Nevus of the Ciliary Body or Choroid 251
Melanocytoma of the Iris, Ciliary Body, or Choroid 254
Iris Melanoma 254
Melanoma of the Ciliary Body or Choroid 259
    Diagnostic Evaluation 260
    Differential Diagnosis 264
    Classification 267
    Metastatic Evaluation 268
    Treatment 270
    Prognosis and Prognostic Factors 273

Pigmented Epithelial Tumors of the Uvea and Retina 275
    Adenoma and Adenocarcinoma. 275
    Acquired Hyperplasia 276
    Combined Hamartoma. 276

18 Angiomatous Tumors 277
Hemangiomas 277
    Choroidal Hemangiomas 277
    Retinal Angiomas. 280
Arteriovenous Malformation 283

19 Retinoblastoma 285
Genetic Counseling 285
Diagnostic Evaluation. 287
    Clinical Examination 291
    Differential Diagnosis 291
Classification. 294
Associated Conditions 296
    Retinocytoma 296
    Trilateral Retinoblastoma 296
Treatment 297
    Enucleation 297
    Chemotherapy. 298
    Photocoagulation and Hyperthermia 299
    Cryotherapy 300
    External-Beam Radiation Therapy 300
    Plaque Radiotherapy (Brachytherapy) 300
    Targeted Therapy 301
Spontaneous Regression 301
Prognosis 301

20 Secondary Tumors of the Eye. 305
Metastatic Carcinoma 305
    Primary Tumor Sites. 305
    Mechanisms of Metastasis to the Eye 306
    Clinical Evaluation 306
    Ancillary Tests 308
    Other Diagnostic Factors 310
    Prognosis 311
    Treatment 312
Direct Intraocular Extension 312

21 Lymphomatous Tumors 313
Intraocular Lymphoma 313
    Clinical Evaluation 313
    Pathologic Studies 314
    Treatment 315
    Prognosis 315

Uveal Lymphoid Infiltration 315
    Clinical Evaluation 315
    Pathologic Studies 315
    Treatment 316
    Prognosis 316

22 Ocular Manifestations of Leukemia 317

23 Rare Tumors 319
Medulloepithelioma 319
Leiomyomas, Neurilemomas, and Neurofibromas 319

Appendix: American Joint Committee on Cancer (AJCC) Definitions
    and Staging of Ocular Tumors, 2002 321
Basic Texts 331
Related Academy Materials 333
Credit Reporting Form 335
Study Questions 339
Answers 347
Index 351

General Introduction

The Basic and Clinical Science Course (BCSC) is designed to meet the needs of residents and practitioners for a comprehensive yet concise curriculum of the field of ophthalmology. The BCSC has developed from its original brief outline format, which relied heavily on outside readings, to a more convenient and educationally useful self-contained text. The Academy updates and revises the course annually, with the goals of integrating the basic science and clinical practice of ophthalmology and of keeping ophthalmologists current with new developments in the various subspecialties.

The BCSC incorporates the effort and expertise of more than 80 ophthalmologists, organized into 13 Section faculties, working with Academy editorial staff. In addition, the course continues to benefit from many lasting contributions made by the faculties of previous editions. Members of the Academy's Practicing Ophthalmologists Advisory Committee for Education serve on each faculty and, as a group, review every volume before and after major revisions.

Organization of the Course

The Basic and Clinical Science Course comprises 13 volumes, incorporating fundamental ophthalmic knowledge, subspecialty areas, and special topics:

1. Update on General Medicine
2. Fundamentals and Principles of Ophthalmology
3. Clinical Optics
4. Ophthalmic Pathology and Intraocular Tumors
5. Neuro-Ophthalmology
6. Pediatric Ophthalmology and Strabismus
7. Orbit, Eyelids, and Lacrimal System
8. External Disease and Cornea
9. Intraocular Inflammation and Uveitis
10. Glaucoma
11. Lens and Cataract
12. Retina and Vitreous
13. Refractive Surgery

In addition, a comprehensive Master Index allows the reader to easily locate subjects throughout the entire series.

References

Readers who wish to explore specific topics in greater detail may consult the journal references cited within each chapter and the Basic Texts section at the back of the book. These references are intended to be selective rather than exhaustive, chosen by the BCSC faculty as being important, current, and readily available to residents and practitioners.

Related Academy educational materials are also listed in the appropriate sections. They include books, audiovisual materials, self-assessment programs, clinical modules, and interactive programs.

Study Questions and CME Credit

Each volume of the BCSC is designed as an independent study activity for ophthalmology residents and practitioners. The learning objectives for this volume are given on page 1. The text, illustrations, and references provide the information necessary to achieve the objectives; the study questions allow readers to test their understanding of the material and their mastery of the objectives. Physicians who wish to claim CME credit for this educational activity may do so by mail, by fax, or online. The necessary forms and instructions are given at the end of the book.

Conclusion

The Basic and Clinical Science Course has expanded greatly over the years, with the addition of much new text and numerous illustrations. Recent editions have sought to place a greater emphasis on clinical applicability while maintaining a solid foundation in basic science. As with any educational program, it reflects the experience of its authors. As its faculties change and as medicine progresses, new viewpoints are always emerging on controversial subjects and techniques. Not all alternate approaches can be included in this series; as with any educational endeavor, the learner should seek additional sources, including such carefully balanced opinions as the Academy's Preferred Practice Patterns.

The BCSC faculty and staff are continuously striving to improve the educational usefulness of the course; you, the reader, can contribute to this ongoing process. If you have any suggestions or questions about the series, please do not hesitate to contact the faculty or the editors.

The authors, editors, and reviewers hope that your study of the BCSC will be of lasting value and that each Section will serve as a practical resource for quality patient care.

Objectives

Upon completion of BCSC Section 4, *Ophthalmic Pathology and Intraocular Tumors*, the reader should be able to

- describe a structured approach to understanding major ocular conditions based on a hierarchical framework of topography, disease process, general diagnosis, and differential diagnosis
- summarize the steps in handling ocular specimens for pathologic study, including obtaining, dissecting, processing, and staining tissues
- explain the basic principles of special procedures used in ophthalmic pathology, including immunohistochemistry, flow cytometry, molecular pathology, and diagnostic electron microscopy
- communicate effectively with the pathologist regarding types of specimens, processing, and techniques appropriate to the clinical situation
- summarize the histopathology of common ocular conditions
- correlate clinical and pathological findings
- list the steps in wound healing in ocular tissues
- summarize current information about the most common primary tumors of the eye
- identify those ophthalmic lesions that indicate systemic disease and/or are potentially life-threatening
- provide useful genetic information to families affected by retinoblastoma
- assess current and new treatment modalities for ocular tumors in terms of patient prognosis and ocular functioning

Introduction

This volume of the Basic and Clinical Science Course (BCSC), Section 4, *Ophthalmic Pathology and Intraocular Tumors*, is divided into 2 parts: Part I, Ophthalmic Pathology; and Part II, Intraocular Tumors: Clinical Aspects. Although these are 2 distinct disciplines, there is overlap, and it is critically important for the sight and life of the patient that the physician understand both the clinical and pathologic aspects of ocular neoplasia. The importance of correlating the clinical findings of other ophthalmic disciplines, such as cornea and retina, with the corresponding pathologic findings should not be neglected.

Part I, Ophthalmic Pathology, uses a hierarchy that moves from general to specific to help derive a differential diagnosis for a specific tissue. This concept was introduced by Curtis E. Margo, MD, and Hans E. Grossniklaus, MD, in the book *Ocular Histopathology: A Guide to Differential Diagnosis*, and it may be used as an organizational framework for the study of ophthalmic pathology.

Part II, Intraocular Tumors: Clinical Aspects, is a compilation of selected clinical aspects of importance to the general ophthalmologist. Because intraocular tumors may be both vision- and life-threatening, ophthalmologists must be aware of the basic principles of their diagnosis and treatment.

The tables that follow Part II outline the American Joint Committee on Cancer 2002 definitions and staging for the ocular and adnexal tumors discussed elsewhere in the book. These tables are referenced where appropriate throughout the main text.

HISTORICAL INTRODUCTION

The History of Ophthalmic Pathology

The establishment of ocular pathology as an independent science depended, obviously, on the development of our knowledge of the normal anatomy of the eye. Although animal eyes had been dissected for thousands of years, both Aristotle and Hippocrates held rather vague ideas about ocular anatomy. Only much later did the Greek school of Alexandria establish a formal structure of ocular anatomy. The first reports are by Rufus of Ephesus. He lived at the end of the first and the beginning of the second century AD and worked at least for a time in Egypt. His observations were astute, and, while he still believed that the crystalline lens was the seat of all vision, he wrote excellent descriptions of the anatomy of the eye and the orbit.

His counterpart in Rome was Aulus Cornelius Celsus, who lived from 25 BC to AD 50 and was the first to give us a systematic treatise on ophthalmology. However, he did not contribute anything original on the anatomy of the eye but rather followed the Greek authors in a slavish way.

The high point of anatomical work during the classical time was reached by the Greek physician Claudius Galenus (Galen). Galenus was born in AD 131 in Pergamon (Asia Minor) and died in Rome in AD 201. He was by far the most prominent of the physicians of Rome, and his anatomical descriptions remained in use until Zinn created the modern study of anatomy when he published his book in Gottingen in 1755.

Johann Gottfried Zinn was born in 1727 in Germany and was only 24 years old when he was appointed professor of medicine in Göttingen. At the same time, he became the director of the botanical gardens, and his important contributions to botany led Linnaeus to name a large family of flowers the zinnias. He died before he was 32. For a short time, Zinn was a pupil of the famous Swiss naturalist and physiologist Albrecht von Haller, who first described the cribriform plate and the ophthalmic artery with its branches. Zinn's book has remained the foundation of modern anatomy for the eye. The exact and detailed descriptions have made this work famous. The superb text by Zinn was later complemented by the beautiful atlas published by Samuel Thomas Soemmerring (1755–1830), which appeared in Frankfurt in 1801.

The next advance in normal anatomy study was a book by Julius Arnold that appeared in Leipzig in 1832, when the author was only 29 years old. He already used the microscope but not yet thin tissue sections.

The anatomical studies in the 19th century culminated in the book by Ernst von Brücke, who was born in Berlin and became a professor of physiology and anatomy in Vienna. In 1847 he wrote his anatomical description of the human eye. Von Brücke was the first to use thin sections to investigate the anatomical structures, and he found the longitudinal fibers of the ciliary muscle.

The first book on histology of the eye, written by Samuel Moritz Pappenheim (1811–1882), appeared in Breslau in 1842. The next step forward in this field was made by William Bowman in his book *Lectures on the Parts Concerned in the Operations on the Eye*, which appeared in 1849.

The first indications of a pathologic anatomy concerning vision appeared in the book *Sepulchretum*, published by Theophile Bonet. Bonet, who was born in 1620 in Geneva, died from rabies in his hometown in 1689. The book appeared in 1700 in Lyons. Among the cases described are an optic atrophy due to a brain tumor, a case of syphilis of the frontal bone, a large retinoblastoma, and a chiasmal cyst with optic atrophy.

A more systematic and extensive discussion of ocular pathology was written by Giambattista Morgagni, who first was an assistant to Valsalva (the pupil of Malpighi) in Bologna and then became professor of anatomy in Padua. He published his classic work *De Sedibus et Causis Morborum . . .* in 1761, when he was nearly 80 years old. His 13th letter gives an extensive description of pathologic changes of the visual organ. It contains excellent discussions of the pathologic anatomy of the cataract, vitreous opacities, and traumatic exophthalmos.

The first anatomical examination of diseased eyes occurred in the 18th century. The peculiar structure of the eye required special examination techniques, and these techniques developed slowly. It is therefore not surprising that the first real textbook on general pathologic anatomy, published by Mattias Baillie in London in 1793, does not discuss the visual organ at all.

The first book devoted entirely to ophthalmic pathology was written by James Wardrop (1782–1869), one of the foremost ophthalmologists of his time in the United Kingdom. He was born in Scotland but soon moved to London, where he became a member of the Royal College of Surgeons. After he had successfully treated the eye of a horse that belonged to the Prince Regent, he became the monarch's surgeon, and in 1828 he became surgeon to King George IV. His essays on the morbid anatomy of the human eye appeared in 1808, and a second volume was added in 1818. In his book Wardrop summarized numerous quotations from the world literature, adding valuable and important personal observations.

Although Wardrop was recognized for his scientific contributions, his personal life soon brought him into conflict with the establishment. As a convinced liberal, he was an ardent supporter of the Reform Movement, and his abrasive personality made him many enemies, especially at court. He withdrew from public life at an early age, hardly ever attended medical meetings, and was practically forgotten.

Albrecht von Graefe tells of being at a banquet in London in 1850. Seated next to him was James Wardrop. After they had introduced themselves, von Graefe asked Wardrop whether the author of the book on retinoblastoma, which had appeared in 1809, was his father or grandfather; Wardrop smiled and explained that he himself was the grandfather. Julius Hirschberg, a well-known ophthalmologist and historian, regarded Wardrop's books on pathology as a rich source of new and important facts destined to be of continuing value.

The second textbook on ocular pathologic anatomy was published by Dr. Matthias Johannes Albrecht Schoen in Hamburg in 1828. Schoen was born and practiced in that city. The book is complete in its contents and extremely well organized.

The third textbook was published by Friedrich August von Ammon. He was born in Göttingen in 1799 and became professor of pathology and pharmacology in Dresden in 1828. He later became surgeon to the court of Saxony. Many feel that von Ammon's contribution inaugurated the modern era of the study of pathologic anatomy of the eye.

Von Ammon's book was followed by a few important monographs, including one by John Dalrymple in English (1849–1852), one by Alan Williams Sichel in French (1852–1859), and one by George Theodor Ruete in German (1854–1860).

Heinrich Müller (1820–1864), a professor in Würzburg, is considered the founder of pathologic histology of the eye. He described the microscopic anatomy of the eye and its pathologic alterations. Müller made a number of important anatomical discoveries: the glial cells in the retina, the annular part of the ciliary muscle, and the smooth eyelid muscles are all named after him. At the same time, R. Albert Kolliker, one of the foremost histologists of his time, and Rudolf Virchow, the creator of modern pathology, worked at the University of Würzburg. It is not surprising that this university became the focal point of modern pathologic anatomy.

Müller attracted numerous pupils, but with his death and with Virchow's move to Berlin, Vienna became the center of ocular pathology. Here Karl Freiherr von Rokitansky pioneered in modern pathology. One of his pupils, the pathologist Carl Wedl, dedicated 10 years of his life to the study of ocular pathology. He published his famous atlas in 1861 in collaboration with the ophthalmologist Stellwag von Carion. Wedl greatly influenced the clinicians of that time, especially Carl Ferdinand Ritter von Arlt, the teacher of Ernst Fuchs (1851–1930), whose numerous contributions to ophthalmic pathology are well known.

A second center developed in Paris. Poncet de Cluny (died 1899) was one of the most prominent pupils of Louis Antoine Ranvier. The first French textbook on pathologic anatomy was published by Panas and André Rochon-Duvigneaud (1898).

The first histologic eye examinations in London were reported by J. W. Hulke (1859). This compilation was soon followed by the works of Edward Nettleship, the excellent textbook by J. Herbert Parsons, and the monograph by E. Treacher Collins and H. Stephen Mayou.

In Italy the science was taken up first by C. de Cincentiis (1872) and later by C. Circincione. Later German textbooks were by Adolf Alt of Toronto (1880), Wedl and Bock of Vienna (1886), and Otto Haab of Zurich (1890).

Ophthalmic pathology developed into a specialty in the 20th century. Jonas Stein Friedenwald (1897–1955) at Johns Hopkins combined scientific investigative skills and eye pathology to become a role model for experimental eye pathologists. Frederick Verhoeff (1874–1968) can be considered the father of American ophthalmic pathology. Verhoeff was the first ophthalmologist to graduate from the Johns Hopkins medical school, and he became the pathologist at the Massachusetts Eye and Ear Infirmary. He studied under Fuchs and Parsons and was their American counterpart. By midcentury, Norman Ashton (1913–2001), a general pathologist, had become the director of the Department of Pathology at Moorfields Hospital in London. Ashton used his general pathology training in diagnostic and experimental eye pathology. Ashton's American counterpart was Lorenz E. Zimmerman (1920–), a general pathologist who became director of the Department of Ophthalmic Pathology at the Armed Forces Institute of Pathology. Zimmerman has directly or indirectly trained many of the ophthalmic pathologists currently practicing in the United States and worldwide. Other prominent American eye pathologists who worked during the middle of the 20th century included Frederick C. Blodi (1917–1994), Michael Hogan (1907–1975), and Georgiana Dvorak-Theobald (1884–1971). The rich heritage of ophthalmic pathology has served as a basis for the clinical practice of ophthalmology and as a liaison between experimental and clinical ophthalmology.

PART I

Ophthalmic Pathology

CHAPTER 1

Introduction to Part I

The purpose of BCSC Section 4, *Ophthalmic Pathology and Intraocular Tumors,* is to provide a general overview of the fields of ophthalmic pathology and ocular oncology. Although there is some overlap between the 2 fields, it is useful to approach specific disease processes from the standpoint of 2 separate disciplines. This book contains numerous illustrations of entities commonly encountered in an ophthalmic pathology laboratory and in the practice of ocular oncology. In addition, important, but less common, entities are included for teaching purposes. For more comprehensive reviews of ophthalmic pathology and ocular oncology, the reader is referred to the excellent textbooks listed in Basic Texts at the end of this volume.

Part I of this text provides a framework for the study of ophthalmic pathology, with the following hierarchical organizational paradigm (explained in detail in the next section): topography, disease process, general diagnosis, differential diagnosis. Chapter 2 briefly covers basic principles and specific aspects of wound repair as it applies to ophthalmic tissues, which exhibit distinct responses to trauma, including end-stage processes such as phthisis bulbi. Chapter 3 discusses specimen handling, including orientation and dissection, and emphasizes the critical communication between the ophthalmologist and the pathologist. Although most ophthalmic pathology specimens are routinely processed and slides are stained with hematoxylin and eosin (H&E), special procedures are used in selected cases. Chapter 4 details several of these procedures, including immunohistochemical staining, flow cytometry, polymerase chain reaction (PCR), and electron microscopy. Also discussed are indications in some instances for special techniques in obtaining the specimen, such as fine-needle aspiration biopsy, and special ways of preparing slides for examination, such as frozen sections. Chapters 5 through 15 apply the organizational paradigm to specific anatomical locations.

Organization

Chapters 5 through 15 are each devoted to a particular ocular structure. Within the chapter, the text is organized from general to specific, according to the following hierarchical framework:

- topography
- disease process

- general diagnosis
- differential diagnosis

Topography

The microscopic evaluation of a specimen, whether on a glass slide or depicted in a photograph, should begin with a description of any normal tissue. For instance, the topography of the cornea is characterized by nonkeratinized stratified squamous epithelium, Bowman's layer, stroma, Descemet's membrane, and endothelium. By recognizing a particular structure, such as Bowman's layer or Descemet's membrane, in a biopsy specimen, an examiner might be able to identify the topography in question as cornea. It may not be possible, however, to identify the specific tissue source from the topography present on a glass slide or in a photograph. For example, a specimen showing the topographic features of keratinized stratified squamous epithelium overlying dermis with dermal appendages may be classified as skin; however, unless specific eyelid structures such as a tarsal plate are identified, that skin is not necessarily from the eyelid. See BCSC Section 2, *Fundamentals and Principles of Ophthalmology,* for a review of ophthalmic anatomy.

Disease Process

After identifying a tissue source, the pathologist should attempt to categorize the general disease process. These processes include

- congenital anomaly
- inflammation
- degeneration and dystrophy
- neoplasia

Congenital anomaly

Congenital anomalies usually involve abnormalities in size, location, organization, or amount of tissue. An example of congenitally enlarged tissue is congenital hypertrophy of the retinal pigment epithelium (CHRPE) (see Figs 11-5 and 17-10). Many congenital abnormalities may be classified as choristomas or hamartomas.

A *choristoma* consists of normal, mature tissue at an abnormal location. It occurs when 1 or 2 embryonic germ layers form mature tissue that is abnormal for a given topographic location. An example of a choristoma is a *dermoid:* skin that is otherwise normal and mature present at the abnormal location of the limbus. A tumor made up of tissue derived from all 3 embryonic germ layers is called a *teratoma* (Fig 1-1).

In contrast, the term *hamartoma* describes an exaggerated hypertrophy and hyperplasia (abnormal amount) of mature tissue at a normal location. An example of a hamartoma is a *cavernous hemangioma,* an encapsulated mass of mature venous channels in the orbit.

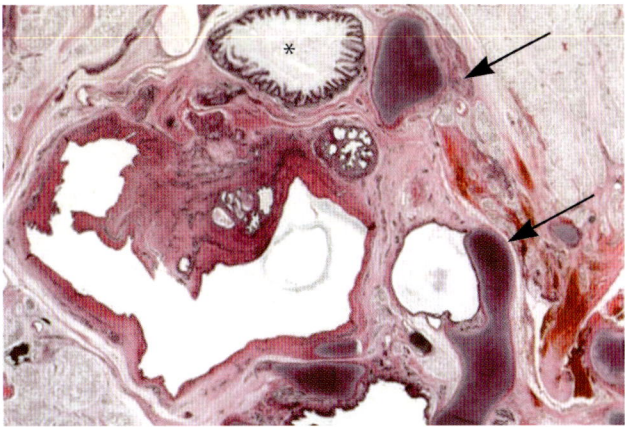

Figure 1-1 Orbital teratoma with tissue from 3 germ layers. Note gastrointestinal mucosa *(asterisk)* and cartilage *(arrows)* in the tumor. *(Courtesy of Hans E. Grossniklaus, MD.)*

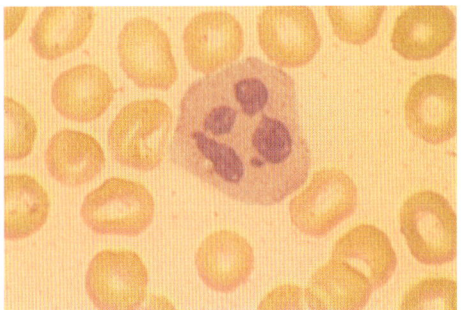

Figure 1-2 Polymorphonuclear leukocyte with multilobulated nucleus. *(Courtesy of Hans E. Grossniklaus, MD.)*

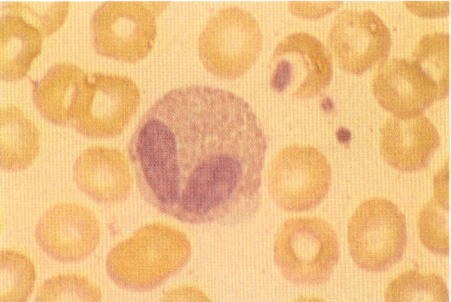

Figure 1-3 Eosinophil with bilobed nucleus and intracytoplasmic eosinophilic granules. *(Courtesy of Hans E. Grossniklaus, MD.)*

Inflammation

The next disease process in the schema, inflammation, is classified in several ways. It may be acute or chronic in onset and focal or diffuse in location. Chronic inflammation is subdivided further as either granulomatous or nongranulomatous. For example, a bacterial corneal ulcer is generally an acute, focal, nongranulomatous inflammation, whereas sympathetic ophthalmia is a chronic, diffuse, granulomatous inflammation.

Polymorphonuclear leukocytes (PMNs), eosinophils, and basophils all circulate in the blood and may be present in tissue in early phases of the inflammatory process (Figs 1-2, 1-3, 1-4). The types of leukocytes present at the site of inflammation vary according to the inflammatory response. PMNs, also known as *neutrophils,* typify acute inflammatory cells and can be recognized by a multisegmented nucleus and intracytoplasmic granules. They may be present in a variety of acute inflammatory processes; for example, they are associated with bacterial infection and found in the walls of blood vessels in some forms of vasculitis. *Eosinophils* have bilobed nuclei and prominent intracytoplasmic eosinophilic granules. They are commonly found in allergic reactions, although they may also be present in chronic inflammatory processes such as sympathetic ophthalmia. *Basophils* contain basophilic intracytoplasmic granules. *Mast cells* are the tissue-bound equivalent of the bloodborne basophils.

Inflammatory cells that are relatively characteristic of chronic inflammatory processes include monocytes (Fig 1-5) and lymphocytes (Fig 1-6). *Monocytes* may migrate from the intravascular space into tissue, in which case they are classified as *histiocytes,* or *macrophages.* Histiocytes have eccentric nuclei and abundant eosinophilic cytoplasm. In some instances, histiocytes may take on the appearance of epithelial cells, with abundant eosinophilic cytoplasm and sharp cell borders, becoming known in the process as *epithelioid histiocytes.* Epithelioid histiocytes may form a ball-like aggregate known as a *granuloma,* the sine qua non for granulomatous inflammation. These granulomas may contain only histologically intact cells ("hard" tubercles, Fig 1-7), or they may exhibit necrotic centers ("caseating" granulomas, Fig 1-8). Epithelioid histiocytes may merge to form a syncytium

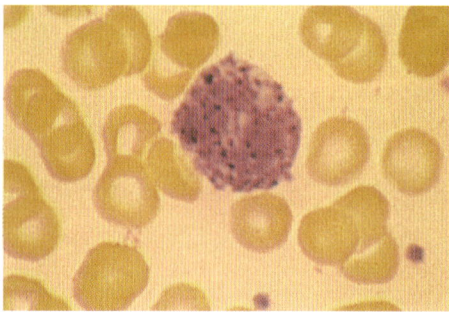

Figure 1-4 Basophil with intracytoplasmic basophilic granules. *(Courtesy of Hans E. Grossniklaus, MD.)*

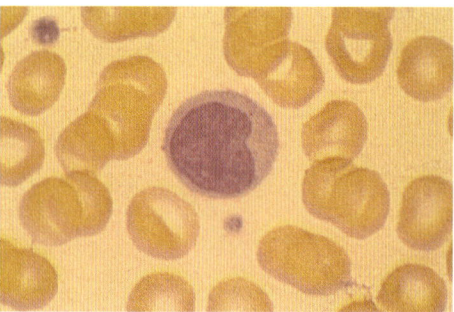

Figure 1-5 Monocyte with indented nucleus. *(Courtesy of Hans E. Grossniklaus, MD.)*

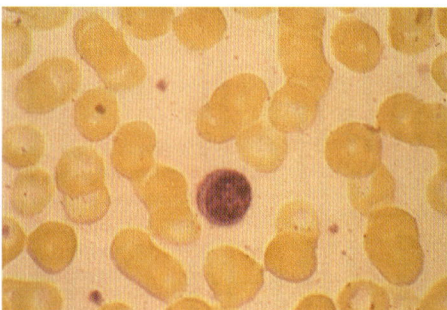

Figure 1-6 Lymphocyte with small, hyperchromatic nucleus and scant cytoplasm. *(Courtesy of Hans E. Grossniklaus, MD.)*

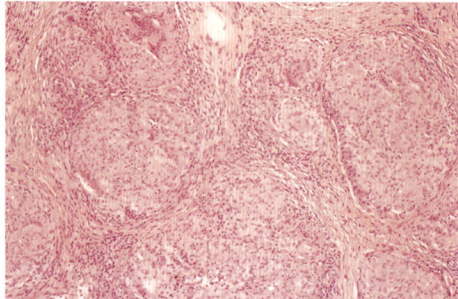

Figure 1-7 Noncaseating granulomas, or "hard" tubercles, are formed by aggregates of epithelioid histiocytes. *(Courtesy of Hans E. Grossniklaus, MD.)*

CHAPTER 1: Introduction to Part I • 15

with multiple nuclei known as a *multinucleated giant cell*. Giant cells formed from histiocytes come in several varieties, including

- Langhans cells, characterized by a horseshoe arrangement of the nuclei (Fig 1-9)
- Touton giant cells, which have an annulus of nuclei surrounded by a lipid-filled clear zone (Fig 1-10)
- foreign body giant cells, with haphazardly arranged nuclei (Fig 1-11)

Lymphocytes are small cells with round, hyperchromatic nuclei and scant cytoplasm. Circulating lymphocytes infiltrate tissue in all types of chronic inflammatory processes. These cells terminally differentiate in the thymus *(T cells)* or bursa equivalent *(B cells)*, although it is not possible to distinguish between B and T lymphocytes with routine histologic stains. B cells may produce immunoglobulin and differentiate into *plasma cells,* with eccentric "cartwheel," or "clockface," nuclei and a perinuclear halo corresponding to the Golgi apparatus. These cells may become completely distended with immunoglobulin and

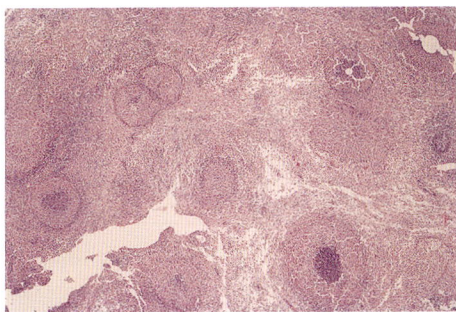

Figure 1-8 Granulomas with necrotic centers are classified as caseating granulomas. *(Courtesy of Hans E. Grossniklaus, MD.)*

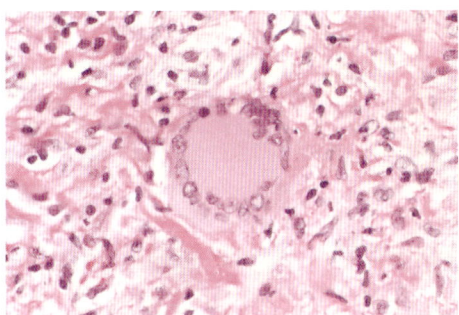

Figure 1-9 Langhans giant cell.

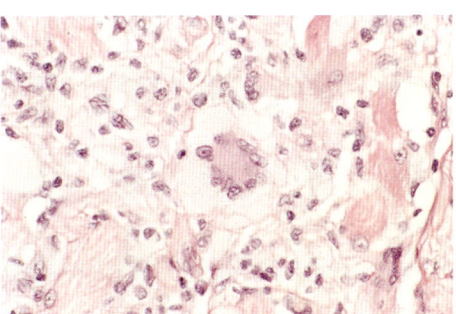

Figure 1-10 Touton giant cell.

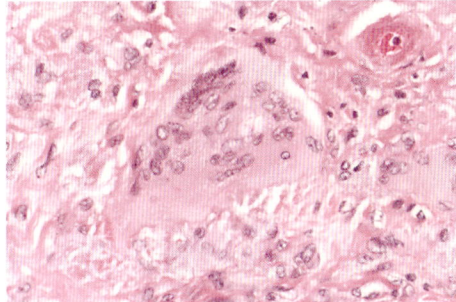

Figure 1-11 Foreign body giant cell.

16 • Ophthalmic Pathology and Intraocular Tumors

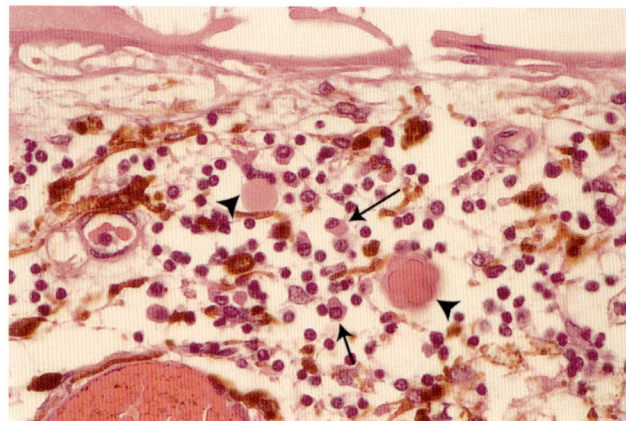

Figure 1-12 This aggregate of plasma cells *(arrows)* is associated with Russell bodies *(arrowheads)*. *(Courtesy of Hans E. Grossniklaus, MD.)*

form *Russell bodies*, which may be extracellular (Fig 1-12). BCSC Section 9, *Intraocular Inflammation and Uveitis*, discusses the cells involved in the inflammatory process in depth in Part I, Immunology.

Degeneration and dystrophy

The term *degeneration* refers to a wide variety of deleterious tissue changes that occur over time. Degenerative processes are not usually associated with a proliferation of cells; rather, there is often an accumulation of acellular material or a loss of tissue mass. Extracellular deposits may result from cellular overproduction of normal material or metabolically abnormal material. These processes, which have a variety of pathologic appearances, may occur in response to an injury or an inflammatory process. As used in this book, "degeneration" is an artificial category used to encompass a wide variety of disease processes. Various categories of diseases, such as those due to vascular causes, normal aging or involutional causes, and trauma, could be considered separately. However, in order to efficiently convey the hierarchical scheme used in this book, these causes are lumped under the rubric of "degeneration." *Dystrophies* are defined as bilateral, symmetric, inherited conditions that appear to have little or no relationship to environmental or systemic factors.

Degeneration of tissue may be seen in conjunction with other general disease processes. Examples include calcification of the lens (degeneration) in association with a congenital cataract (congenital anomaly); corneal amyloid (degeneration) in association with trachoma (inflammation); and orbital amyloid (degeneration) in association with a lymphoma (neoplasm). The ophthalmic manifestations of diabetes mellitus can be classified as degenerative changes associated with a metabolic disease.

Neoplasia

A *neoplasm* is a stereotypic, monotonous new growth of a particular tissue phenotype. Neoplasms can occur in either benign or malignant forms. Examples found in particular tissues include

- adenoma (benign) versus adenocarcinoma (malignant) in glandular epithelium

- topography + *oma* (benign) versus topography + *sarcoma* (malignant) in soft tissue
- hyperplasia/infiltrate (benign) versus leukemia/lymphoma (malignant) in hematopoietic tissue

Some neoplastic proliferations are called *borderline,* in that they are difficult to classify histologically as benign or malignant. Although most of the neoplasms illustrated and discussed in this text are classified as benign or malignant, the reader should be aware that tissue evaluation in a particular disease can give only a static portrait of a dynamic process. Thus, it may be impossible to determine whether the process will ultimately be benign or malignant, and in some instances "indeterminate" or "borderline" is a legitimate interpretation. Table 1-1 summarizes the origin, general classification of benign versus malignant, and growth pattern of neoplasms originating in various tissues.

The growth patterns described in Table 1-1 are shown in Figure 1-13. General histologic signs of malignancy include cellular pleomorphism, necrosis, hemorrhage, and mitotic activity.

Table 1-1 Classification of Neoplasia

Tissue Origin	Benign	Malignant	Growth Pattern
Epithelium	Hyperplasia/adenoma	Carcinoma Adenocarcinoma	Cords Tubules
Soft tissue	Topography + *oma*	Topography + *sarcoma*	Coherent sheets
Hematopoietic tissue	Hyperplasia/infiltrate	Leukemia Lymphoma	Loosely arranged

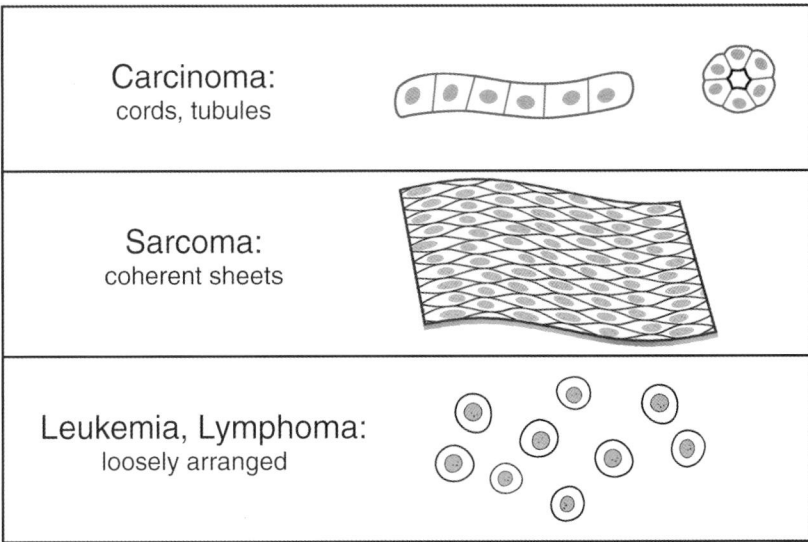

Figure 1-13 General classification and growth patterns of malignant tumors. *(Illustration by Christine Gralapp.)*

General Diagnosis

After considering the topography and disease process, the examiner formulates the general diagnosis. Recognizing a tissue *index feature* is a critical step in arriving at the general diagnosis. Index features are morphologic identifiers that help to define the disease process more specifically. Examples include the presence of pigment in a pigmented neoplasm, necrosis in a necrotizing granulomatous inflammation, and accumulation of smudgy extracellular material in a smudgy eosinophilic corneal degeneration. The index feature should differentiate the particular specimen from others demonstrating the same general disease process. For instance, retinoblastoma and melanoma are both intraocular malignant neoplasms; the former is a retinal malignancy, and the latter is a uveal tract malignancy. Other index features for distinguishing between these lesions could be "small, round, blue cell tumor" for the retinoblastoma and "melanocytic proliferation" for the melanoma. Although the most basic index features can be recognized without great difficulty, it takes experience and practice to identify subtle index features.

Differential Diagnosis

After the examiner has distinguished a key index feature and formulated a general diagnosis, developing a differential diagnosis is the next step. The differential diagnosis is a

Table 1-2 Organizational Paradigm for Ophthalmic Pathology

Topography
Conjunctiva
Cornea
Anterior chamber/trabecular meshwork
Sclera
Lens
Vitreous
Retina
Uveal tract
Eyelids
Orbit
Optic nerve

Disease Process
Congenital anomaly
   Choristoma versus hamartoma
Inflammation
   Acute versus chronic
   Focal versus diffuse
   Granulomatous versus nongranulomatous
Degeneration (includes dystrophy)
Neoplasia
   Benign versus malignant
   Epithelial versus soft tissue versus hematopoietic

General Diagnosis
Index feature

Differential Diagnosis
Limited list

limited list of specific conditions resulting from pathologic processes that were identified in the general diagnosis. For instance, the differential diagnosis based on the features of noncaseating granulomatous inflammation of the conjunctiva includes sarcoidosis, foreign body, fungus, and mycobacterium. The differential diagnosis of melanocytic proliferation of the conjunctiva includes nevus, primary acquired melanosis, and melanoma.

Readers are encouraged to practice working through the hierarchical framework by verbalizing each step in sequence while examining a pathologic specimen. Chapters 5 through 15 of this book provide tissue-specific examples of the differential diagnoses for each of the 4 disease process categories. The expanded organizational paradigm is shown in Table 1-2.

CHAPTER 2

Wound Repair

General Aspects of Wound Repair

Wound healing, though a common physiologic process, requires a complicated sequence of tissue events. The purpose of wound healing is to restore the anatomical and functional integrity of an organ or tissue as quickly and perfectly as possible. Repair may take a year, and the result of wound healing is a scar with variable consequences (Fig 2-1). A series of reactions follows a wound, including an acute inflammatory phase, regeneration/repair, and contraction:

- The *acute inflammatory phase* may last from minutes to hours. Blood clots quickly in adjacent vessels in response to tissue activators. Neutrophils and fluid enter the extracellular space. Macrophages remove debris from the damaged tissues, new vessels form, and fibroblasts begin to produce collagen.
- *Regeneration* is the replacement of lost cells; this process occurs only in tissues composed of labile cells (eg, epithelium), which undergo mitosis throughout life. *Repair* is the restructuring of tissues by granulation tissue that matures into a fibrous scar.
- Finally, *contraction* causes the reparative tissues to shrink so that the scar is smaller than the surrounding uninjured tissues.

Healing in Specific Ocular Tissues

The processes summarized in the following sections are also discussed in other volumes of the BCSC series: Section 7, *Orbit, Eyelids, and Lacrimal System;* Section 8, *External Disease and Cornea;* Section 9, *Intraocular Inflammation and Uveitis;* Section 11, *Lens and Cataract;* and Section 12, *Retina and Vitreous.* See also the appropriate chapters in this volume for a specific topography.

Cornea

A corneal *abrasion,* a painful but rapidly healing defect, is limited to the surface corneal epithelium, although Bowman's layer and superficial stroma may also be involved. Within an hour of injury the parabasilar epithelial cells begin to slide and migrate across the denuded area until they touch other migrating cells; then *contact inhibition* stops further migration. Simultaneously, the surrounding basal cells undergo mitosis to supply additional cells to

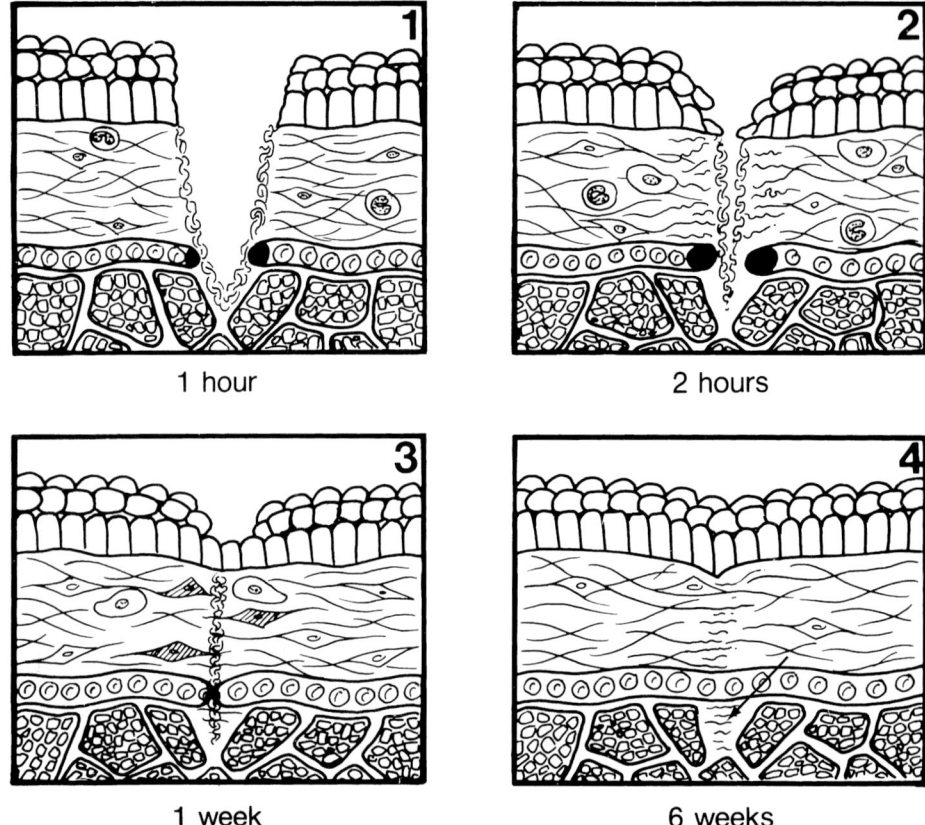

Figure 2-1 Sequence of general wound healing with an epithelial surface. **1,** The wound is created. Blood clots in the vessels; neutrophils migrate to the wound; the wounded edges begin to disintegrate. **2,** The wound edges are reapposed with the various tissue planes in good alignment. The epithelium is lost over the wound but starts to migrate. The subcutaneous fibroblasts enlarge and become activated. Fibronectin is deposited at the wound edges. The blood vessels begin to produce buds. **3,** The epithelium seals the surface. Fibroblasts and blood vessels enter the wound and lay down new collagen. Much of the debris is removed by macrophages. **4,** As the scar matures, the fibroblasts subside. Newly formed blood vessels recanalize. New collagen strengthens the wound, which contracts. Note that the striated muscle cells (permanent cells) at bottom are replaced by scar *(arrow).*

cover the defect. Although a large corneal abrasion is usually sealed within 24 hours, complete healing, which includes restoration of the full thickness of epithelium (4–6 layers) and re-formation of the anchoring fibrils, takes 4–6 weeks. The epithelial cells are labile; that is, some are continuously active mitotically and thus are able to completely replace the lost cells. If a thin layer of anterior cornea is lost with the abrasion, the shallow crater will be filled by epithelium, forming a facet.

Corneal stromal healing is avascular. Unlike with other tissues, healing in the corneal stroma occurs by means of fibrosis rather than by fibrovascular proliferation. This avascular aspect of corneal wound healing is critical to the success of penetrating keratoplasty as well as photorefractive keratectomy (PRK), laser in situ keratomileusis (LASIK), laser epithelial keratomileusis (LASEK), and other corneal refractive surgical procedures.

Following a central corneal wound, neutrophils are carried to the site by the tears (Fig 2-2), and the edges of the wound swell. Healing factors derived from vessels are not present. The matrix glycosaminoglycans, which in the cornea are keratan sulfate and chondroitin sulfate, disintegrate at the edge of the wound. The fibroblasts of the stroma become activated, eventually migrating across the wound, laying down collagen and fibronectin. The direction of the fibroblasts and collagen is not parallel to stromal lamellae. Hence, cells are directed anteriorly and posteriorly across a wound that is always visible microscopically as an irregularity in the stroma and clinically as an opacity. If the wound edges are separated, the gap is not completely filled by proliferating fibroblasts, and a partially filled crater results.

Both the epithelium and the endothelium are critical to good central wound healing. If the epithelium does not cover the wound within days, the subjacent stromal healing is limited and the wound is weak. Growth factors from the epithelium stimulate and sustain

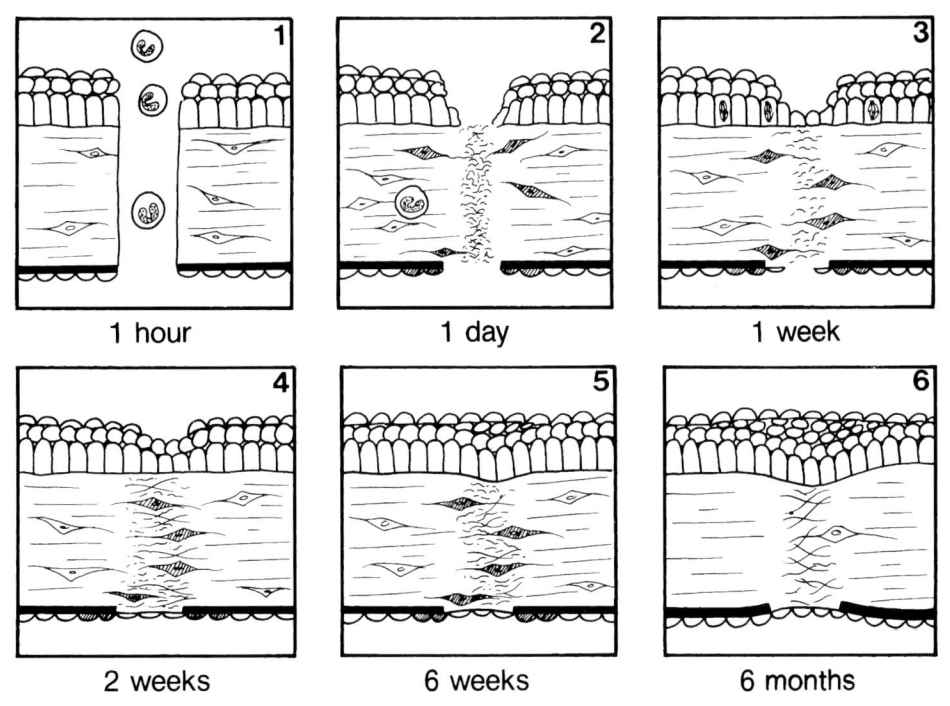

Figure 2-2 Clear corneal wound. **1,** The tear film carries neutrophils with lysozymes to the wound within an hour. **2,** With closure of the incision, the wound edge shows early disintegration and edema. The glycosaminoglycans at the edge are degraded. The nearby fibroblasts are activated. **3,** At 1 week, migrating epithelium and endothelium partially seal the wound; fibroblasts begin to migrate and supply collagen. **4,** Fibroblast activity and collagen and matrix deposition continue. The endothelium, sealing the inner wound, lays down new Descemet's membrane. **5,** Epithelial regeneration is complete. Fibroblasts fill the wound with type I collagen and repair slows. **6,** The final wound contracts. The collagen fibers are not parallel with the surrounding lamellae. The number of fibroblasts decreases.

healing. The endothelial cells adjacent to the wound slide across the posterior cornea; a few cells are replaced through mitotic activity. Endothelium lays down a new thin layer of Descemet's membrane. If the internal margin of the wound is not covered by Descemet's membrane, stromal fibroblasts may continue to proliferate into the anterior chamber as fibrous ingrowth, or the posterior wound may remain permanently open. The initial fibrillar collagen is replaced by stronger collagen in the late months of healing. Bowman's layer does not regenerate when incised or destroyed. In an ulcer, the surface is covered by epithelium, but little of the lost stroma is replaced by fibrous tissue. Modification of the healing process by use of topical antimetabolites, such as 5-fluorouracil and mitomycin C, may be desirable in certain clinical situations (see BCSC Section 10, *Glaucoma*, Chapter 8).

Sclera

The sclera differs from the cornea in that the collagen fibers are randomly distributed rather than laid down in orderly lamellae, and the glycosaminoglycan is dermatan sulfate. Sclera is relatively avascular and hypocellular. When stimulated by wounding, the episclera migrates down the scleral wound, supplying vessels, fibroblasts, and activated macrophages. The final wound contracts, creating a pinched-in appearance. If the adjacent uvea is damaged, uveal fibrovascular tissue may enter the scleral wound, resulting in a scar with a dense adhesion between uvea and sclera. Indolent episcleral fibrosis produces a dense coat around an extrascleral foreign body such as a scleral buckle.

Limbus

The limbus is a complex region of corneal, scleral, and episcleral tissues. Wounds of the limbus cause swelling in the cornea and shrinking of the sclera (Fig 2-3). Healing involves episcleral ingrowth and clear corneal fibroblastic migration. Collector channels in the sclera do not contribute to the healing. Alterations in surgical technique between clear corneal and limbal incisions may produce different healing responses. Differences include

- the potential for vascular ingrowth from episcleral vessels into a limbal wound and the absence of vascularity of a clear corneal wound
- surface remodeling of epithelium over a clear corneal wound that does not occur over a limbal wound

Uvea

Under ordinary circumstances, wounds of the iris do not stimulate a healing response in either the stroma or the epithelium. Though richly endowed with blood vessels and fibroblasts, the iridic stroma does not produce granulation tissue to close a defect. The pigmented epithelium may be stimulated to migrate in some circumstances, such as excessive inflammation, but its migration is usually limited to the subjacent surface of the lens capsule, where subsequent adhesion of epithelial cells occurs. When fibrovascular tissue forms, it usually does so on the anterior surface of the iris as an exuberant and aberrant membrane (eg, rubeosis iridis) that may cross iridectomy or pupillary openings. The fibrovascular tissue may arise from the iris, the chamber angle, or the cornea.

CHAPTER 2: Wound Repair • 25

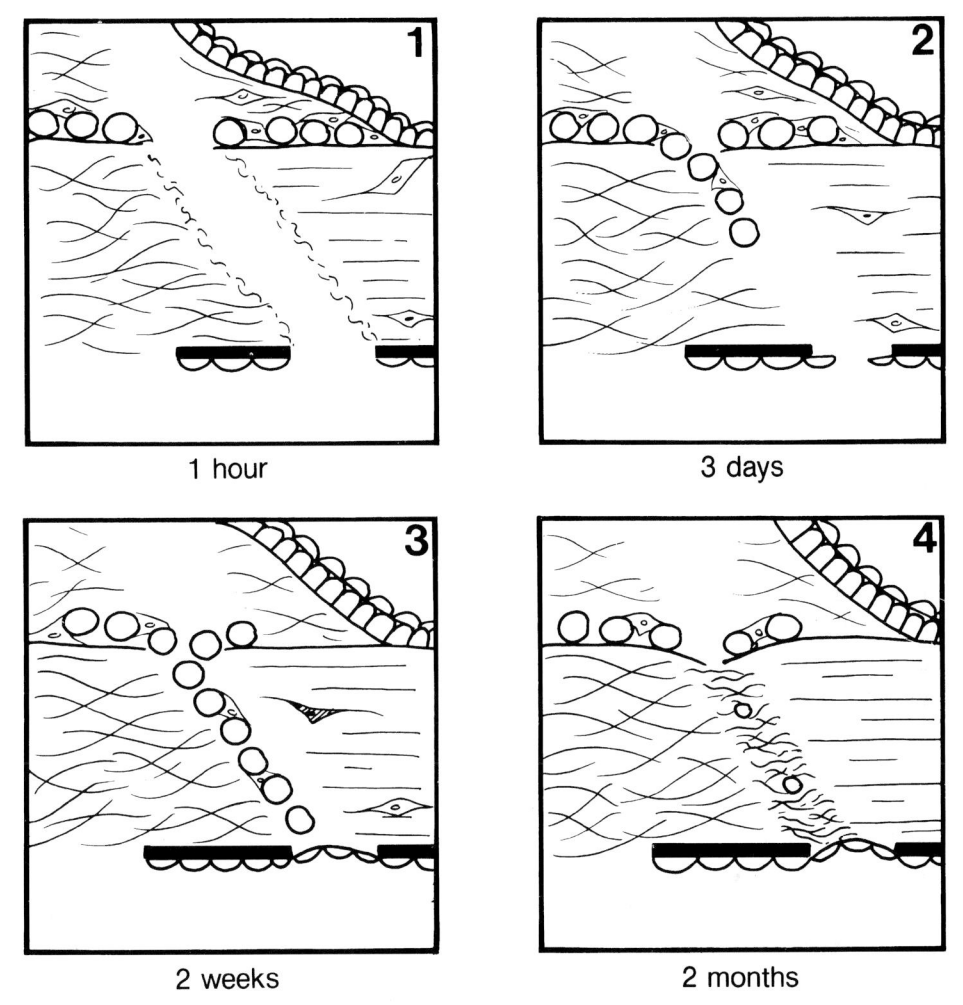

Figure 2-3 Limbal wound. **1,** The limbal wound with a conjunctival flap passes through episclera externally and enters the globe through Descemet's membrane and endothelium. Sclera is on the left and cornea on the right. The wound edge shows early disintegration. Neutrophils and macrophages are omitted in this diagram. **2,** Episcleral vessels and fibroblasts migrate down the wound. Some activity is present in the corneal fibroblasts. **3,** Episcleral fibrovascular migration in the wound is stopped at the endothelium crossing the internal margin of the incision. **4,** The number of vessels decreases in the late stage of healing. Irregular collagen fibers and matrix fill the contracting wound.

Stroma and melanocytes of the iris, ciliary body, and choroid do not regenerate after injury. Debris is removed, and a thin fibrous scar develops that appears white and atrophic clinically.

Dunn SP. Iris repair: putting the pieces back together. *Focal Points: Clinical Modules for Ophthalmologists.* San Francisco: American Academy of Ophthalmology; 2002, module 11.

Lens

Small rents in the lens capsule are sealed by nearby lenticular epithelial cells. When posterior synechiae make the lenticular epithelium anoxic or hypoxic, a metaplastic response occurs, producing fibrous plaques intermixed with basement membrane.

Retina

The retina is made of permanent cells that do not regenerate when fatally injured. Instead, a glial plug pulls the retina together after closure. Surgical techniques to close openings in the peripheral retina are successful when the neurosensory retina and retinal pigment epithelium (RPE) are destroyed (eg, cryotherapy, photocoagulation) and the surrounding tissues form an adhesive, atrophic scar.

Retinal scars are produced by glia rather than fibroblasts. After inflammatory cells have cleared away the debris, the tissues most damaged by the therapeutic modality remain as a thin, atrophic area in the center of the scar. Increasing numbers of residual viable cells ring the zone of greatest destruction. Adhesion between the residual neurosensory retina and Bruch's membrane develops according to the size of the original wound and the type of injury. The internal limiting membrane and Bruch's membrane provide the architectural planes for glial scarring. Adhesions from the internal limiting membrane to Bruch's membrane may incorporate a rare residual glial cell, and variable numbers of retinal cells and RPE may be present between the membranes. If the wound has damaged Bruch's membrane, choroidal fibroblasts and vessels may participate in the formation of the final scar. The end result is a metaplastic collagenous plaque in the sub–neurosensory retina and sub-RPE areas. The RPE usually proliferates rather exuberantly in such scars, giving rise to the dense black clumps seen clinically in scars of the fundus.

Vitreous

The vitreous has few cells and no blood vessels. Nonetheless, in conditions that cause vitreal inflammation, mediators stimulate the formation of membranes composed of new vessels and the proliferation of glial and fibrous tissue. With contraction of these membranes, the retina becomes distorted and detached.

Eyelid, Orbit, and Lacrimal Tissues

The rich blood supply of the skin of the eyelids supports rapid and complete healing. On about the third day after injury to the skin, myofibroblasts derived from vascular pericytes migrate around the wound and actively contract, resulting in a volumetric decrease in the size of the wound. Early invasion of ocular wounds by myofibroblasts does not occur, and the resultant early contraction does not happen. The eyelid and orbit are compartmentalized by intertwining fascial membranes enclosing muscular, tendinous, fatty, lacrimal, and ocular tissues that are distorted by scarring. Exuberant contracting distorts muscle action, producing dysfunctional scars. The striated muscles of the orbicularis oculi and extraocular muscles are made of permanent cells that do not regenerate, but the viable cells may hypertrophy. Contraction of tissue may occur after injury, hence the shrunken appearance of eyelids and globe following a crushing injury to the orbit.

Histologic Sequelae of Ocular Trauma

The anterior chamber angle structures, especially the trabecular beams, are vulnerable to distortion of the anterior globe. *Cyclodialysis* results from disinsertion of the longitudinal muscle of the ciliary muscle from the scleral spur (Fig 2-4). This condition can lead to hypotony because the aqueous of the anterior chamber now has free access to the suprachoroidal space, and, because the blood supply to the ciliary body is diminished, the production of aqueous is decreased.

Traumatic recession of the anterior chamber angle is a rupture of the face of the ciliary body (Fig 2-5). A plane of relative weakness starts at the ciliary body face and extends posteriorly between the longitudinal muscles of the ciliary body and the more centrally located oblique and circular muscle fibers. Concurrent damage to the trabecular meshwork may lead to glaucoma. The oblique and circular muscle fibers will usually atrophy, changing the overall shape of the cross-sectional appearance of the ciliary body from triangular to fusiform. The ciliary process will appear posteriorly and externally displaced as defined by a line drawn through the scleral spur parallel to the visual axis. In normal eyes, this line intersects the first ciliary process. These changes are also shown in Figure 7-10 in Chapter 7.

The uveal tract is attached to the sclera at 3 points: the scleral spur, the internal ostia of the vortex veins, and the peripapillary tissue. This anatomical arrangement is the basis of the evisceration technique and explains the vulnerability of the eye to expulsive choroidal hemorrhage. The borders of the dome-shaped choroidal hemorrhage are defined by the position of the vortex veins and the scleral spur (Fig 2-6).

An *iridodialysis* is a rupture of the iris at the thinnest portion of the diaphragm, the iris base, where it inserts into the supportive tissue of the ciliary body (Fig 2-7; see also Fig 7-11). Only a small amount of supporting tissue surrounds the iris sphincter. If the sphincter muscle is ruptured, contraction of the remaining muscle will create a notch at the pupillary border. The iris diaphragm may be lost completely through a relatively small limbal rupture associated with 360° iridodialysis.

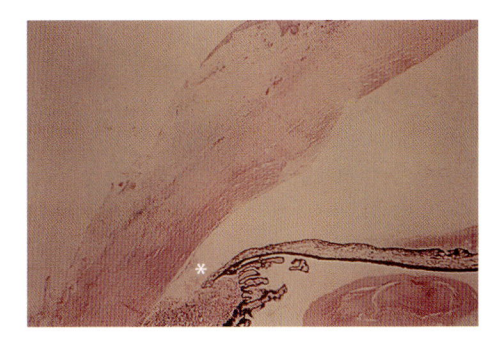

Figure 2-4 Cyclodialysis shows disinsertion of ciliary body muscle from the scleral spur *(asterisk)*. *(Courtesy of Hans E. Grossniklaus, MD.)*

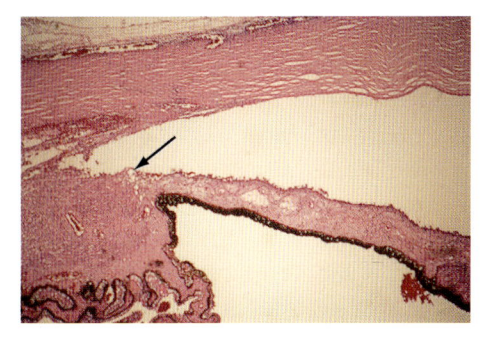

Figure 2-5 Angle recession shows a torn ciliary body muscle *(arrow)*. *(Courtesy of Hans E. Grossniklaus, MD.)*

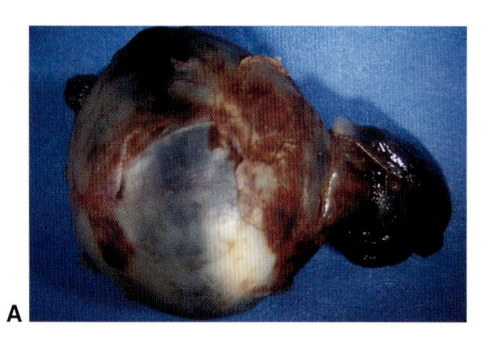

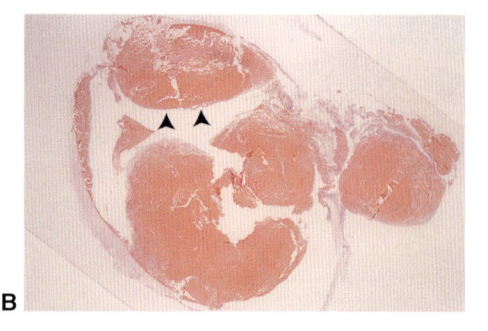

28 • Ophthalmic Pathology and Intraocular Tumors

Figure 2-6 **A,** This eye developed an expulsive hemorrhage after a corneal perforation. **B,** The intraocular choroidal hemorrhage is dome shaped *(arrowheads),* delineated by the insertion of the choroid at the scleral spur. *(Courtesy of Hans E. Grossniklaus, MD.)*

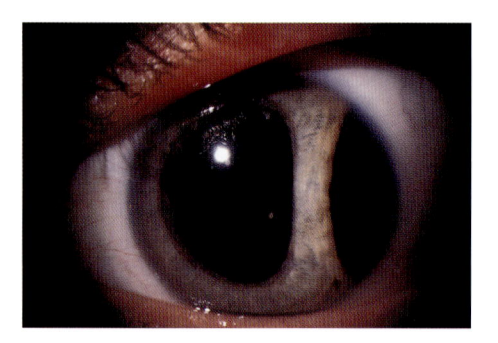

Figure 2-7 Iridodialysis shows a tear in the base of the iris. *(Courtesy of Hans E. Grossniklaus, MD.)*

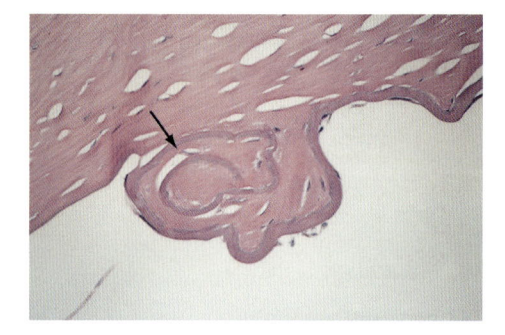

Figure 2-8 A break in Descemet's membrane in keratoconus shows anterior curling of Descemet's membrane toward the corneal stroma *(arrow). (Courtesy of Hans E. Grossniklaus, MD.)*

A *Vossius ring* appears when compression and rupture of iris pigment epithelial cells against the anterior surface of the lens occurs, depositing a ring of melanin pigment concentric to the pupil.

A *cataract* may form immediately if the lens capsule is ruptured. The lens capsule is thinnest at the posterior pole, a point farthest away from the lens epithelial cells. The epithelium of the lens may be stimulated by trauma to form an anterior lenticular fibrous plaque. The lens zonular fibers are points of relative weakness; if they are ruptured, displacement of the lens can be partial (subluxation) or complete (luxation). Focal areas of zonular rupture may allow formed vitreous to enter the anterior chamber.

Rupture of Descemet's membrane may occur after minor trauma (eg, in keratoconus, Fig 2-8) or major trauma (eg, after forceps injury, Fig 2-9). *Rupture of Bruch's membrane* can occur after compressive injuries (choroidal rupture); the rupture is often concentric to the optic disc. Ruptures of Bruch's membrane itself are not as functionally significant as the accompanying rupture of the overlying retina, which is usually undetectable clinically. A rupture of Bruch's membrane may also permit choroidal neovascularization by allowing the choroidal vasculature access to the sub–neurosensory retina space.

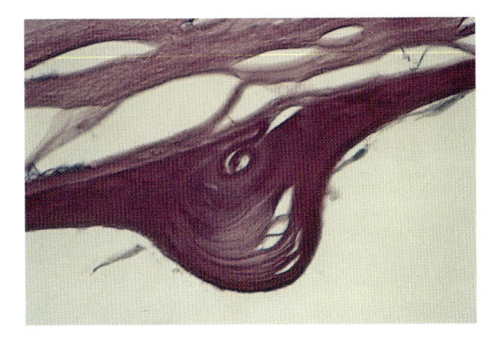

Figure 2-9 A break in Descemet's membrane as a result of forceps injury shows anterior curling of the original membrane and production of a secondary thickened membrane. *(Courtesy of Hans E. Grossniklaus, MD.)*

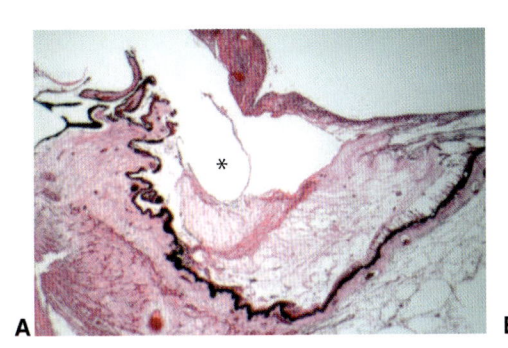

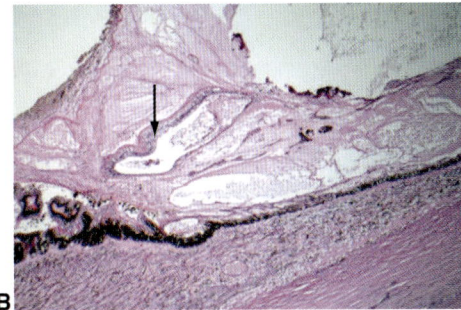

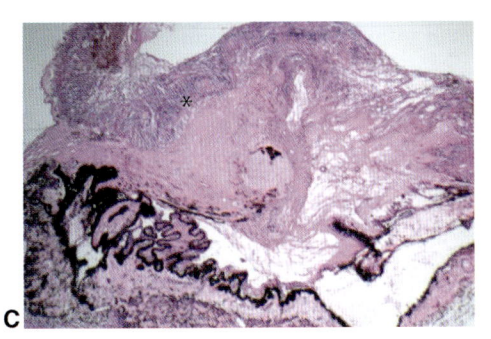

Figure 2-10 Anterior proliferative vitreoretinopathy (PVR). **A,** Traction of the vitreous base on the peripheral retina and ciliary body epithelium *(asterisk)*. **B,** Incorporation of peripheral retinal and ciliary body tissue into the vitreous base *(arrow)*. **C,** Proliferation of incorporated tissue in the vitreous base *(asterisk)*. *(Courtesy of Hans E. Grossniklaus, MD.)*

Retinal dialysis is most likely to develop in the inferotemporal or superonasal quadrant. The retina is anchored anteriorly to the nonpigmented epithelium of the pars plana. This union is reinforced by the attachment of the vitreous, which straddles the ora serrata. Deformation of the eye can result in a circumferential tear of the retina at the point of attachment of the ora or immediately posterior to the point of attachment of the vitreous base (Fig 2-10). Vitreoretinal traction may cause tears in a retina weakened by necrosis.

Intraocular *fibrocellular proliferation* may occur after a penetrating injury. Such proliferation may lead to vitreous/subretinal/choroidal hemorrhage; traction retinal detachment; proliferative vitreoretinopathy (PVR), including anterior PVR; hypotony; and ultimately phthisis bulbi. Formation of proliferative intraocular membranes may

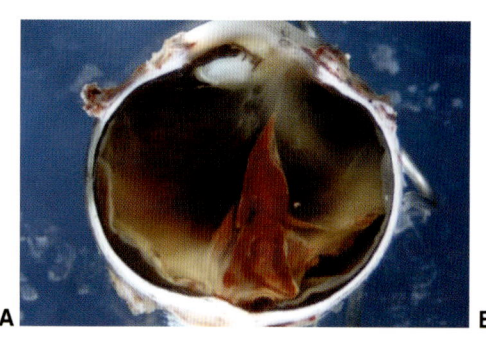

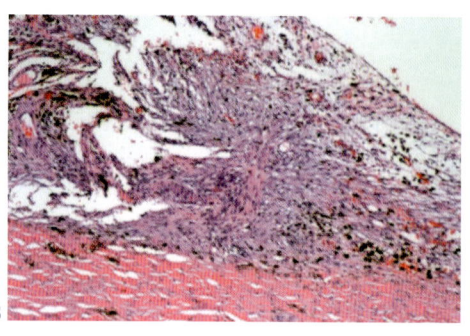

Figure 2-11 Focal posttraumatic choroidal granulomatous inflammation. **A,** Enucleated eye with a projectile causing a perforating limbal injury that extends to the posterior choroid. **B,** Microscopic examination shows a focus of choroidal granulomatous inflammation. *(Courtesy of Hans E. Grossniklaus, MD.)*

affect the timing of vitreoretinal surgery. The timing of the drainage of a ciliochoroidal hemorrhage is based on lysis of the blood clot (10–14 days). Hemosiderin forms at approximately 72 hours after hemorrhage. Sequelae of intraocular hemorrhage include siderosis bulbi, cholesterosis, and hemoglobin spherulosis.

Choroidal rupture may occur after direct or indirect injury to the globe. This results in granulation tissue proliferation and scar formation. Choroidal neovascularization may occur in an area of a choroidal rupture. A subset of direct choroidal ruptures, those usually occurring after a projectile injury, may result in *focal posttraumatic choroidal granulomatous inflammation* (Fig 2-11). This may be related to foreign material introduced into the choroid. A chorioretinal rupture and necrosis is known as *sclopetaria*.

> Wilson MW, Grossniklaus HE, Heathcote JG. Focal posttraumatic choroidal granulomatous inflammation. *Am J Ophthalmol.* 1996;121:397–404.

Commotio retinae (Berlin edema) often complicates blunt trauma to the eye. Most prominent in the macula, commotio retinae can affect any portion of the retina. Originally, the retinal opacification seen clinically was thought to result from retinal edema (extracellular accumulation of fluid), but experimental evidence shows that a disruption in the architecture of the photoreceptor elements causes the loss of retinal transparency.

Phthisis bulbi is defined as atrophy, shrinkage, and disorganization of the eye and intraocular contents. Not all eyes rendered sightless by trauma become phthisical. If the nutritional status of the eye and near-normal intraocular pressure (IOP) are maintained during the repair process, the globe will remain clinically stable. However, blind eyes are at high risk of repeated trauma with cumulative destructive effects. Slow, progressive functional decompensation may also prevail. Many blind eyes pass through several stages of atrophy and disorganization into the end stage of phthisis bulbi:

- *Atrophia bulbi without shrinkage* (Fig 2-12). Initially, the size and shape of the eye are maintained. The atrophic eye often has elevated IOP. The following structures are most sensitive to loss of nutrition: the lens, which becomes cataractous; the retina, which atrophies and becomes separated from the RPE by serous fluid accumulation; and the aqueous outflow tract, where anterior and posterior synechiae develop.

CHAPTER 2: Wound Repair • 31

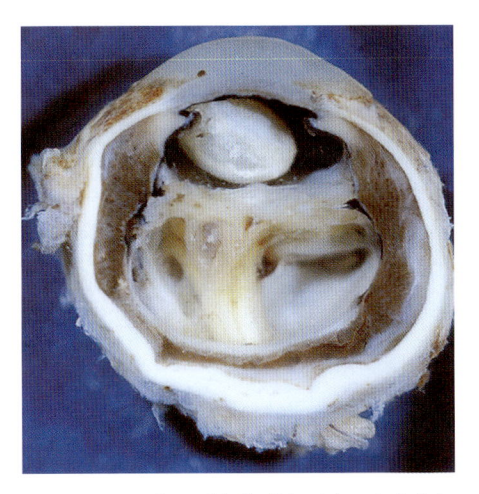

Figure 2-12 Atrophia bulbi without shrinkage. Note the dense cyclitic membrane and the corresponding detachment of the ciliary body.

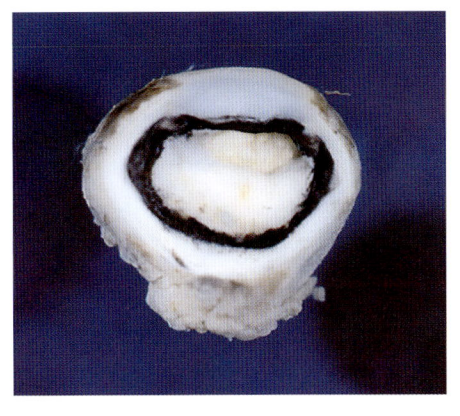

Figure 2-13 Phthisis bulbi. The size of the globe is markedly reduced, the sclera is thickened, and the contents of the eye are totally disorganized.

- *Atrophia bulbi with shrinkage.* The eye becomes soft because of ciliary body dysfunction and progressive diminution of IOP. The globe becomes smaller and assumes a squared-off configuration as a result of the influence of the 4 rectus muscles. The anterior chamber collapses. Associated corneal endothelial cell damage results initially in corneal edema followed by opacification from degenerative pannus, stromal scarring, and vascularization. Most of the remaining internal structures of the eye will be atrophic but recognizable histologically.
- *Atrophia bulbi with disorganization (phthisis bulbi)* (Fig 2-13). The size of the globe shrinks from a normal average diameter of 24–26 mm to an average diameter of 16–19 mm. Most of the ocular contents become disorganized. In areas of preserved uvea, the RPE proliferates and drusen may be seen. Extensive calcification of Bowman's layer, lens, retina, and drusen usually occurs. Osseous metaplasia of the RPE may be a prominent feature. The sclera becomes massively thickened, particularly posteriorly

CHAPTER 3

Specimen Handling

Communication

Communication with the pathologist before, during, and after surgical procedures is an essential aspect of quality patient care. The final histologic diagnosis reflects successful collaborative work between clinician and pathologist. The ophthalmologist should provide a relevant and reasonably detailed clinical history when the specimen is submitted to the laboratory. This history facilitates clinicopathologic correlation and enables the pathologist to provide the most accurate interpretation of the specimen. The clinical history portion of the pathology request form, therefore, should not be neglected, even in "routine" cases.

Where there is an ongoing relationship between a pathologist and an ophthalmologist, communication usually can be accomplished through the pathology request form and the pathology report. However, if a malignancy is suspected or if the biopsy will be used to establish a critical diagnosis, direct and personal communication between the ophthalmic surgeon and the pathologist can be essential. This preoperative consultation allows the surgeon and pathologist to discuss the best way to submit a specimen. For example, the pathologist may wish to have fresh tissue for immunohistochemical stains and molecular diagnostic studies, glutaraldehyde-fixed tissue for electron microscopy, and formalin-fixed tissue for routine paraffin embedding. If the tissue is simply submitted in formalin, the opportunity for a definitive diagnosis may be lost. Communication between clinician and pathologist is especially important in ophthalmic pathology, where specimens are often very small and require very careful handling. Biopsies may be incisional, in which only a portion of the tumor is sampled, or excisional, in which the entire lesion is removed. (See BCSC Section 7, *Orbit, Eyelids, and Lacrimal System*, Chapter 11, for further discussion.)

Any time a previous biopsy has been performed at the site of the present pathology, the sections of the previous biopsy should be requested and reviewed with the pathologist who will interpret the second biopsy. The surgical plan may be altered substantially if the initial biopsy was thought to represent, for example, a basal cell carcinoma when in fact the disease was a sebaceous carcinoma. In addition, the pathologist will be able to interpret intraoperative frozen sections more accurately when the case has been reviewed in advance.

34 • Ophthalmic Pathology and Intraocular Tumors

If substantial disagreement arises between the clinical diagnosis and the histopathologic diagnosis, the ophthalmologist should contact the pathologist directly and promptly to resolve the discrepancy. Mislabeling of pathology specimens or reports through a simple typing error, for example, can have serious consequences. Merely correcting the patient age on the pathology request form may change the interpretation of melanotic lesions of the conjunctiva. Benign pigmental melanotic lesions in children may have a similar histologic appearance to malignant melanotic lesions in adults. Whether the patient is age 4 or age 44 makes a tremendous difference in interpretation.

Finally, the ophthalmologist who makes an effort to consult with the pathologist prior to surgery sends a clear signal both of special interest in the case and of respect for the contribution of the pathologist. This collaborative approach will ultimately benefit the patient by rendering the correct diagnosis in the most efficient manner.

Orientation

Globes may be oriented according to the location of the extraocular muscles and of the long posterior ciliary artery and nerve, which are located in the horizontal meridian. The medial, inferior, lateral, and superior rectus muscles insert progressively farther from the limbus. Locating the insertion of the inferior oblique muscle is very helpful in distinguishing between a right and a left eye (Fig 3-1). The inferior oblique inserts temporally over the macula, with its fibers running inferiorly. Once the laterality of the eye is determined, the globe may be transilluminated and dissected.

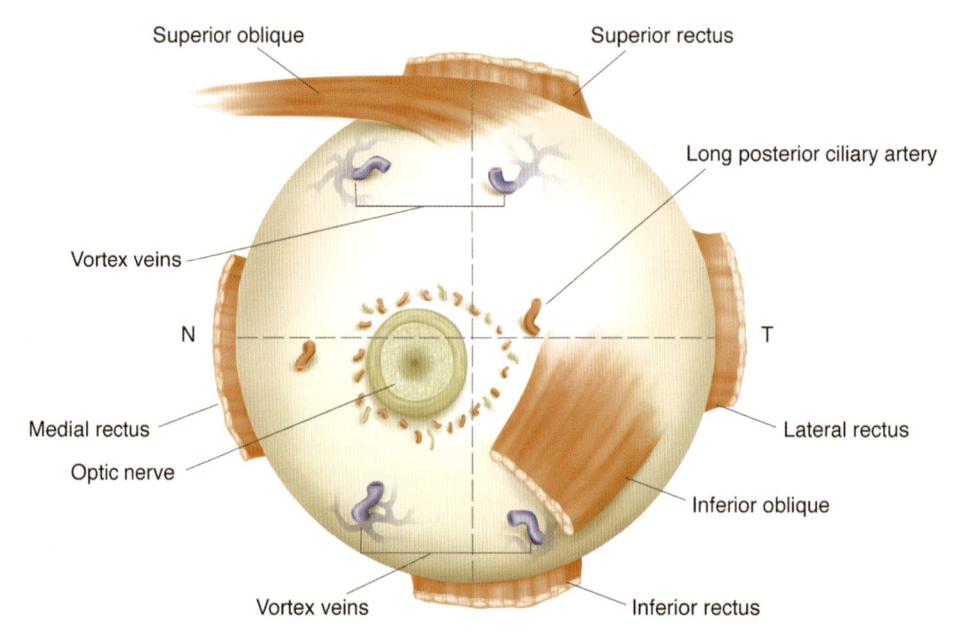

Figure 3-1 Posterior view of right globe. *(Modified by Cyndie Wooley from illustration by Thomas A. Weingeist, PhD, MD.)*

CHAPTER 3: Specimen Handling • 35

Transillumination

Eyes are transilluminated with bright light prior to gross dissection. This helps to identify intraocular lesions such as a tumor that blocks the transilluminated light and casts a shadow (Fig 3-2A). The shadow can be outlined with a marking pencil on the sclera (Fig 3-2B). This outline can then be used to guide the gross dissection of the globe so that the center of the section will include the maximum extent of the area of interest (Figs 3-2C to 3-2E).

Gross Dissection

A globe is opened so as to display as much of the pathologic change as possible on a single slide. The majority of eyes are cut so that the pupil and optic nerve are present in the same section, the *PO section*. The meridian, or clock-hour, of the section is determined by the

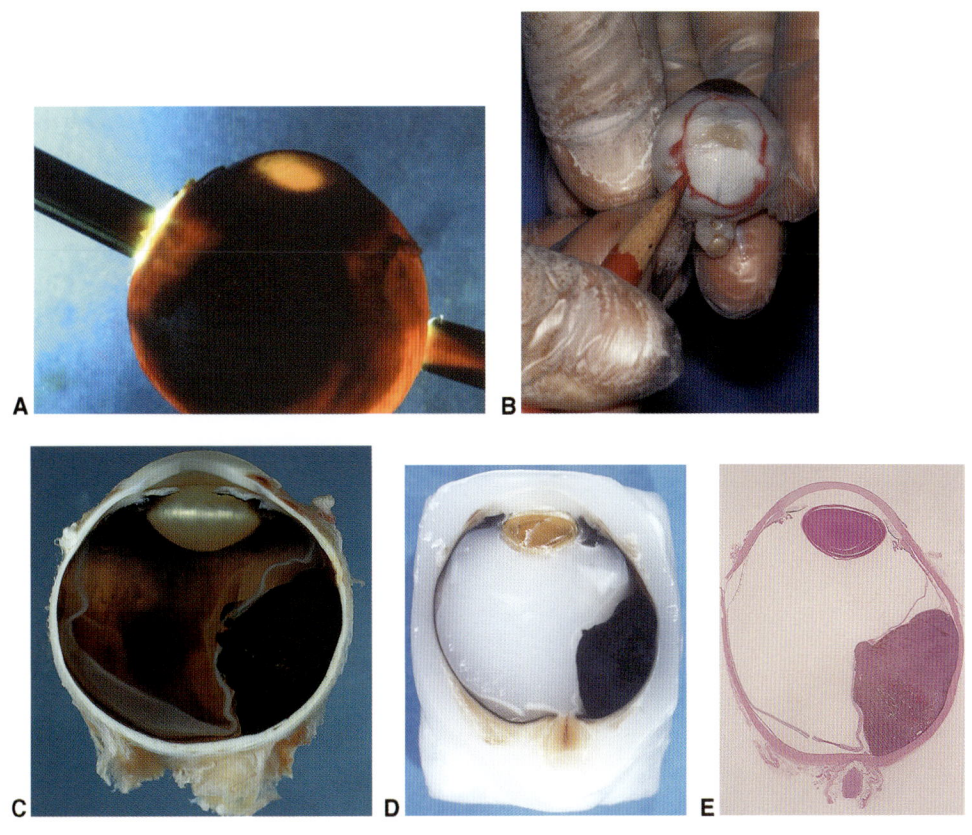

Figure 3-2 Preparation of an intraocular tumor specimen. **A,** Transillumination shows blockage to light secondary to an intraocular tumor. **B,** The area of blockage to light is marked with a marking pencil. **C,** The opened eye shows the intraocular tumor that was demonstrated by transillumination. **D,** The paraffin-embedded eye shows the intraocular tumor. **E,** The H&E-stained section shows that the maximum extent of the tumor demonstrated by transillumination is in the center of the section, which includes the pupil and optic nerve. *(Courtesy of Hans E. Grossniklaus, MD.)*

36 • Ophthalmic Pathology and Intraocular Tumors

unique features of the case, such as the presence of an intraocular tumor or a history of previous surgery or trauma. In routine cases, with no prior surgery or intraocular neoplasm, most eyes are opened in the horizontal meridian, which includes the macula in the same section as the pupil and optic nerve (Fig 3-3). Globes with a surgical or nonsurgical wound should be opened so the wound will be perpendicular to, and included in, the PO section, which often means opening the globe vertically. Globes with intraocular tumors are opened in a way (horizontal, vertical, or oblique) that places the center of the tumor as outlined by transillumination in the PO section.

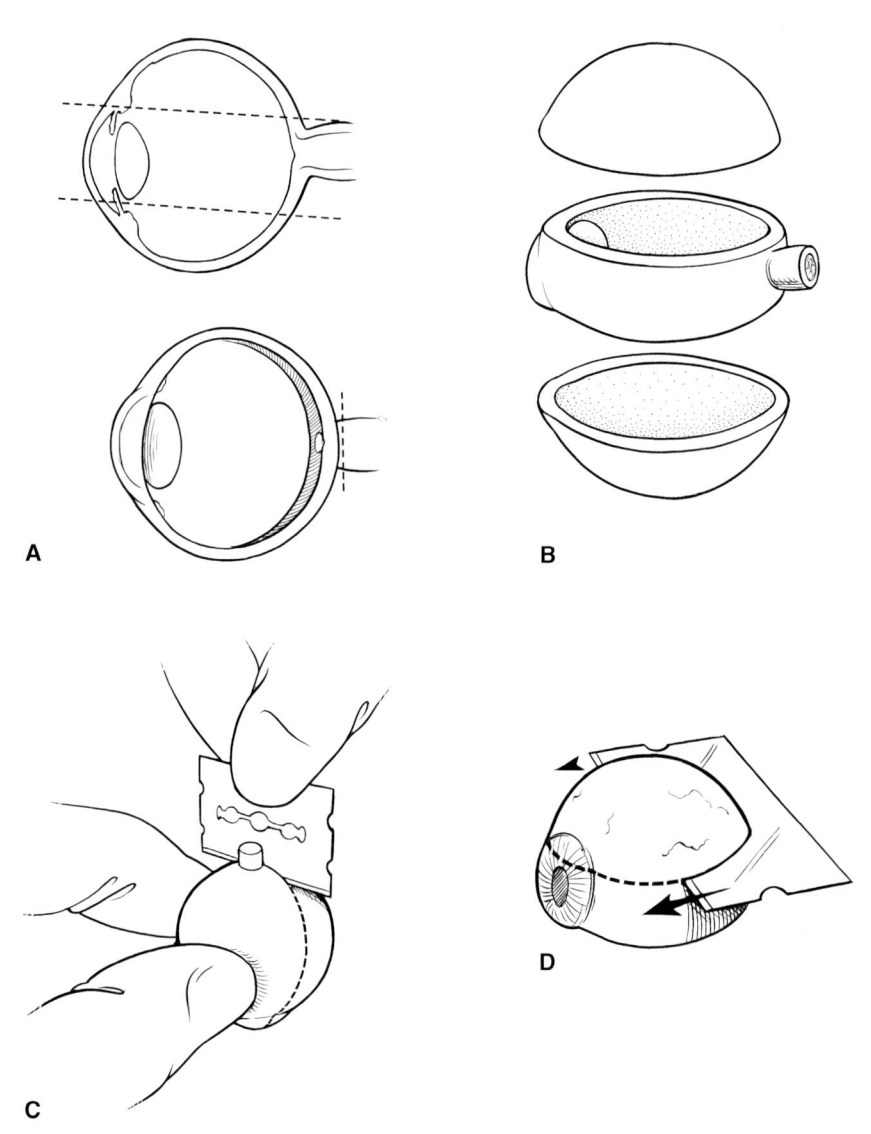

Figure 3-3 **A,** The goal of sectioning is to obtain a pupil–optic nerve (PO) section that contains the maximum area of interest. **B,** Two caps, or *calottes*, are removed to obtain a PO section. **C,** The first cut is generally performed from posterior to anterior. **D,** The second cut will yield the PO section. *(Illustration by Christine Gralapp.)*

The globe can also be opened coronally with separation of the anterior and posterior compartments. The tumor can be visualized directly with this technique, and a section including the maximum extent of the tumor may then be obtained.

Processing and Staining

Fixatives

The most commonly used fixative is 10% neutral buffered formalin. Formalin is a 40% solution of formaldehyde in water that stabilizes protein, lipid, and carbohydrates and prevents postmortem enzymatic destruction of the tissue (autolysis). In specific instances, other fixatives may be preferred, such as glutaraldehyde for electron microscopy and ethyl alcohol for cytologic preparations. Table 3-1 lists examples of some commonly used fixatives.

Formalin diffuses rather quickly through tissue. Because most of the functional tissue of the eye is within 2–3 mm of the surface, it is not necessary or desirable to open the eye. Opening the eye prior to fixation may damage or distort sites of pathology, making histologic interpretation difficult or impossible. The adult eye measures approximately 24 mm in diameter, and formalin diffuses at a rate of approximately 1 mm/hr; therefore, globes should be fixed at least 12 hours prior to processing. It is generally desirable to suspend an eye in formalin in a volume of approximately 10:1 for at least 24 hours prior to processing to ensure adequate fixation. Different institutions may use different protocols, and preoperative consultation is critical.

Tissue Processing

The infiltration and embedding process removes most of the water from the tissue and replaces the water with paraffin. Organic solvents used in this process will dissolve lipid and may dissolve some synthetic materials. Routine processing usually dissolves intraocular lenses made of polymethylmethacrylate (PMMA), polypropylene, and silicone, although the PMMA may fall out during sectioning. Silk, nylon, and other synthetic sutures do not dissolve during routine processing. Specimens are routinely processed through increasing concentrations of alcohol followed by xylene or another clearing agent prior to infiltration with paraffin. Alcohol dehydrates water and xylene replaces alcohol prior to paraffin infiltration. The paraffin mechanically stabilizes the tissue, making possible the cutting of sections.

Table 3-1 Common Fixatives Used in Ophthalmic Pathology

Fixative	Color	Examples of Use
Formalin	Clear	Routine fixation of all tissues
Bouin solution	Yellow	Small biopsies
B5	Clear	Lymphoproliferative tissue (eg, lymph node)
Glutaraldehyde	Clear	Electron microscopy
Ethanol/methanol	Clear	Crystals (eg, urate crystals of gout)
Michel fixative	Light pink	Immunofluorescence
Zenker acetic fixative	Orange	Muscle differentiation

The processing of even a "routine" specimen usually takes a day. Thus, it is unreasonable for a surgeon to expect an interpretation of a specimen sent for permanent sections to be available on the same day as the biopsy. Techniques for the rapid processing of special surgical pathology material are generally reserved for biopsy specimens that require emergent handling. Because the quality of histologic preparation after rapid processing is usually inferior to that of standard processed tissue, it should not be requested routinely. Surgeons should communicate directly with their pathologists about the availability and shortcomings of these techniques.

Tissue Staining

Tissue sections are usually cut at 4–6 μm. A tissue adhesive is sometimes used to secure the thin paraffin section to a glass slide. The cut section is colorless except for areas of indigenous pigmentation, and various tissue dyes—principally hematoxylin and eosin (H&E) and periodic acid–Schiff (PAS)—are used to color the tissue for identification (Fig 3-4). Other histochemical stains used in ophthalmic pathology are alcian blue or colloidal iron for acid mucopolysaccharides, Congo red for amyloid, Gram stain for bacteria, Masson trichrome for collagen, Gomori methenamine silver stain for fungi, and oil red O for lipid. A small amount of resin is placed over the stained section and covered with a thin glass coverslip to protect and preserve it. Table 3-2 lists some common stains and gives examples of their use in ophthalmic pathology.

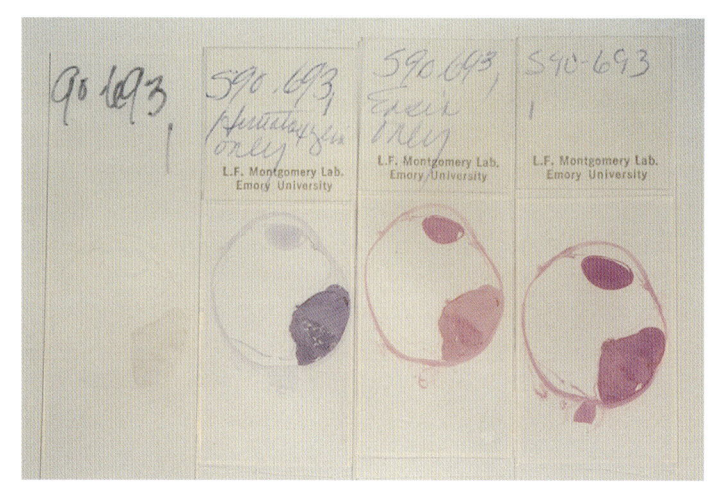

Figure 3-4 The section of paraffin-embedded tissue at the far left is colorless except for mild indigenous pigmentation in the tissue. Moving to the right are shown slides stained with hematoxylin only, eosin only, and both hematoxylin and eosin. *(Courtesy of Hans E. Grossniklaus, MD.)*

Table 3-2 **Common Stains Used in Ophthalmic Pathology**

Stain	Material Stained: Color	Example
Hematoxylin and eosin (H&E)	Nucleus: blue Cytoplasm: red	General tissue stain (Fig 3-2E)
Periodic acid–Schiff (PAS)	Neutral mucopolysaccharide: magenta	Fungi (Fig 6-6)
Alcian blue	Acid mucopolysaccharide: blue	Cavernous optic atrophy (Fig 15-8)
Alizarin red	Calcium: red	Band keratopathy
Colloidal iron	Acid mucopolysaccharide: blue	Macular dystrophy (Fig 6-14)
Congo red	Amyloid: orange, red-green dichroism	Lattice dystrophy (Fig 6-16)
Ziehl-Neelsen	Acid-fast organisms: red	Atypical mycobacterium
Gomori methenamine silver	Fungal elements: black	*Candida, Aspergillus*
Crystal violet	Amyloid: purple, violet	Lattice dystrophy
Gram stain (tissue Brown & Brenn [B&B] or Brown & Hopps [B&H] stain)	Bacteria Positive: blue Negative: red	Bacterial infection (Fig 5-6C)
Masson trichrome	Collagen: blue	Granular dystrophy (Fig 6-15)
	Muscle: red	Red deposits
Perls Prussian blue	Iron: blue	Hemosiderosis bulbi (Fig 6-19B)
Thioflavin T (ThT)	Amyloid: fluorescent yellow	Lattice dystrophy
Verhoeff–van Gieson	Elastic fibers: black	Temporal artery elastic layer
von Kossa	Calcium phosphate salts: black	Band keratopathy (Fig 6-8)

CHAPTER 4

Special Procedures

New technologies have contributed to improvements in the diagnosis of infectious agents and tumors as well as to the classification of tumors, especially the non–Hodgkin lymphomas (NHLs), childhood tumors, and sarcomas. Use of a more extensive test menu of paraffin-active monoclonal antibodies for immunohistochemistry; molecular cytogenetic studies, including standard cytogenetics; multicolor fluorescence in situ hybridization (FISH); polymerase chain reaction (PCR); and locus-specific FISH; as well as developments in high-resolution techniques, including microarray gene expression profiling and array comparative genomic hybridization (CGH), allow a more accurate diagnosis and more precise definition of biomarkers of value in risk stratification and prognosis. The ophthalmic surgeon is responsible for appropriately obtaining and submitting tissue for evaluation and consulting with the ophthalmic pathologist. See Table 4-1 for a checklist of important considerations when submitting tissue for pathologic consultation.

Immunohistochemistry

Pathologists making a diagnosis take advantage of the property that a given cell can express specific antigens. The immunohistochemical stains commonly used in ophthalmic pathology work because a primary antibody binds to a specific antigen in or on a cell, and because that antibody is linked to a chromogen, usually through a secondary antibody (Fig 4-1). The color product of the chromogens generally used in ophthalmic pathology is brown or red in tissue sections, depending on the chromogen selected for use (Fig 4-2). Red chromogen is especially helpful in working with ocular pigmented tissues and melanomas because it differs from the brown melanin (see Fig 4-7).

The precise cell or cells that display the specific antigen can be identified using these methods. Many antibodies are used routinely for diagnosis, treatment, and prognosis:

- cytokeratins for lesions composed of epithelial cells (adenoma, carcinoma)
- desmin, myoglobin, or actin for lesions with smooth muscle or skeletal muscle features (leiomyoma, rhabdomyoma)
- S-100 protein for lesions of neuroectodermal origin (schwannoma, neurofibroma, melanoma)
- HMB-45 and Melan A for melanocytic lesions (nevus, melanoma)

Table 4-1 Checklist for Requesting an Ophthalmic Pathologic Consultation

Routine Specimens (Cornea, pterygium, eyelid lesions, and so on)
1. Fill out requisition form
   a. Sex and age of patient
   b. Location of lesion (laterality and exact location)
   c. Previous biopsies of the site and diagnosis
   d. Pertinent clinical history
   e. Clinical differential diagnosis
   f. Ophthalmologist phone and fax numbers
2. Specimen submitted in adequately sealed container with
   a. ample amount of 10% formalin (at least 5 times the size of the biopsy)
   b. label with patient's name and location of biopsy
3. Drawing/map of site of biopsy for orientation of margins (eyelid lesions for margins, en bloc resections of conjunctiva, scleral, and ciliary body/iris tumors)

Frozen Sections
1. If possible, previous communication with ophthalmic pathologist
2. Fill out specific frozen section requisition form, specifying the reason for submitting tissue, such as
   a. Margins
   b. Diagnosis
   c. Adequacy of sampling
   d. Obtaining tissue for molecular diagnosis (retinoblastoma, rhabdomyosarcoma, metastatic neuroblastoma, etc) or flow cytometry
3. Map/diagram of lesion indicating margins and orientation
4. Labeling of tissue (ink, sutures) to orient according to the diagram (for margins)

FNAB and Cytology
1. Previous communication with ophthalmic pathologist to discuss
   a. Logistics of the biopsy
      i. Possible adequacy check during the biopsy (intraocular tumors)
      ii. Fixative to be used
      iii. Fresh tissue for possible molecular diagnosis
   b. Fill out specific cytology form

Molecular Techniques and Electron Microscopy
1. Previous communication with ophthalmic pathologist to discuss
   a. Differential diagnosis
   b. Fixative (fresh vs alcohol vs glutaraldehyde vs other)
   c. Logistics of the biopsy
      i. Time and date (availability of specialized personnel)

- chromogranin and synaptophysin for neuroendocrine lesions (metastatic carcinoid [see Fig 4-2], small cell carcinoma)
- leukocyte common antigen for lesions of hematopoietic origin (leukemia, lymphoma)
- Her2Neu and c-Kit for prognosis and treatment (metastatic breast carcinoma, mastocytosis)

These antibodies vary in their specificity and sensitivity. Specificities and sensitivities of new antibodies are continually being evaluated (for examples, see the online immunohistology query system at www.immunoquery.com). Automated equipment and antigen retrieval techniques are currently used to increase sensitivity and decrease turnaround

CHAPTER 4: Special Procedures • 43

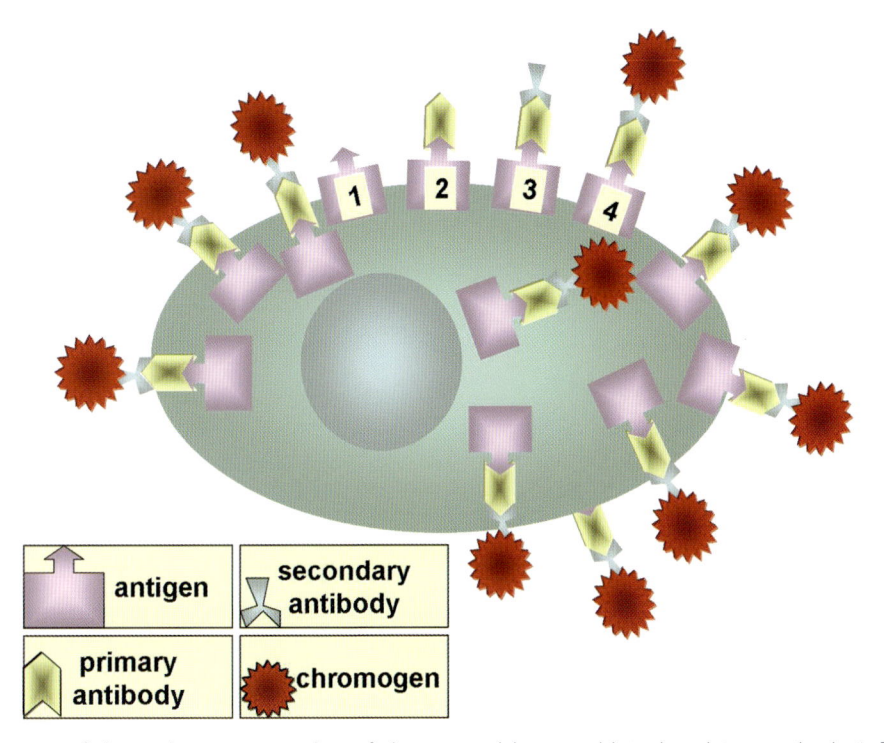

Figure 4-1 Schematic representation of the general immunohistochemistry method. *1,* The cellular antigen is recognized by the specific primary antibody, *2*. A secondary antibody, *3,* directed against the primary antibody reacts with the enzymatic complex to create the chromogen, *4*. The final product allows the visualization of the cell containing the antigen. *(Courtesy of Patricia Chévez-Barrios, MD.)*

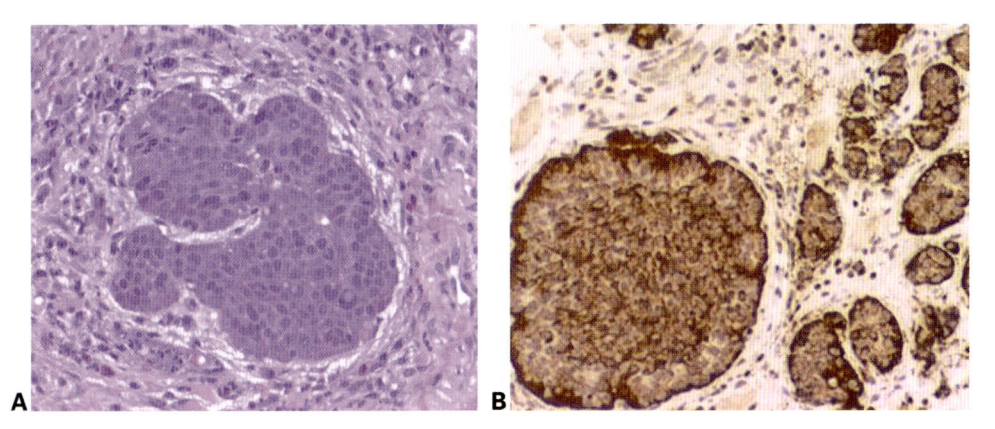

Figure 4-2 A metastatic carcinoid to the orbit seen by H&E **(A)** shows bland epithelial characteristics. **B,** Chromogranin antibody highlights the neuroendocrine nature of the cells. *(Courtesy of Patricia Chévez-Barrios, MD.)*

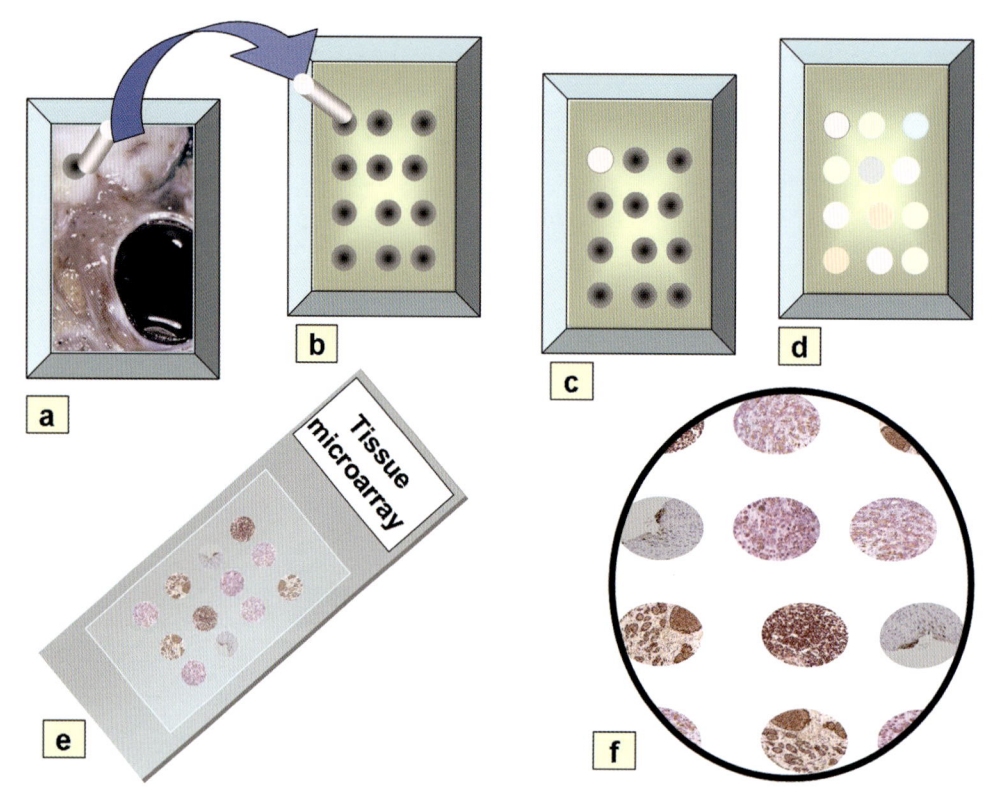

Figure 4-3 Tissue microarrays are constructed with small core biopsies of different tumors/tissues. A core is obtained from the donor paraffin block of the tumor (a). A recipient paraffin block is prepared, creating empty cores (b). The cores are incorporated into the slots (c) until all are occupied (d). Glass slides are prepared and stained with a selected antibody (e). Microscopic examination reveals the different staining patterns of each core (f). *(Courtesy of Patricia Chévez-Barrios, MD.)*

time. Protein expression is presently evaluated, for research purposes mainly, in large series of tumors and tissues included in tissue microarrays (TMAs). Tissue microarrays are paraffin blocks constructed with multiple cores of different tumors/tissues, including positive controls. Microscopic slides are prepared from these blocks and immunohistochemistry performed on a single slide for the entire group of samples (Fig 4-3).

Flow Cytometry, Molecular Pathology, and Diagnostic Electron Microscopy

Flow Cytometry

Flow cytometry is used to analyze the physical and chemical properties of particles or cells moving in single file in a fluid stream (Fig 4-4, *a*). An example of flow cytometry is immunophenotyping of leukocytes. The cells need to be fresh (unfixed). Fluorochrome-labeled specific antibodies bind to the surface of lymphoid cells, and a suspension of labeled

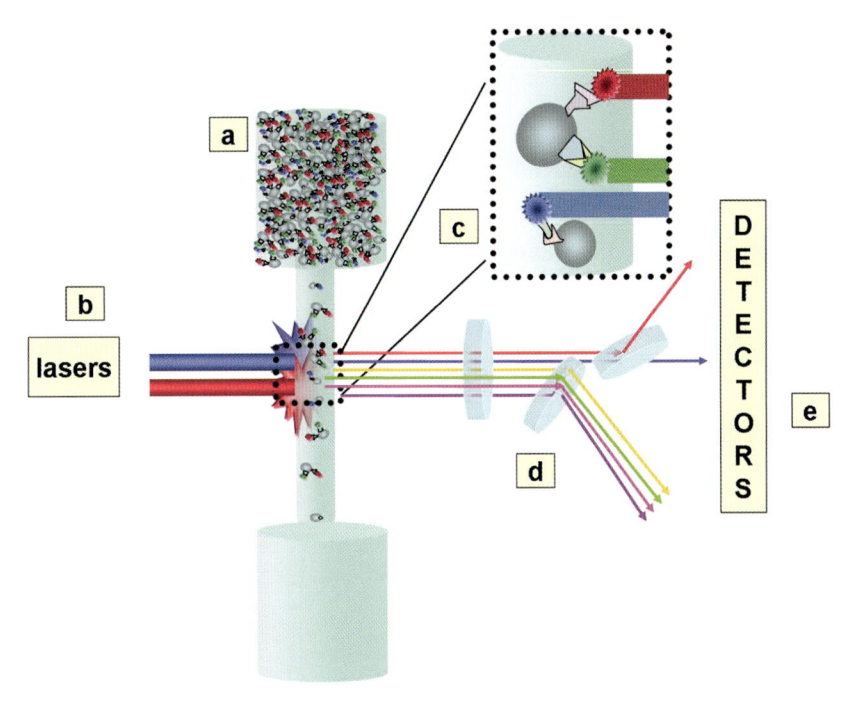

Figure 4-4 Flow cytometry analyzes particles or cells moving in single file in a fluid stream *(a)*. Fluorochrome-labeled specific antibodies bind to the surface of cells, and a suspension of labeled cells is sequentially illuminated by a laser *(b)*. As the excited fluorochrome returns to its resting energy level, a specific wavelength of light is emitted *(c)* that is sorted by wavelength *(d)* and received by a photodetector *(e)*. This signal is then converted to electronic impulses, which are in turn analyzed by computer software. *(Courtesy of Patricia Chévez-Barrios, MD.)*

cells is sequentially illuminated by a light source (usually argon laser) for approximately 10^{-6} second (Fig 4-4, *b*). As the excited fluorochrome returns to its resting energy level, a specific wavelength of light is emitted (Fig 4-4, *c*) that is sorted by wavelength stream (Fig 4-4, *d*) and received by a photodetector (Fig 4-4, *e*). This signal is then converted to electronic impulses, which are in turn analyzed by computer software. The results may be imaged by a multicolored dot-plot histogram (Fig 4-5). The most common use of flow cytometry in clinical practice is for immunophenotyping hematopoietic proliferations. This procedure may be performed on vitreous, aqueous, or ocular adnexal tissue.

In addition, multiple antibodies and cellular size can be analyzed, and the relative percentages of cells may be displayed. For example, CD4 (helper T cells), CD8 (suppressor T cells), both $CD4^+$ and $CD8^+$, or either $CD4^+$ or $CD8^+$ may be displayed for a given lymphocytic infiltrate. The advantage of this method is that it actually shows the percentages of particular cells in a specimen. Disadvantages are the failure to show the location and distribution of these cells in tissue and the possibility of sampling errors. Depending on the number of cells in the sample and on clinical information, the flow cytometrist chooses the panel of antibodies to be tested. Flow cytometric data should therefore be used as an adjunct to morphologic H&E and sometimes immunohistochemistry interpretation. Flow cytometric analysis is particularly useful for the evaluation of lymphoid proliferations.

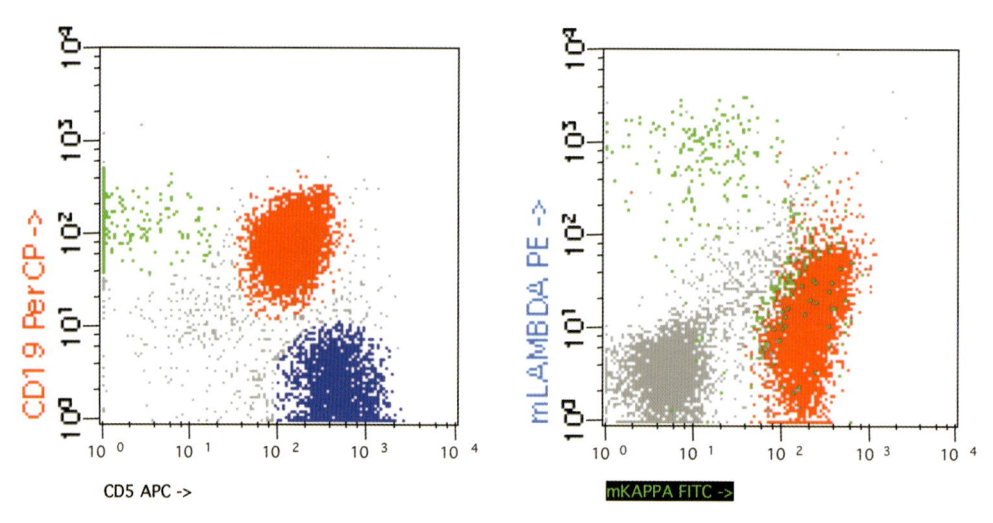

Figure 4-5 Flow cytometry scatter graphs showing a clonal population of CD19⁺ kappa restricted lymphocytes. Note that most of the CD19⁺ cells fail to express lambda light chains. *(Courtesy of Patricia Chévez-Barrios, MD.)*

Molecular Pathology

Molecular pathology techniques are used increasingly in diagnostic ophthalmic pathology and extensively in experimental pathology. A common molecular biological technique is the *polymerase chain reaction (PCR)*, which amplifies a single strand of nucleic acid thousands of times, enabling recognition (Fig 4-6). Techniques used in diagnostic pathology are presented in brief in Table 4-2. Molecular pathology is used to identify tumor-promoting or tumor-inhibiting genes (CGH, PCR, array CGH), such as the retinoblastoma gene; and viral DNA or RNA strands, such as those seen in herpesviruses and Epstein-Barr virus (PCR, in situ hybridization [ISH]). The clinical relevance of detecting a PCR product depends on numerous variables, including the primers selected, the laboratory controls, and the demographic considerations. Therefore, PCR should be used to derive supplementary information for making a clinicopathologic diagnosis. For further information about the PCR technique, see Part III, Genetics, in BCSC Section 2, *Fundamentals and Principles of Ophthalmology*.

Leukemias, lymphomas, and soft tissue tumors represent a heterogeneous group of lesions whose classification continues to evolve as a result of advances in cytogenetic and molecular techniques. In the last decade, traditional diagnostic approaches were supplemented by the successful application of these newer techniques (see Table 4-2) to formalin-fixed, paraffin-embedded tissue, making it possible to subject a broader range of clinical material to molecular analysis. Thus, molecular genetics has already become an integral part of the workup in tumors, such as pediatric orbital tumors (rhabdomyosarcomas, neuroblastoma, peripheral neuroectodermal tumors [PNET]), that demonstrate characteristic translocations. Based on the results, treatment can be directed and prognostic features associated with certain mutations and translocations.

The evolution of molecular pathology techniques has made it possible not only to recognize the presence or absence of a strand of nucleic acid but also to demonstrate the localization in the specific cells (FISH, ISH).

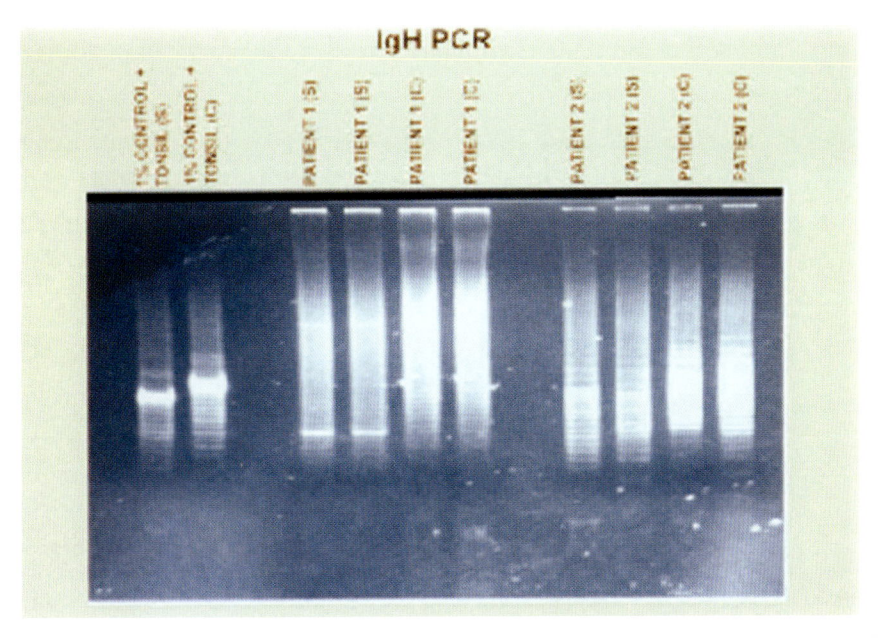

Figure 4-6 A patient's conjunctival lymphoid infiltrate was evaluated by PCR for clonality. PCR of the patient's infiltrate demonstrated a clonal band of IgH gene rearrangement in the lanes labeled "Patient 1 (S)." *(Courtesy of Hans E. Grossniklaus, MD.)*

Hicks J, Mierau GW. The spectrum of pediatric tumors in infancy, childhood, and adolescence: a comprehensive review with emphasis on special techniques in diagnosis. *Ultrastruct Pathol.* 2005;29:175–202.

Oostlander AE, Meijer GA, Ylstra B. Microarray-based comparative genomic hybridization and its applications in human genetics. *Clin Genet.* 2004;66:488–495.

Diagnostic Electron Microscopy

Diagnostic electron microscopy is used primarily to indicate the cell of origin of a tumor of questionable differentiation rather than to distinguish between benign and malignant processes. Although immunopathologic studies are less expensive and performed more rapidly than diagnostic electron microscopy, in some cases, diagnostic electron microscopy complements immunopathologic studies. Once again, the surgeon should consult with the pathologist before surgery to determine whether diagnostic electron microscopy might play a role in the study of a particular tissue specimen.

Special Techniques

Fine-Needle Aspiration Biopsy

Fine-needle aspiration biopsy (FNAB) has been used instead of excisional biopsy by non-ophthalmic surgeons and pathologists. It is especially useful if the physician performing the biopsy can grasp the lesion (usually between the thumb and forefinger) and make several passes with the needle to obtain representative areas. In the practice of general

Table 4-2 Summary of Molecular Techniques Used in Diagnostic Pathology

Technique	Year	Method	Advantages	Disadvantages
Karyotyping	1950s	Chromosomes treated to spread apart and arrange into pairs	Identification of specific chromosomal abnormalities	1. Need for dividing cells 2. Resolution limitations; cannot detect small aberrations
Chromosomal banding	1960s	Metaphase chromosomes stained, producing patterns of dark and light bands along the length of each chromosome	Gross chromosomal abnormalities, both numerical and structural, studied more easily	1. Need for dividing cells 2. Resolution limitations; cannot detect small aberrations
Fluorescence in situ hybridization (FISH)	1980s	Chromosome region-specific, fluorescent-labeled DNA probes (cloned pieces genomic DNA) able to detect their complementary DNA sequences	1. Localization in the lesion of positive cells 2. Fluorescent signal easily detected in fresh or fixed tissue	1. Known type and location of expected aberrations 2. Limited number of chromosomal loci at one time
Polymerase chain reaction (PCR)	1980s	Amplification of a single strand of nucleic acid thousands of times, enabling recognition	Quality snap-frozen tissue (optimal) and archival paraffin-embedded tissue	1. Variable success rate of DNA extraction 2. Contamination with other nucleic acid material
Reverse transcriptase-polymerase chain reaction (RT-PCR)	1990s	Detection of specific chimeric RNA transcripts	Quality snap-frozen tissue (optimal) and archival paraffin-embedded tissue	1. Variable success rate of RNA extraction 2. Contamination with other nucleic acid material
"Real time" quantitative RT-PCR	1999	Measurement of PCR-product accumulation during the exponential phase of the PCR reaction using a dual-labeled fluorogenic probe	Direct detection of PCR-product formation by measuring the increase in fluorescent emission continuously during the PCR reaction	Variable success rate of RNA extraction
Comparative genomic hybridization (CGH)	1990s	Genomic DNAs of test (patient) and reference (normal) samples, labeled green and red, respectively.	1. Detects and maps alterations in copy number of DNA sequences	Inability to detect mosaicism, balanced chromosomal translocations, inversions, and whole-genome ploidy changes

(Continued)

Table 4-2 (continued)

Technique	Year	Method	Advantages	Disadvantages
		Normal chromosomes = yellow (red + green) with ratio of 1. Deleted regions = red with ratio <1. Amplified regions = green with ratio >1.	2. Analyzes all chromosomes in a single experiment and no dividing cells required	
Microarray-based CGH (array CGH)	2000s	Differentially labeled test and reference DNAs, hybridized to cloned fragments, genomic DNA or cDNA, which are spotted on a glass slide (the array). The DNA copy number aberrations measured by detecting intensity differences in the hybridization patterns	High resolution	1. Inability to detect aberrations not resulting in copy number changes 2. Limited in its ability to detect mosaicism

surgical pathology, FNAB is very useful in assessing enlarged lymph nodes, thyroid nodules, salivary gland masses, and breast masses.

Intraocular FNAB may be useful in distinguishing between primary uveal tumors and metastases. The procedure is performed under direct visualization through a dilated pupil. Iris tumors may be accessible for FNAB during slit-lamp biomicroscopy. However, FNAB alone cannot reliably predict the prognosis of a uveal melanoma because the sample with intraocular FNAB is limited. Intraocular FNAB may also enable tumor cells to escape the eye; this possibility is an area of some controversy. In general, properly performed, FNAB does not pose a risk for seeding a tumor, but retinoblastoma is a notable exception. FNAB of a possible retinoblastoma lesion, if indicated, should be performed by an *ophthalmic oncologist* with ample experience in making the diagnosis and performing the procedure.

The cells obtained through FNAB can be processed through cytospin, liquid base cytology, or cell block (Fig 4-7). Cell block allows the pathologist to employ special stains, immunohistochemistry, and in situ hybridization, if necessary.

Some orbital surgeons have used FNAB in the diagnosis of orbital lesions, especially presumed metastases to the orbit and optic nerve tumors. However, because it is difficult to make several passes at different angles through an intraorbital tumor, FNAB of orbital masses may not adequately sample representative areas of the tumor. Specific indications

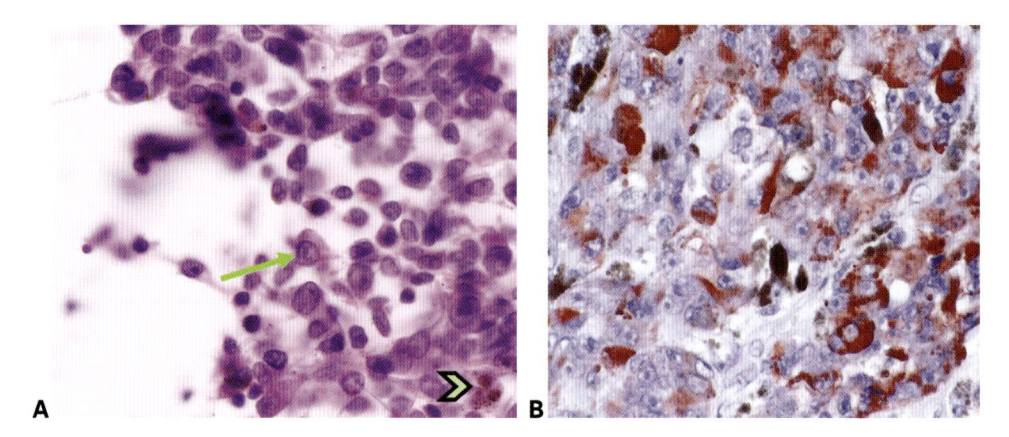

Figure 4-7 Fine-needle aspiration biopsy (FNAB) of choroidal tumor. **A,** Cytologic liquid-based preparation displays prominent nucleoli *(arrow)* and some brown pigment *(arrowhead)* suggestive of melanoma. **B,** Cell block of the aspirated cells, stained with HMB-45 using a red chromogen, is positive, confirming the diagnosis of melanoma. Notice the difference between the red chromogen and the brown melanin. *(Courtesy of Patricia Chévez-Barrios, MD.)*

for when and when not to perform intraocular or intraorbital FNAB are beyond the scope of this discussion, but some of these indications are discussed in Part II of this book, Intraocular Tumors: Clinical Aspects. Ophthalmic FNAB should be performed only when an ophthalmic pathologist or cytologist experienced in the preparation and interpretation of these specimens is available. The surgeon should be prepared to treat the patient appropriately when the FNAB results become known.

> Cohen VM, Dinakaran S, Parsons MA, Rennie IG. Transvitreal fine needle aspiration biopsy: the influence of intraocular lesion size on diagnostic biopsy result. *Eye.* 2001;15(Pt 2):143–147.
> Shields JA, Shields CL, Ehya H, Eagle RC Jr, De Potter P. Fine-needle aspiration biopsy of suspected intraocular tumors. The 1992 Urwick Lecture. *Ophthalmology.* 1993;100:1677–1684.

Frozen Section

Permanent sections (tissue that is processed after fixation through alcohols and xylenes, embedded in paraffin, and sectioned) are always preferred in ophthalmic pathology because of the inherent small size of samples. If the lesion is too small, it could be lost during frozen sectioning. A frozen section (tissue that is snap-frozen and immediately sectioned in a cryostat) is indicated when the results of the study will affect management of the patient in the operating room. For example, the most frequent indication for a frozen section is to determine whether the resection margins are free of tumor, especially in eyelid carcinomas. Appropriate orientation of the specimen (through drawings of the excision site, labeled margins, or margins of the excised tissue that are tagged with sutures or other markers) is crucial when submitting tissue for margin evaluation.

Two techniques are used for accessing the margins in eyelid carcinomas (basal cell carcinoma, squamous cell carcinoma, and sebaceous carcinoma): regular frozen sections and Mohs micrographic surgery. Mohs surgery preserves tissue while obtaining free margins. Eyelid lesions, especially those located in the canthal areas, require tissue conservation to maintain adequate cosmetic results and function. Other frequent indications for frozen sections are to determine whether the surgeon has biopsied representative material for diagnosis (metastasis) and to submit fresh tissue for flow cytometry and molecular genetics (sarcomas, lymphomas, and so on). Frozen sections are not indicated merely to satisfy the curiosity of the surgeon or the patient's family; the utilization of frozen sections is carefully monitored by most hospital quality assurance committees. Surgeons must keep in mind that the use of frozen sections is a time-intensive and costly process.

It is considered inappropriate to order frozen sections and then to proceed with a case before receiving the results from the pathologist. To ensure adequate understanding of the case and facilitate the best possible results for the patient, the surgeon should communicate with the pathologist ahead of time if a frozen section is anticipated.

> Chévez-Barrios P. Frozen section diagnosis and indications in ophthalmic pathology. *Arch Pathol Lab Med.* 2005;129:1626–1634.

CHAPTER 5

Conjunctiva

Topography

The conjunctiva is a mucous membrane lining the posterior surface of the eyelids and the anterior surface of the globe as far as the limbus. It can be subdivided into *palpebral, forniceal,* and *bulbar* sections. The conjunctiva consists of stratified, nonkeratinizing squamous epithelium that is flat and regular without goblet cells in the epibulbar area and, at the limbus, may be slightly pigmented (Fig 5-1A). In the palpebral area, the epithelium is thickened and covers nests of lymphocytes, vessels, and some lymphoid follicle in children and young adults (Fig 5-1B). The squamous epithelium is interspersed with mucus-containing goblet cells, which are most numerous in the fornices and plica semilunaris (Fig 5-1C, 5-1D). The epithelial layer covers a substantia propria that is thickest in the fornices and thinnest covering the tarsus. Constituents of this stromal layer include loosely arranged collagen fibers; vessels; nerves; and resident lymphocytes, plasma cells, and mast cells. In the medial canthal area, the conjunctiva forms a vertical fold, the *plica semilunaris,* and medial to this is the *caruncle.* The caruncle is covered by nonkeratinizing stratified squamous epithelium, and within the stroma are sebaceous glands, hair follicles, and accessory lacrimal glands. BCSC Section 8, *External Disease and Cornea,* also discusses the conjunctiva in depth.

Congenital Anomalies

Choristomas

Choristomas are congenital proliferations of histologically mature tissue elements not normally present at the site of occurrence. Examples include

- limbal dermoid
- dermolipoma
- ectopic lacrimal gland
- episcleral osseous choristoma

Dermoids are firm, dome-shaped, white-yellow papules at or straddling the limbus in the inferotemporal quadrant. Size varies from a few millimeters to more than 1 cm. They may occur in isolation or, particularly when bilateral, as a manifestation of a congenital

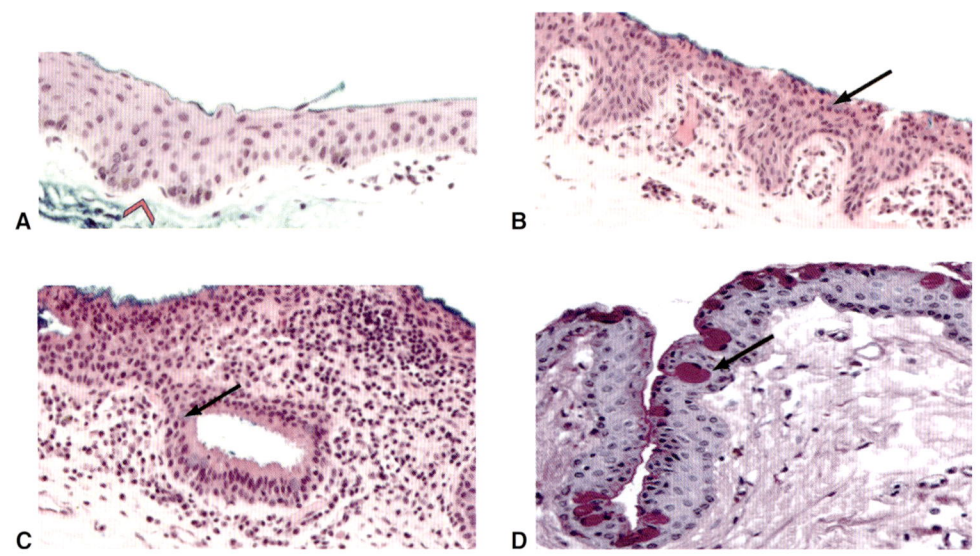

Figure 5-1 A, Epibulbar conjunctiva with regular, nonkeratinizing squamous epithelium with areas of light basal pigmentation at the limbus *(arrowhead).* **B,** Palpebral conjunctiva with thickened epithelium covering vessels and inflammatory cells and containing some goblet cells *(arrow).* **C,** Conjunctiva at the fornix may contain pseudoglands of Henle, infoldings of conjunctiva with abundant goblet cells *(arrow).* **D,** Periodic acid–Schiff (PAS) stain highlights the mucinous origin of the goblet cells *(arrow). (Courtesy of Patricia Chévez-Barrios, MD.)*

complex such as Goldenhar syndrome or linear nevus sebaceous syndrome. A dermoid recapitulates the tissues of the skin; that is, it contains epidermis and dermis, including dermal adnexal structures. The surface epithelium may or may not be keratinized. Figure 6-3, in Chapter 6, shows an example of a corneal dermoid.

Dermolipomas occur more frequently in the superotemporal quadrant toward the fornix and may extend posteriorly into the orbit. A dermolipoma is softer and yellower than a limbal dermoid as a result of the adipose tissue component present in the deeper layers of the choristoma (Fig 5-2). Histopathologically, it also differs from a dermoid in that the dermal adnexal structures are often absent. Dermolipomas may also be associated with Goldenhar syndrome or linear nevus sebaceous syndrome.

Complex choristomas, in addition to having the features of a dermoid or dermolipoma, include other tissues such as cartilage, bone, and lacrimal gland. Clinically, they usually are indistinguishable from dermoids or dermolipomas.

Spencer WH, ed. *Ophthalmic Pathology: An Atlas and Textbook.* Vol 1. 4th ed. Philadelphia: Saunders; 1996:chap 2.

Hamartomas

Hamartomas, in contrast to choristomas, are overgrowths of mature tissue normally present at that site. In the conjunctiva, the most common variety of hamartoma is *hemangioma,* although a hemangioma can also be considered to be a true neoplasm. Although it may involve only the conjunctiva, typically the hemangioma is also present in the eyelid, face,

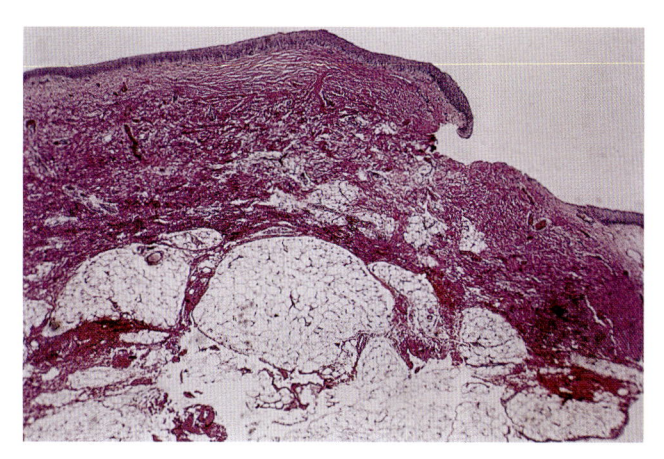

Figure 5-2 A dermolipoma differs from a dermoid in that adnexal structures are often absent and significant amounts of mature adipose tissue are present in the deeper aspect of the choristoma. *(Courtesy of Harry H. Brown, MD.)*

and orbit. Congenital hemangiomas are detected at or shortly after birth as elevated, soft, red-purple nodules that may continue to grow in the first year of life before stabilizing. The majority of cases then begin a slow process of involution, resulting in complete regression. Intervention is necessary only when vision or ocular integrity is compromised. The histopathologic appearance varies depending on the stage at which the tissue is excised. Early, actively growing hemangiomas show a cellular proliferation of plump endothelial cells forming solid nests and cords within the connective tissue stroma. Mitotic figures are often present. In fully developed hemangiomas, the endothelial cells flatten, forming easily recognizable capillary lumina. In the involutional phase, the lobules of capillary proliferation are replaced by fibrous tissue.

Inflammations

Because the conjunctiva is an exposed surface, a variety of organisms, toxic agents, and allergens can initiate an inflammatory response known as *conjunctivitis*. Clinically, the response can be subdivided into acute or chronic conjunctivitis, according to the time frame of signs and symptoms. *Acute conjunctivitis* has a rapid onset of redness and irritation. Mucus production is particularly prominent in the acute phase and, in concert with the sloughing of necrotic epithelium and outpouring of acute inflammatory cells and fibrin, a surface membrane may form. A true membrane is formed when the underlying epithelium is ulcerated and granulation tissue forms beneath the fibrinopurulent exudate; attempts to remove a true membrane will result in petechial hemorrhages. However, if the underlying epithelium remains intact, removal does not cause bleeding and the surface material is known as a *pseudomembrane*.

The signs and symptoms of *chronic conjunctivitis* develop more insidiously. The inflammatory response is composed predominantly of lymphocytes and plasma cells, often causing localized nodules with infoldings of surface epithelium *(pseudoglands of Henle)*.

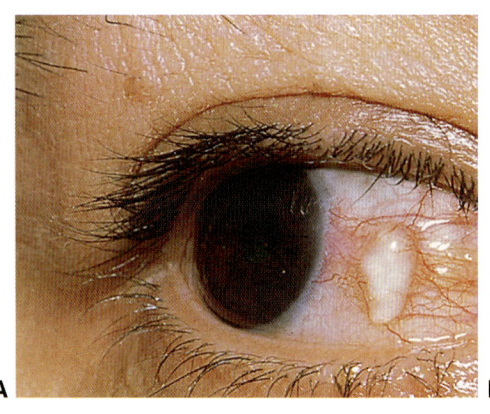

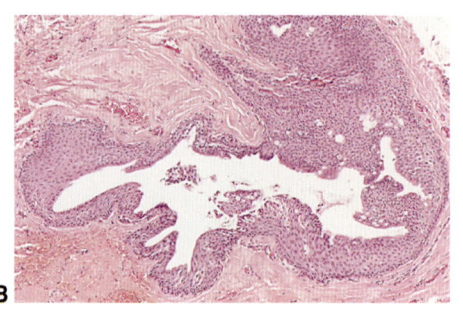

Figure 5-3 A, Epithelial inclusion cysts may follow conjunctival trauma. **B,** The cyst is lined by nonkeratinizing, stratified squamous epithelium, consistent with conjunctiva.

Although more commonly a sequela of trauma, epithelial inclusion cysts and calcification of inspissated secretions may also occur in the postinflammatory period (Fig 5-3).

Papillary versus Follicular Conjunctivitis

Conjunctivitis may be further subdivided into papillary and follicular types, according to the macroscopic and microscopic appearance of the conjunctiva (Fig 5-4). Neither is pathognomonic for a particular disease entity. *Papillary conjunctivitis* shows a cobblestone arrangement of flattened nodules with a central vascular core (Fig 5-5). It is most commonly associated with an allergic immune response, as in vernal and atopic keratoconjunctivitis, or is a response to a foreign body such as a contact lens or ocular prosthesis. Papillae coat the tarsal surface of the upper eyelid and may reach large size *(giant papillary conjunctivitis).* Limbal papillae may occur in vernal keratoconjunctivitis *(Horner-Trantas dots).* The histopathologic appearance is identical, regardless of the cause: closely packed, mesa-like nodules lined by conjunctival epithelium, with numerous eosinophils, lymphocytes, and plasma cells in the stroma surrounding a central vascular channel. Mast cells may also be conspicuous.

Follicular conjunctivitis is seen in a variety of conditions, including those caused by pathogens such as viruses; bacteria; chlamydiae; and toxins, including ocular topical medications (antiglaucomatous, over-the-counter ophthalmic decongestants, and so on; Fig 5-6). In contrast to papillae, follicles are small, dome-shaped nodules without a prominent central vessel. Histopathologically, they are composed of aggregates of lymphocytes and plasma cells in the superficial stroma between the tarsus and the fornix or within the palpebral and bulbar conjunctiva. Lymphocytes may form germinal centers within the follicles, complete with tingible body macrophages (histiocytes containing ingested intracytoplasmic nuclear debris).

Blondeau P, Rousseau JA. Allergic reactions to brimonidine in patients treated for glaucoma. *Can J Ophthalmol.* 2002;37:21–26.

Soparkar CN, Wilhelmus KR, Koch DD, Wallace GW, Jones DB. Acute and chronic conjunctivitis due to over-the-counter ophthalmic decongestants. *Arch Ophthalmol.* 1997;115:34–38.

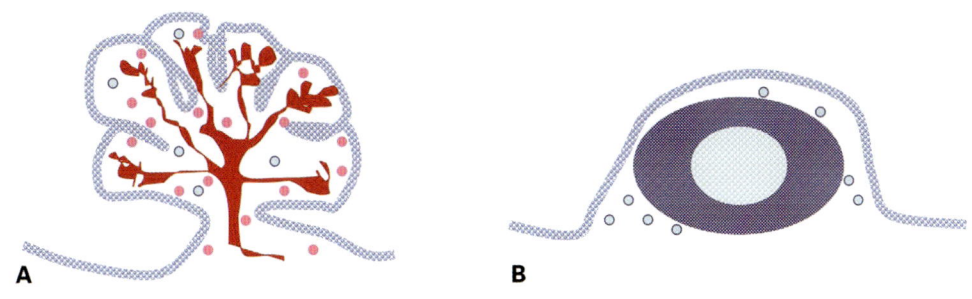

Figure 5-4 Schematic representation of papillary and follicular conjunctivitis. **A,** In papillary conjunctivitis, the conjunctival epithelium *(pale blue)* covers fibrovascular cores with blood vessels *(red)*, and the stroma contains eosinophils *(pink)* and lymphocytes and plasma cells *(dark blue)*. **B,** In follicular conjunctivitis, the conjunctival epithelium covers lymphocytes, forming follicles with paler follicular centers *(dark blue with central pale blue)*, and the surrounding stroma contains lymphocytes and plasma cells *(dark blue)*. *(Courtesy of Patricia Chévez-Barrios, MD.)*

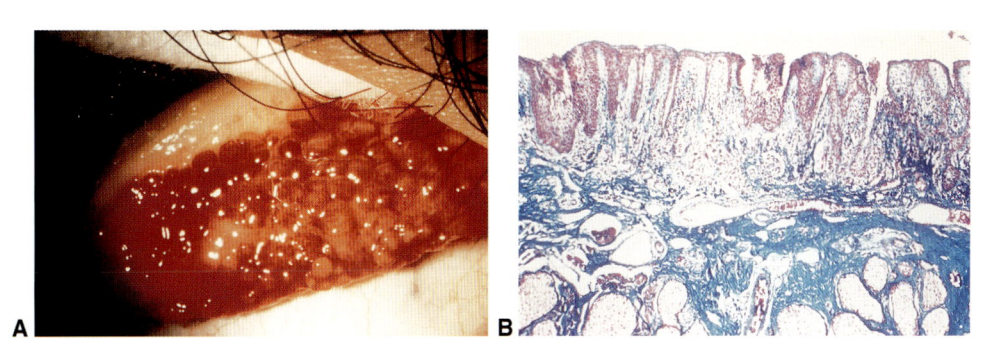

Figure 5-5 A, Papillae efface the normal palpebral conjunctival surface and form a confluent cobblestone pattern. **B,** Low-power photomicrograph highlights the closely packed, flat-topped papillae with central fibrovascular cores (trichrome stain). *(Courtesy of Harry H. Brown, MD.)*

Infectious Conjunctivitis

A wide variety of pathogens may infect the conjunctiva, including viruses, bacteria, fungi, and chlamydiae. The most common offending agents in children are bacterial *(Haemophilus influenzae)* and, in adults, viral; the usual culprits are adenovirus and the herpesviruses (simplex and zoster). Viral infections, in addition to inciting a follicular conjunctivitis, often affect the cornea, resulting in ulcers in herpetic disease and subepithelial infiltrates in adenoviral disease.

Bacterial infections cause about 50% of the cases of conjunctivitis in children and 5% of the cases in adults. See BCSC Section 8, *External Disease and Cornea,* for additional information on current pathogens.

When the conjunctiva alone is infected, fungi are rarely the inciting pathogen. *Rhinosporidium seeberi,* which may cause an isolated conjunctivitis, is seen most often in areas such as India and Southeast Asia.

Chlamydiae are obligate intracellular pathogens, among which *Chlamydia trachomatis* is a major cause of ocular infection, particularly in the Middle East. Serotypes A, B,

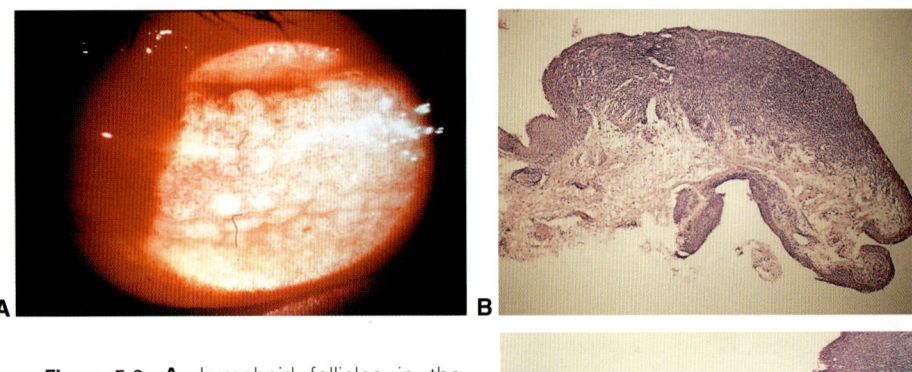

Figure 5-6 A, Lymphoid follicles in the bulbar conjunctiva obscure the underlying congested conjunctival vasculature and cause an irregular light reflex. **B** and **C,** Nodular lymphoid aggregates may develop germinal centers. *(Part A courtesy of Hans E. Grossniklaus, MD; parts B and C courtesy of Harry H. Brown, MD.)*

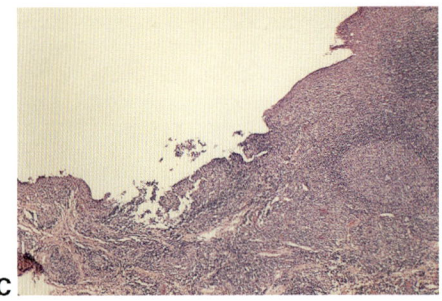

and C are associated with trachoma; serotypes D through K cause neonatal and adult inclusion conjunctivitis. *Microsporida* is another group of obligate intracellular parasites that may cause conjunctivitis, keratitis, or keratoconjunctivitis, particularly in patients with acquired immunodeficiency syndrome (AIDS). Exfoliative cytology of conjunctival or corneal epithelium (Giemsa stain) may be useful in demonstrating these intracellular organisms (Fig 5-7).

> Kane KY, Meadows S, Ellis MR. Clinical inquiries. When should acute nonvenereal conjunctivitis be treated with topical antibiotics? *J Fam Pract.* 2002;51:312.
> Wald ER. Conjunctivitis in infants and children. *Pediatr Infect Dis J.* 1997;16:S17–20.

Noninfectious Conjunctivitis

Sarcoidosis may involve any ocular tissues, including the conjunctiva. It manifests as small, tan nodules, primarily within the forniceal conjunctiva. Conjunctival biopsy can be a simple, expedient way of providing pathologic correlation in this systemic disease. Histopathologically, granulomas (aggregates of epithelioid histiocytes) are present within the conjunctival stroma with a variable, but usually minimal, cuff of lymphocytes and plasma cells. Multinucleated giant cells may or may not be present within the granuloma. Central necrosis is not characteristic and, if present, should suggest other causes of granulomatous inflammation, such as infection with mycobacteria, fungi, spirochetes, or parasites. Bacteria such as *Francisella tularensis* (tularemia) and *Bartonella henselae* (cat-scratch disease) are other considerations; these usually are accompanied by microabscesses. The diagnosis of sarcoidosis is tenable only when supported by clinical findings and after other causes of granulomatous inflammation have been excluded by histochemical stains and/or, most

CHAPTER 5: Conjunctiva • 59

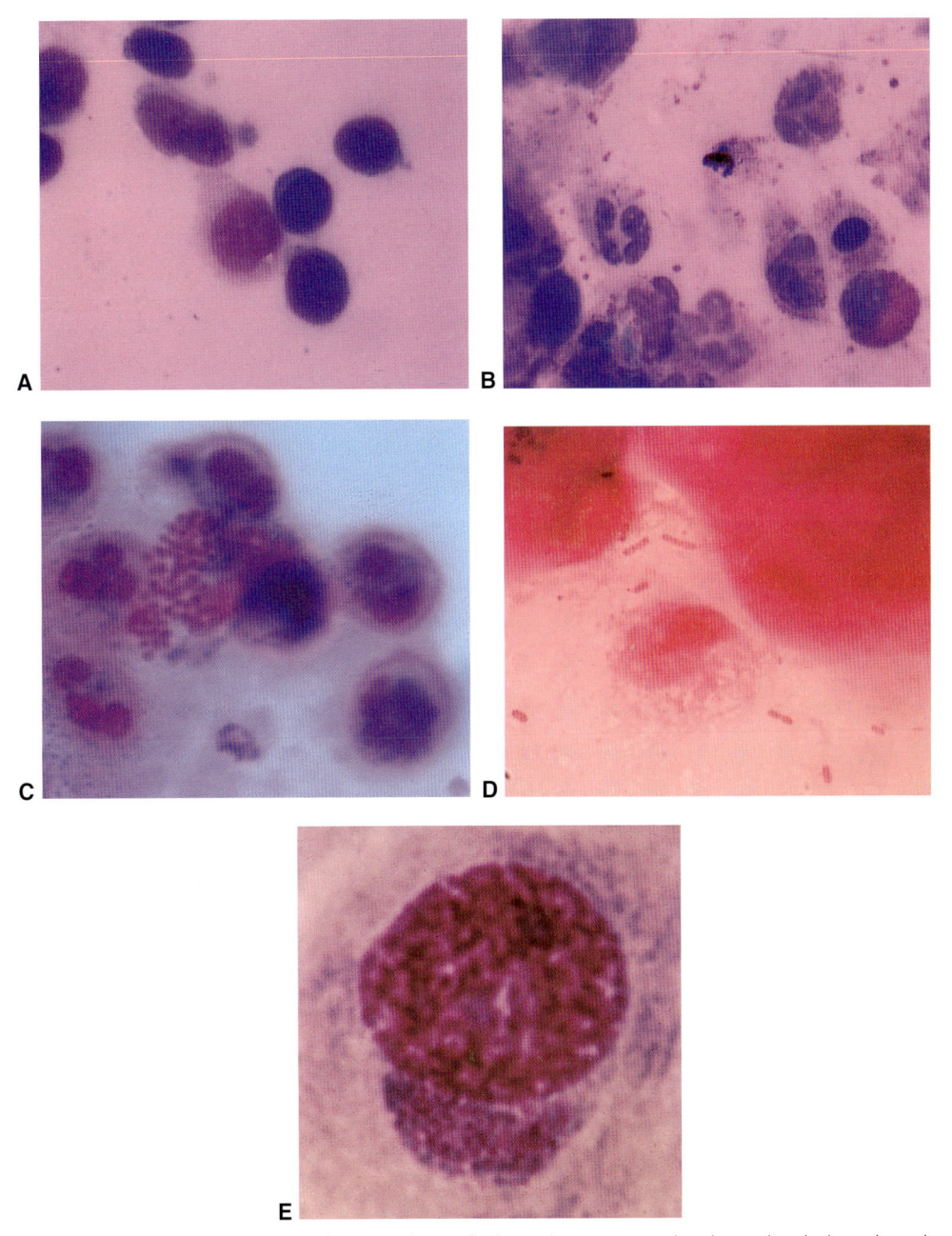

Figure 5-7 Exfoliative conjunctival cytology. **A,** Lymphocytes predominate in viral conjunctivitis. **B,** A mixture of polymorphonuclear leukocytes and eosinophils is typical of vernal conjunctivitis. **C,** Gram stain reveals the polymorphonuclear leukocyte response to gonococcal conjunctivitis. Note the intracellular, gram-negative diplococci. **D,** A case of *Moraxella lacunata* angular conjunctivitis demonstrating the bacilli, which often are found in pairs. **E,** *Chlamydia*, conjunctival scraping, Giemsa stain. The inclusion body, composed of multiple chlamydial organisms, can be seen capping the nucleus. A distinct space separates the inclusion body from the nuclear chromatin. Occasionally, crushing the cells during specimen preparation may cause chromatin to stream through a defect in the nuclear membrane, resulting in an appearance similar to that of a chlamydial inclusion body.

60 • Ophthalmic Pathology and Intraocular Tumors

importantly, by culture. BCSC Section 9, *Intraocular Inflammation and Uveitis,* discusses sarcoidosis in greater detail. See also Chapter 12 in this volume.

Granulomatous conjunctivitis in association with preauricular lymphadenopathy is known as *Parinaud oculoglandular syndrome.* This condition is discussed in BCSC Section 6, *Pediatric Ophthalmology and Strabismus,* and Section 8, *External Disease and Cornea.*

As an exposed surface, the conjunctiva is vulnerable to contact with foreign bodies. Some may be transient and/or inert, whereas others may become embedded and incite a foreign-body reaction, identifiable as a granuloma surrounding the foreign object. Multinucleated giant cells are common. Viewing the slide under polarized light may be helpful in identifying the type of offending foreign material.

Degenerations

Pinguecula and Pterygium

A *pinguecula* is a small, yellowish gray nodule, often bilateral, situated at the nasal or temporal limbus (Fig 5-8). It is seen in individuals with prolonged exposure to sunlight and is therefore more common with advancing years. The overlying epithelium is often thinned but may be acanthotic (thickened) or dysplastic. The stromal collagen shows fragmentation and basophilic degeneration called *elastotic degeneration* because the degenerated collagen will stain positively with a histochemical stain for elastic fibers such as the Verhoeff–van Gieson stain (see Fig 5-8). However, pretreatment of the slide with elastase does not diminish the staining.

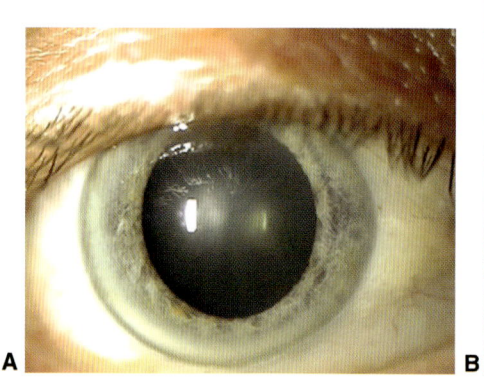

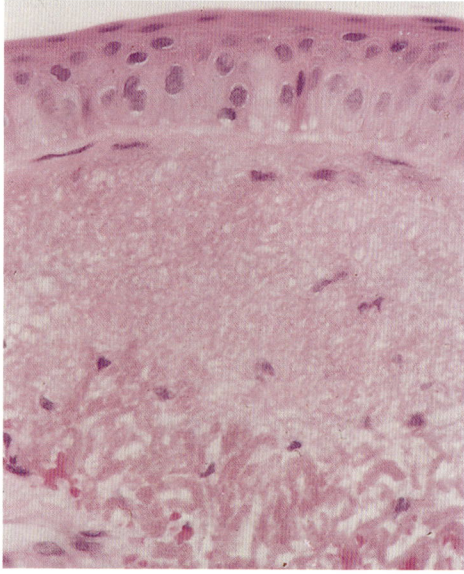

Figure 5-8 **A,** Pinguecula forms a dome-shaped yellow nodule adjacent to the limbus. **B,** Pinguecula showing the basophilic hue of elastotic degeneration, a type of collagen degeneration caused by ultraviolet light. A pterygium specimen would be similar except that a portion of Bowman's layer could be represented in the section. *(Part B courtesy of Hans E. Grossniklaus, MD.)*

A *pterygium* has similar etiology, location, and histologic features, but it encroaches onto the cornea in a winglike fashion (similar to an insect wing; Fig 5-9). Because they can interfere with vision, pterygia are excised when they threaten the visual axis. The destruction of Bowman's layer by the advancing fibrovascular tissue results in a corneal scar. So-called *recurrent pterygia* may completely lack the histopathologic feature of elastotic degeneration and are more accurately classified as an exuberant fibrous tissue response. Some studies have demonstrated that there is mutated p53 expression and loss of heterozygosity and microsatellite instability, especially in recurrent pterygia harboring dysplastic and cancerous epithelium.

> Detorakis ET, Sourvinos G, Tsamparlakis J, Spandidos DA. Evaluation of loss of heterozygosity and microsatellite instability in human pterygium: clinical correlations. *Br J Ophthalmol.* 1998;82:1324–1328.
> Dushku N, Hatcher SL, Albert DM, Reid TW. p53 expression and relation to human papillomavirus infection in pingueculae, pterygia, and limbal tumors. *Arch Ophthalmol.* 1999;117:1593–1599.
> Gans LA. Surgical treatment of pterygium. *Focal Points: Clinical Modules for Ophthalmologists.* San Francisco: American Academy of Ophthalmology; 1996, module 12.

Amyloid Deposits

Amyloid deposition in the conjunctiva is most commonly a primary localized process seen in healthy young and middle-aged adults. Less often, it occurs secondary to preexisting, long-standing inflammation, such as with trachoma, or as an ocular manifestation of a systemic disease such as multiple myeloma. Deposits within the stroma cause a nodular or diffuse waxy, rubbery thickening of any portion of the conjunctiva (Fig 5-10). Amyloid is an eosinophilic, extracellular, hyaline-appearing substance within the stroma, often in a perivascular distribution. Congo red stain tints amyloid an orange-red, but amyloid deposits viewed with polarized light and a rotating analyzer polarization filter also exhibit dichroism (see Fig 5-10); that is, they change from orange-red to green-yellow as the analyzer is rotated. Other useful staining methods include crystal violet and thioflavin T. When describing amyloid deposits involving the eyelid, the physician should specify the location of the

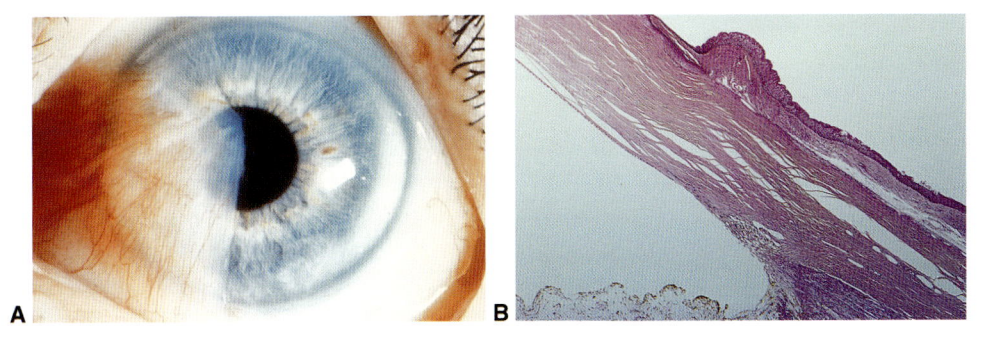

Figure 5-9 **A,** Pterygium is so named because of its winglike configuration across the corneal surface. **B,** Histologically, a pterygium differs from a pinguecula only in the encroachment onto the cornea and the destruction of Bowman's layer. *(Courtesy of Hans E. Grossniklaus, MD.)*

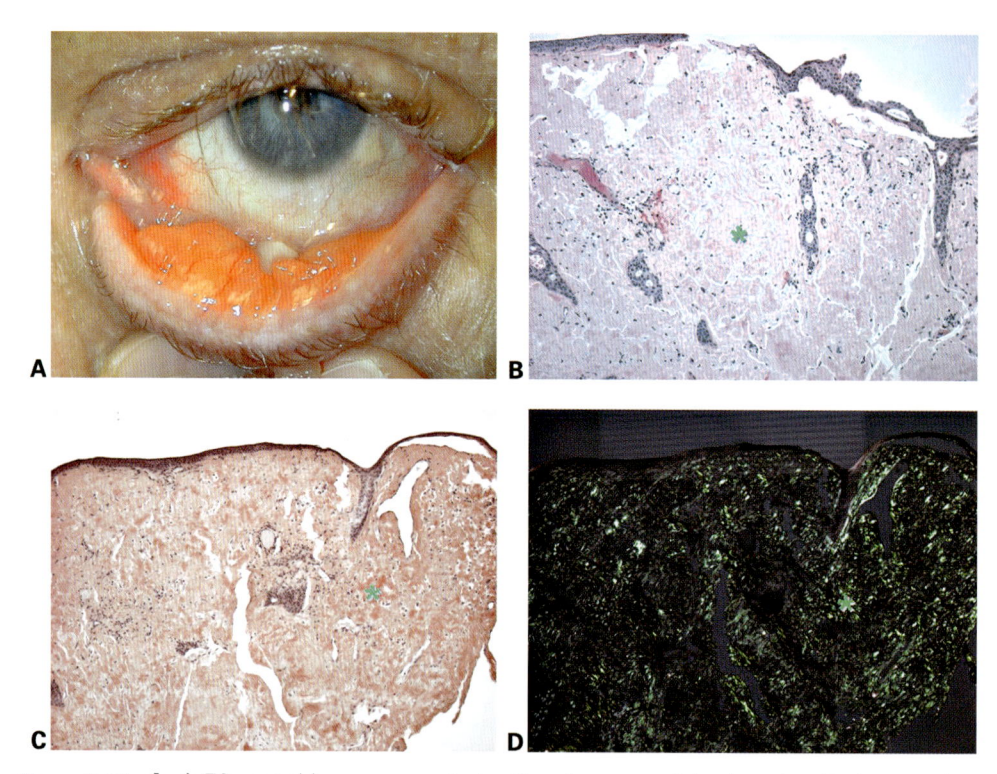

Figure 5-10 **A,** A 70-year-old man presented with a lower eyelid subconjunctival mass that was found to be an amyloid deposit. **B,** Amyloidosis characterized by extracellular amorphous eosinophilic material in the substantia propria of the conjunctiva *(asterisk).* **C,** Congo red stain shows the amyloid staining orange-red *(asterisk).* **D,** Under polarization, amyloid displays dichroism with the characteristic apple green color *(asterisk). (Part A courtesy of John B. Holds, MD; parts B, C, D courtesy of Nasreen A. Syed, MD.)*

deposit: amyloid deposits affecting the skin of the eyelid usually reflect a systemic condition, whereas amyloid deposits affecting the palpebral conjunctiva usually indicate localized pathology.

Neoplasia

Epithelial Lesions

Squamous papillomas are exophytic, pink-red, strawberry-like papillary growths with a biphasic age distribution, growth pattern, and site of involvement (Fig 5-11). In children they are most commonly multiple and pedunculated, involving the fornix, caruncle, or eyelid margin. In adults they are usually single and sessile, occurring at the limbus. Limbal papillomas cannot be clinically distinguished from precancerous dysplasia or invasive squamous cell carcinoma; they require excision for histopathologic diagnosis (Fig 5-12).

Human papillomavirus (HPV) has been detected in both pediatric and adult papillomas: HPV subtype 6 in the former and subtype 16 in the latter. The histopathologic examination of papillomas demonstrates papillary fibrovascular fronds covered by acanthotic squamous

CHAPTER 5: Conjunctiva • 63

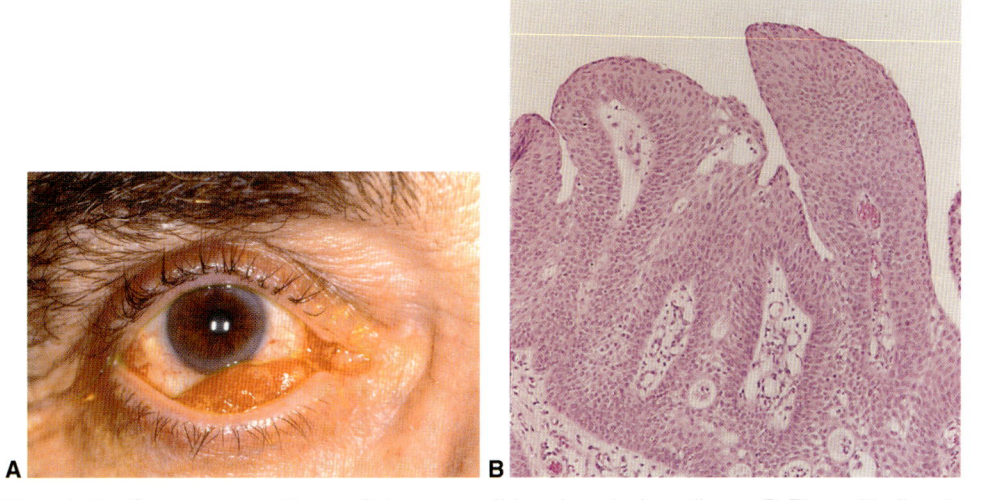

Figure 5-11 Squamous papilloma. **A,** Lower eyelid conjunctival papilloma. **B,** The epithelium is acanthotic and draped over fibrovascular cores. *(Part A courtesy of John B. Holds, MD.)*

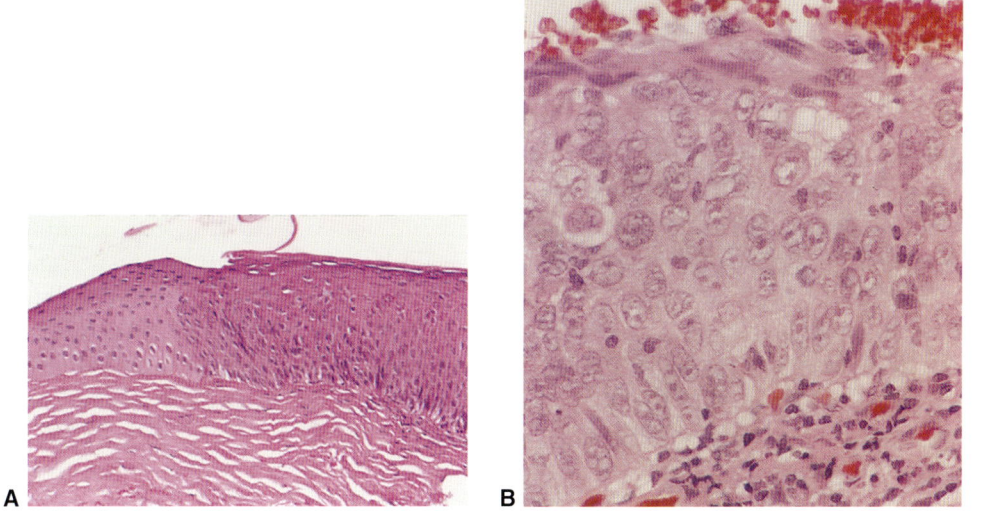

Figure 5-12 Conjunctival dysplasia. **A,** Note the sharp demarcation between normal and abnormal epithelium. The abnormal epithelial cells are confined to the lower half of the conjunctival epithelial thickness. **B,** This is carcinoma in situ, showing full-thickness abnormalities. Because of the difficulties in distinguishing between partial- and full-thickness abnormalities, the term *conjunctival intraepithelial neoplasia (CIN)* is used to describe the spectrum of abnormalities in these conditions.

epithelium. Pediatric papillomas often have an admixture of goblet cells and neutrophils within the epithelium. A chronic inflammatory infiltrate may occupy the stroma. Adult papillomas may exhibit various degrees of epithelial dysplasia, characterized by nuclear enlargement, increased nuclear-to-cytoplasmic ratio, loss of architectural maturation toward the epithelial surface, and mitotic figures above the basal epithelial layer.

Hereditary benign intraepithelial dyskeratosis (HBID) is a rare autosomal dominant disorder with incomplete penetrance. It is characterized by bilateral limbal conjunctival plaques combined with similar changes in the oral mucosa. The clinical and histologic findings are characteristic of HBID. The lesions are characterized histologically by dyskeratosis, acanthosis, parakeratosis, and a variable amount of subepithelial inflammation. Symptoms usually start in early childhood and show a waxing and waning course. HBID was first seen among Haliwa-Saponi Native Americans in North Carolina. It has now been found in other parts of the United States as well as in Europe. Malignant changes of the conjunctival or oral lesions have not been reported.

> Haisley-Royster CA, Allingham RR, Klintworth GK, Prose NS. Hereditary benign intraepithelial dyskeratosis: report of two cases with prominent oral lesions. *J Am Acad Dermatol.* 2001;45:634–636.

Dysplasia of the conjunctival epithelium occurs in other clinical settings. *Dysplasias* are generally classified as focal and well circumscribed or diffuse and poorly demarcated (see Fig 5-12). As mentioned previously, dysplasia may arise in the epithelium covering areas of solar elastosis, similar to actinic keratoses of the skin. The dysplasia is focal and well delineated in this situation, often showing a white, flaky appearance (leukoplakia) caused by surface keratinization. When diffuse dysplasias occur in regions of the conjunctiva not exposed to the sun, the clinical appearance is more gelatinous and less well defined. Human papillomavirus subtype 16 has been demonstrated within some cases of dysplasia as well.

Dysplasia is graded as mild, moderate, or severe, according to the degree of involvement of the epithelium. Mild dysplasia, or *conjunctival intraepithelial neoplasia (CIN)* grade I, is defined as dysplasia confined to the lower third of the conjunctival epithelial thickness. Moderate dysplasia (CIN II) extends into the middle third, and severe dysplasia (CIN III) the upper third (Fig 5-13). The risk of invasive carcinoma developing from conjunctival dysplasia appears to be lower than in its counterpart in the uterine cervix, although it expresses mutated p53 in most of the dysplastic cells. Excision of affected epithelium with cryotherapy of the margins is the standard treatment. Topical mitomycin has shown efficacy as an adjunctive therapy in cases with multifocal or extensive surface involvement.

> Auw-Haedrich C, Sundmacher R, Freudenberg N, et al. Expression of p63 in conjunctival intraepithelial neoplasia and squamous cell carcinoma. *Graefes Arch Clin Exp Ophthalmol.* 2006;244:96–103.
>
> Kemp EG, Harnett AN, Chatterjee S. Preoperative and intraoperative local mitomycin C adjuvant therapy in the management of ocular surface neoplasias. *Br J Ophthalmol.* 2002;86:31–34.

Invasive *squamous cell carcinoma* of the conjunctiva is an uncommon sequela to preexisting dysplasia (Figs 5-14, 5-15). It occurs in older individuals, usually beginning at the limbus, then superficially invading the conjunctival stroma and spreading onto

CHAPTER 5: Conjunctiva • 65

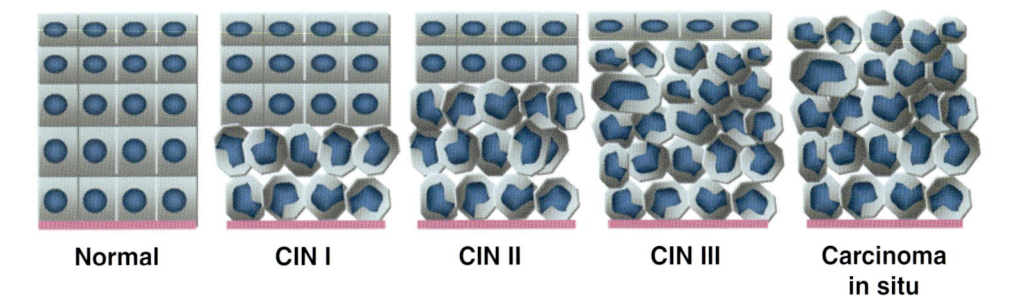

Figure 5-13 Schematic representation of the progression of conjunctival dysplasia. The first panel represents normal epithelium with basement membrane *(pink)*. CIN I is the replacement of the deeper third of the epithelium by dysplastic, pleomorphic (irregular) cells. CIN II replaces half or more of the thickness of the epithelium with dysplastic cells. CIN III replaces almost the full thickness of the epithelium with dysplastic cells, leaving only 1 layer of nondysplastic epithelium. Carcinoma in situ is the complete replacement of epithelium by dysplastic cells, with the basement membrane still intact. *(Courtesy of Patricia Chévez-Barrios, MD.)*

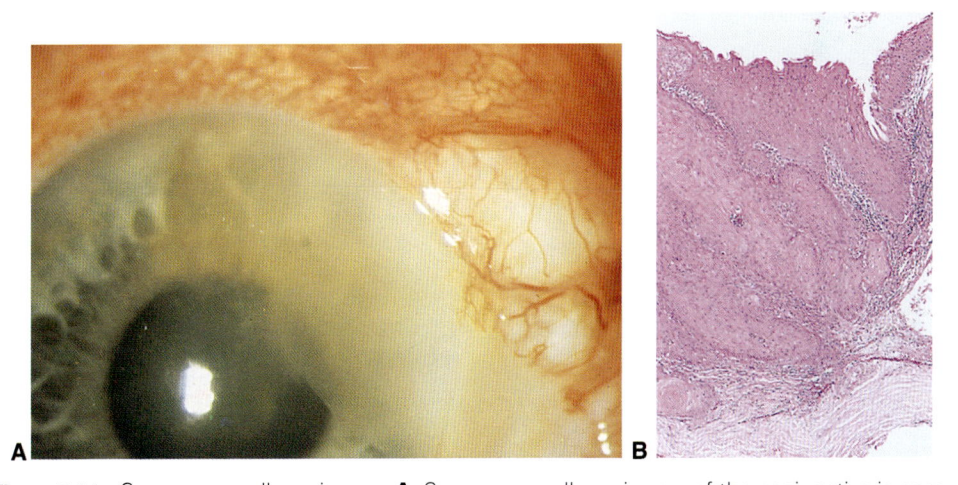

Figure 5-14 Squamous cell carcinoma. **A,** Squamous cell carcinoma of the conjunctiva is commonly centered about the limbus and may spread to involve the corneal epithelium. **B,** The tumor has massively replaced the conjunctival substantia propria. The lamellar eosinophilic fibers at the bottom right of the photograph are sclera. It is unusual for squamous cell carcinoma of the conjunctiva to penetrate the sclera into the eye.

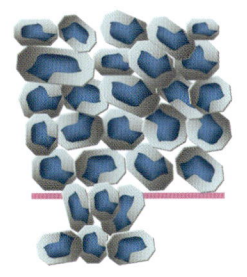

Figure 5-15 Schematic representation of invasive squamous cell carcinoma. Note the full thickness replacement of the epithelium by malignant cells plus the invasion of subepithelial stroma with infiltration through the basement membrane *(pink line)*. *(Courtesy of Patricia Chévez-Barrios, MD.)*

66 • Ophthalmic Pathology and Intraocular Tumors

the corneal surface. Deep invasion of the cornea or sclera and intraocular spread are uncommon complications. Histopathologic examination demonstrates infiltrating nests that have penetrated the epithelial basement membrane and spread into the conjunctival stroma. Tumor cells may be well differentiated and easily recognizable as squamous, moderately differentiated, or poorly differentiated and difficult to distinguish from other malignancies, such as sebaceous carcinoma. Although regional lymph node metastasis is not common, dissemination and death are possible.

Mucoepidermoid carcinoma and *spindle cell carcinoma* are rare variants of squamous cell carcinoma. Both entities are more aggressive neoplasms with higher rates of recurrence and intraocular spread.

For the American Joint Committee on Cancer (AJCC) definitions and staging of carcinoma of the conjunctiva, see Table A-1 in the appendix.

Subepithelial Lesions

Clinically, both benign and malignant lymphoid lesions of the conjunctiva usually show a salmon pink appearance, are relatively flat with a smooth surface, and have a soft consistency (Fig 5-16). Most (approximately two thirds) of conjunctival lymphoid lesions are localized and *not* associated with systemic disease; however, nearly two thirds of lymphomas arising in the preseptal skin eventually show evidence of systemic involvement. Prediction of biological behavior based on clinical, histopathologic, and even immunophenotypic features is not always clear-cut in pathologic diagnosis of lymphoproliferative disorders of the conjunctiva. See also Chapter 14 on lymphoid lesions of the orbit and BCSC Section 7, *Orbit, Eyelids, and Lacrimal System.*

Histopathologic features favoring a diagnosis of *reactive lymphoid hyperplasia* include the presence of lymphoid follicles with germinal centers and an admixture of plasma cells and mature, small lymphocytes in the surrounding stroma (Fig 5-17). *Russell bodies,* eosinophilic spherules representing inspissated immunoglobulin, may be present

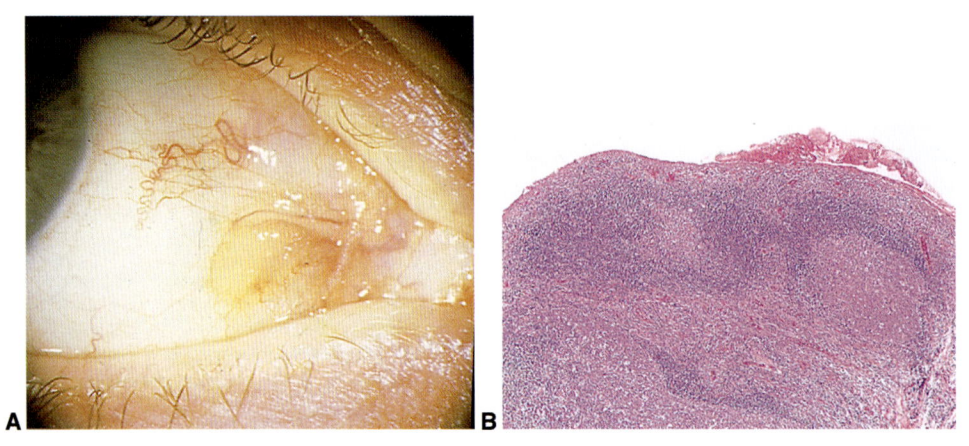

Figure 5-16 Benign reactive lymphoid hyperplasia of the conjunctiva. **A,** Clinical photograph (note the salmon patch). **B,** Note the irregularly shaped germinal centers in the conjunctival substantia propria.

either within plasma cell cytoplasm or extruded into the extracellular milieu. A diffuse sheet of monotonous, small, round or cleaved lymphocytes is more characteristic of a *low-grade malignant lymphoma* (Fig 5-18). *High-grade lymphomas* are readily recognized as malignant by virtue of their nuclear features and their high mitotic rate.

As expected, a histopathologically indeterminate zone exists between reactive hyperplasia and low-grade lymphoma, and ancillary studies may be helpful in classifying proliferations as benign or malignant. Immunophenotypic analysis, either by flow cytometry of fresh, unfixed tissue or by immunoperoxidase staining, may demonstrate B-cell monoclonality by revealing either κ or λ light chain predominance (Fig 5-19). More sophisticated molecular techniques may show monoclonality by revealing immunoglobulin gene rearrangements within tumor cells. However, although these advanced techniques are helpful, they are not definitive: not all lesions demonstrating monoclonality will behave in a malignant fashion that results in systemic disease. Other factors, such as host immune response, are important in determining clinical behavior of the lesion.

Albert DM, Jakobiec FA, eds. *Principles and Practice of Ophthalmology.* 2nd ed. Philadelphia: Saunders; 2000.

Shields CL, Shields JA, Carvalho C, Rundle P, Smith AF. Conjunctival lymphoid tumors: clinical analysis of 117 cases and relationship to systemic lymphoma. *Ophthalmology.* 2001;108:979–984.

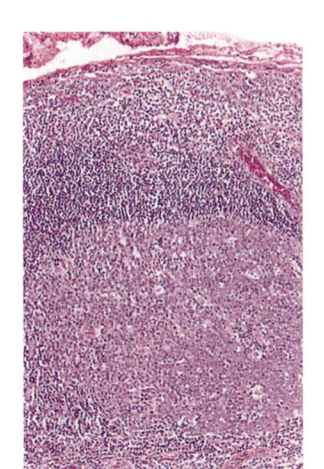

Figure 5-17 Note the large germinal center in this case of benign reactive lymphoid hyperplasia of the conjunctiva.

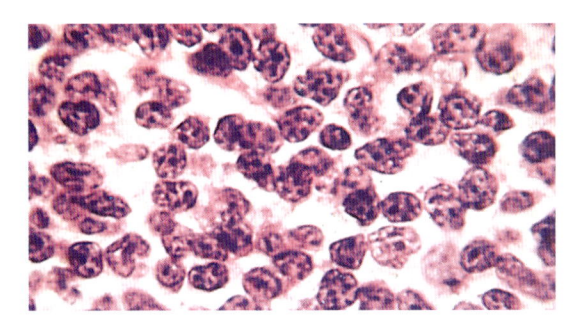

Figure 5-18 Lymphoma composed of sheets of atypical lymphocytes.

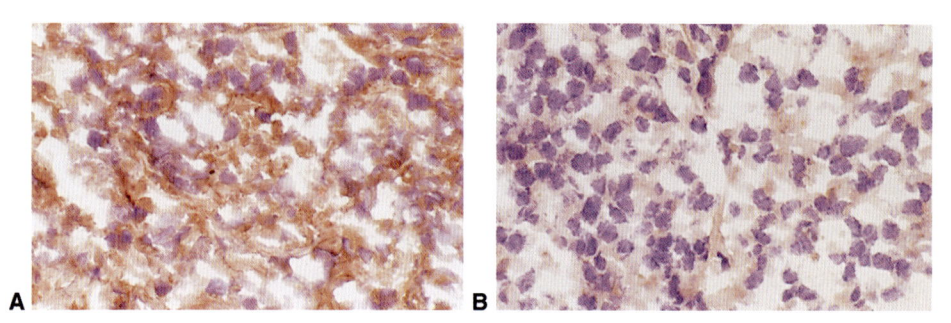

Figure 5-19 Conjunctival lymphoma. **A,** This is an immunoperoxidase stain for λ light chains. Note the diffuse brown staining. **B,** This is an immunoperoxidase stain for κ light chains. The stain is negative. The fact that only λ light stains were demonstrated in this tumor indicates that this is a monoclonal proliferation, consistent with the histologic impression of malignant lymphoma.

Melanocytic Lesions

As with hemangiomas, melanocytic nevi are classified by some authors as hamartomas and by others as neoplasms (Table 5-1). *Conjunctival melanocytic nevi* usually appear on the bulbar conjunctiva in childhood. Analogous to cutaneous melanocytic nevi, conjunctival nevi undergo evolutionary changes. In the initial junctional phase, nevus cells are confined to nests *(theques)* at the interface between the epithelium and the substantia propria. As the nevus evolves, the nests "drop off" into the substantia propria, eventually losing connection with the epithelium and existing solely in the substantia propria. Nevi with both junctional and subepithelial components are designated as *compound nevi;* those without junctional activity are termed *subepithelial* or *stromal nevi.* Subcategories of nevi (eg, Spitz nevus, halo nevus) and other types of nevi (eg, blue nevus) also exist. Epithelial cysts may be encountered within compound and subepithelial nevi (Fig 5-20). Nevi occur only rarely in the palpebral conjunctiva; pigmented lesions in this area are more likely to be primary acquired melanosis or melanoma.

Primary acquired melanosis (PAM) appears as a unilateral flat patch, or patches, of golden brown pigmentation with an irregular margin (Fig 5-21). It is most common in middle-aged persons. The lesions may wax and wane or grow slowly without remission over a period of 10 or more years. It is not possible to predict in which patient PAM is likely to progress to malignant melanoma on clinical grounds alone. However, histologic criteria have been developed to identify patients at high risk for malignancy. *PAM without atypia* denotes hyperplasia of melanocytes without atypical cytologic or architectural features (Fig 5-22A). PAM without atypia does not progress to melanoma. *PAM with atypia* will progress to invasive melanoma in approximately 46% of patients (Fig 5-22B).

Atypia in PAM is defined according to both cytomorphologic and architectural features. Atypical melanocytes show nuclear enlargement as compared with adjacent basal epithelial cells and may be spindled, polygonal, or epithelioid. Architectural features of atypia include lentiginous hyperplasia, intraepidermal migration of individual cells or nests *(pagetoid spread),* or complete replacement of the epithelium, mimicking carcinoma

CHAPTER 5: Conjunctiva • 69

Table 5-1 Clinical Comparison of Conjunctival Pigmentary Lesions

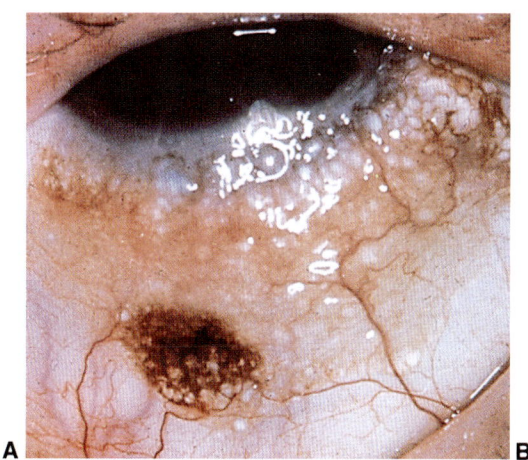

Lesion	Onset	Area	Location	Malignant Potential
Freckle	Youth	Small	Conjunctiva	No
Benign acquired melanosis	Adulthood	Patchy or diffuse	Conjunctiva	No
Conjunctival nevus	Youth	Small	Conjunctiva	Low (conjunctival melanoma)
Ocular and oculodermal melanocytosis	Congenital	Patchy or diffuse	Under conjunctiva	Yes (uveal melanoma)
Primary acquired melanosis	Middle age	Diffuse	Conjunctiva	Yes (conjunctival melanoma)

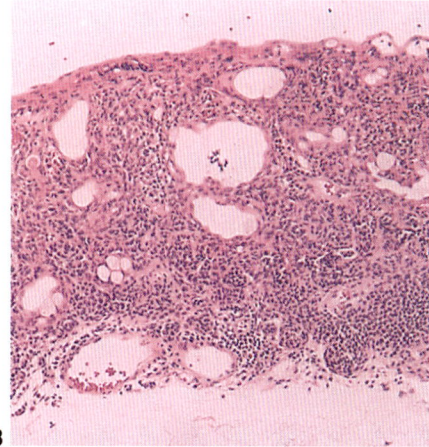

Figure 5-20 A, Compound nevus of the conjunctiva. Note the characteristic cysts. **B,** Histology of a compound conjunctival nevus. Note the cystic epithelial inclusions within the lesion, corresponding with the clinically observed cysts.

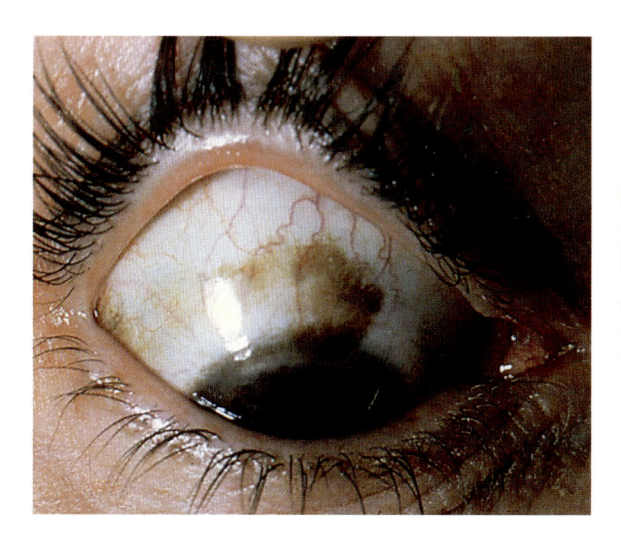

Figure 5-21 Primary acquired melanosis (PAM). Note the flat, patchy pigmentation of the conjunctiva. When examining this patient clinically, the physician should evert the eyelids to exclude involvement of the palpebral conjunctiva.

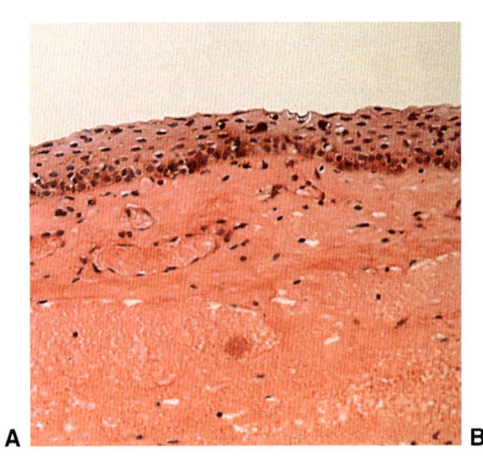

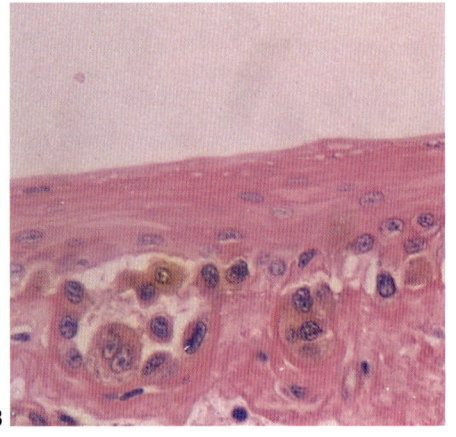

Figure 5-22 A, PAM without atypia. The basilar layer of the conjunctival epithelium is pigmented. There is no histologic evidence of melanocytic atypia. Note that in the term *PAM without atypia,* the word *atypia* refers to histologic findings, not to the clinical presentation. **B,** PAM with atypia. Highly atypical epithelioid melanocytes are present within the epithelium. The patient is at high risk for progression to melanoma.

in situ. Pagetoid spread by epithelioid melanocytes and full-thickness replacement of the epithelium are the most important of these features as predictors of subsequent invasive melanoma (75%–90% of cases). PAM with atypia should be treated by excision if the area is small or by cryotherapy for more extensive areas. Mitomycin C has been shown to cause regression in PAM with atypia and may be considered as an alternative therapy, particularly in extensive or multifocal cases; the efficacy of this treatment remains to be proven in a larger series.

> Demirci H, McCormick SA, Finger PT. Topical mitomycin chemotherapy for conjunctival malignant melanoma and primary acquired melanosis with atypia: clinical experience with histopathologic observations. *Arch Ophthalmol.* 2000;118:885–891.
> Helm CJ. Melanoma and other pigmented lesions of the ocular surface. *Focal Points: Clinical Modules for Ophthalmologists.* San Francisco: American Academy of Ophthalmology; 1996, module 11.

Approximately two thirds of cases of *conjunctival melanoma* arise from PAM with atypia (Fig 5-23A); the remainder develop either from a preexisting nevus or de novo. Tumors are usually nodular growths that may involve any portion of the conjunctiva; those not on the bulbar surface appear to behave more aggressively. Histopathologically, melanomas have diverse cellular morphology from pleomorphic, large, bizarre cells with prominent nucleoli to small, polygonal cells with mild anaplasia to spindle cells without identifiable melanin pigment. Immunohistochemical stains for S-100 protein and HMB-45 may help to identify problematic cases as melanocytic (Fig 5-23B). Conjunctival melanomas are more akin to cutaneous melanoma than to uveal melanoma in behavior.

The overall mortality rate from conjunctival melanoma is 25%. Typically, metastases first develop in parotid or submandibular lymph nodes. Unfavorable prognostic factors,

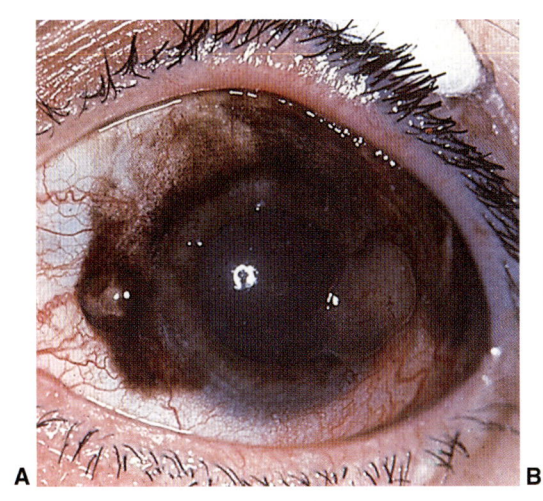

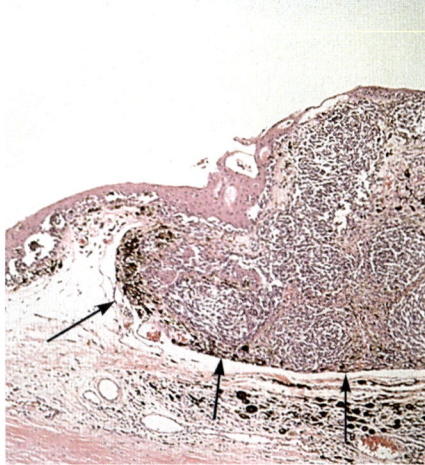

Figure 5-23 A, Melanoma with PAM. Note the melanoma nodule at the 2 o'clock position at the limbus that has appeared on a background of PAM (diffuse, flat, brown pigmentation). **B,** Melanoma with PAM, histologic appearance. Intraepithelial atypical melanocytes (PAM) are present just to the left of the nodule of invasive melanoma *(arrows)*.

in addition to the conjunctival site, as just mentioned, include

- nonepibulbar location, orbital or scleral invasion
- histopathologic identification of pagetoid or full-thickness intraepithelial spread
- involvement of the eyelid skin margin

Tumor thickness can be measured objectively using a calibrated microscope; tumors thicker than 1.8 mm carry a greater risk for dissemination and death than thinner ones. However, even lesions less than 0.8 mm thick have resulted in patient mortality. The treatment for conjunctival melanoma is complete surgical removal. Detailed surgical planning with wide microsurgical excisional biopsy with minimal or no manipulation of the tumor ("no touch" technique) and supplemental alcohol corneal epitheliectomy, followed by conjunctival cryotherapy or brachytherapy, is the currently recommended treatment of choice. Melanomas can spread to regional lymph nodes of the preauricular or parotid and cervical nodes. Sentinel lymph node evaluation at the time of surgery has recently gained favor, as better techniques have evolved that decrease the chances of facial nerve paralysis. Metastases occur to the lungs, liver, skin, and brain.

Melanocytic lesions are discussed and illustrated extensively in Chapter 17. For AJCC definitions and staging of conjunctival melanoma, see Table A-2 in the appendix.

> Albert DM, Jakobiec FA, eds. *Principles and Practice of Ophthalmology.* 2nd ed. Philadelphia: Saunders; 2000.
>
> Missotten GS, Keijser S, De Keizer RJ, De Wolff-Rouendaal D. Conjunctival melanoma in the Netherlands: a nationwide study. *Invest Ophthalmol Vis Sci.* 2005;46:75–82.
>
> Shields CL, Shields JA, Gunduz K, et al. Conjunctival melanoma: risk factors for recurrence, exenteration, metastasis, and death in 150 consecutive patients. *Arch Ophthalmol.* 2000;118:1497–1507.

CHAPTER 6

Cornea

Topography

The normal cornea is composed of 5 layers: epithelium, Bowman's layer, stroma, Descemet's membrane, and endothelium (Fig 6-1). The average adult cornea has a horizontal diameter of 11–12 mm, a vertical diameter of 9–11 mm, and a thickness ranging between 0.52 mm centrally and 0.65 mm peripherally. The cornea is embryologically derived from surface ectoderm and neural crest. BCSC Section 8, *External Disease and Cornea,* discusses the structures and disorders of the cornea in depth.

The normal external surface of the cornea is composed of a stratified, squamous, nonkeratinizing *epithelium* ranging between 5 and 7 cell layers in thickness. The 1–2 most superficial layers consist of flattened cells that are continually exfoliated and replaced by the underlying cells. The deepest epithelial layer is composed of basal cells, where mitotic activity is greatest. The basal cells are attached to the underlying basement membrane by hemidesmosomes and filaments that may be visualized with transmission electron microscopy. The epithelial basement membrane is thin and is best seen with the use of periodic acid–Schiff (PAS) stain.

Bowman's layer is present subjacent to the epithelial basement membrane. This layer is composed of acellular collagen and measures 8–14 nm in thickness. The posterior aspect of Bowman's layer blends imperceptibly with the underlying corneal stroma.

The corneal *stroma* makes up 90% of the total corneal thickness. The elongated collagenous lamellae are arranged in a precise orientation to allow for the orderly passage of light through the cornea. The ground substance, consisting of mucoprotein and glycoprotein, coats each collagen fibril and is responsible for the exact spacing required for corneal clarity.

The next layer, *Descemet's membrane,* is the basement membrane elaborated by the corneal endothelium. The production of Descemet's membrane begins during fetal development and continues throughout adulthood; therefore, the thickness of Descemet's membrane continually increases with age. Descemet's membrane is a true basement membrane, composed primarily of type IV collagen, and is strongly PAS-positive.

The corneal *endothelium* is a single layer derived from the neural crest. The primary function of the endothelium is to maintain corneal clarity by pumping water from the corneal stroma. The number of endothelial cells gradually decreases over time. As the endothelial cell number declines, the remaining cells flatten and elongate to provide coverage of the posterior corneal surface.

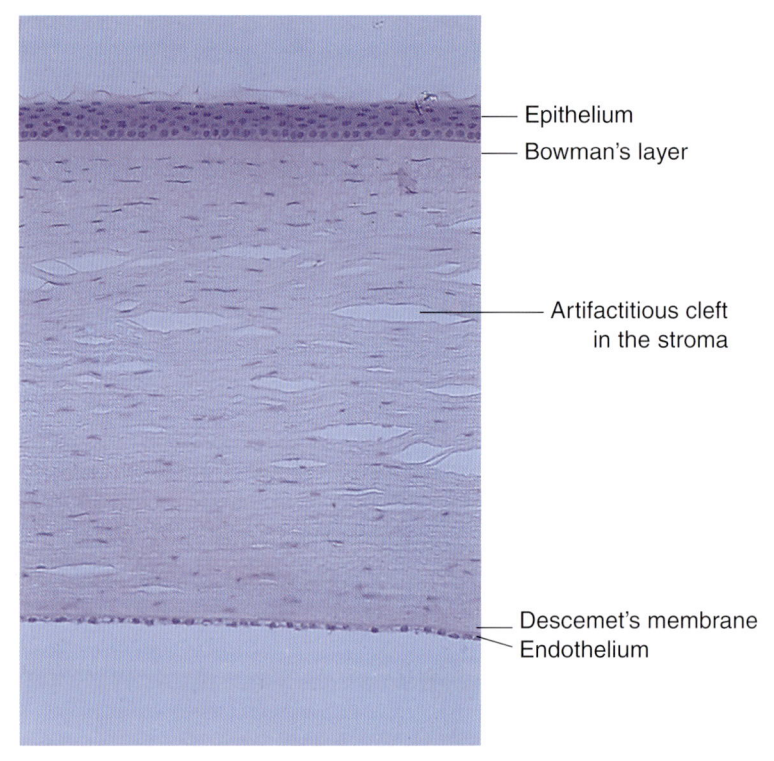

Figure 6-1 The cornea is composed primarily of collagen. Because of dehydration of the tissue during processing for paraffin embedding, multiple areas of separation of the stromal lamellae are evident. If the lamellar separations are absent, corneal edema is suspected. This is an example of a meaningful artifact.

Congenital Anomalies

Congenital Hereditary Endothelial Dystrophy

The 2 forms of congenital hereditary endothelial dystrophy (CHED) causing bilateral congenital corneal edema are the autosomal recessive form and the autosomal dominant form. The more common autosomal recessive form is present at birth, remains stable, and is accompanied by nystagmus. Clinically, the cornea appears bluish white, is 2–3 times the normal thickness, and has a ground-glass appearance. The autosomal dominant form of CHED becomes apparent in the first or second year of life and exhibits slowly increasing edema of the corneal stroma. In these patients, the cornea has the same diffuse, blue-white appearance as in the autosomal recessive form, and patients may experience pain and photophobia (Fig 6-2A). Nystagmus, however, does not develop. The genetic loci for the AD and AR forms of CHED have been mapped to chromosomes 20p11.2-q11.2 and 20p13, respectively.

Despite the distinct clinical differences between autosomal recessive and autosomal dominant CHED, the 2 forms appear similar histologically. The corneal stroma is diffusely edematous, accounting for the marked increase in thickness observed clinically.

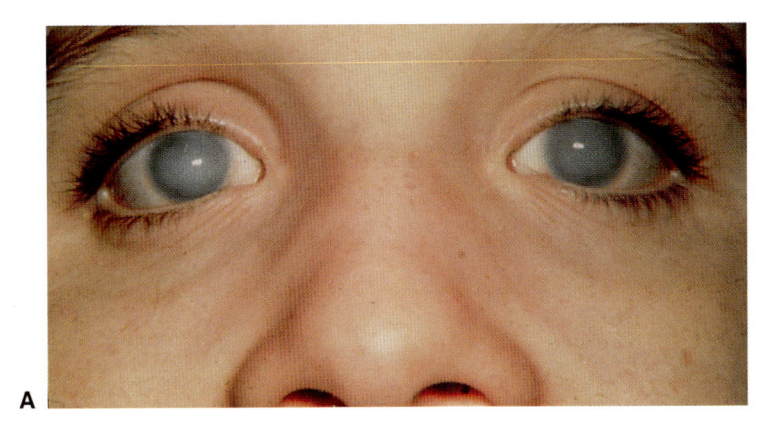

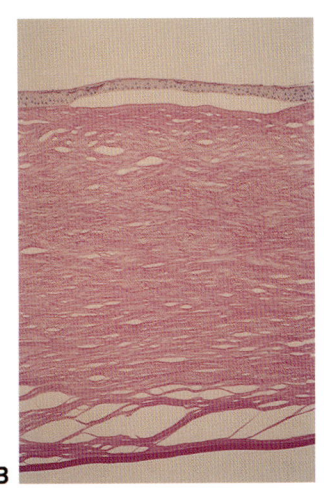

Figure 6-2 Congenital hereditary endothelial dystrophy. **A,** Clinical appearance. **B,** Note diffuse edema of the corneal epithelium and stroma. Descemet's membrane is diffusely thickened. *(Courtesy of Hans E. Grossniklaus, MD.)*

Descemet's membrane appears thickened, but guttae are not present (Fig 6-2B). The endothelium appears atrophic or may be focally absent. The primary abnormality is thought to be a degeneration of endothelial cells during or after the fifth month of gestation. CHED may be considered part of the spectrum of anterior segment dysgenesis abnormalities caused by abnormal differentiation of the neural crest ectoderm that forms the corneal endothelium. No systemic abnormalities are consistently associated with CHED.

> Judisch GF, Maumenee IH. Clinical differentiation of recessive congenital hereditary endothelial dystrophy and dominant hereditary endothelial dystrophy. *Am J Ophthalmol.* 1978;85: 606–612.
>
> Klintworth GK. The molecular genetics of the corneal dystrophies—current status. *Front Biosci.* 2003;8:d687–713.

Dermoid

Dermoid, a type of choristoma that may involve the cornea, is discussed in Chapter 5, Conjunctiva, and depicted in Figure 6-3.

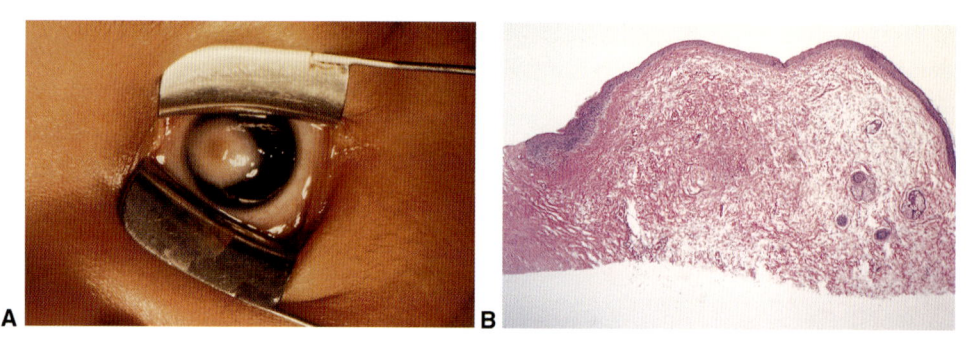

Figure 6-3 Corneal dermoid. **A,** Clinical photograph shows elevated, smooth, tan lesion on corneal surface. **B,** Histopathology shows keratinizing stratified epithelium overlying fibrous stroma containing scattered adnexal structures. *(Courtesy of Hans E. Grossniklaus, MD.)*

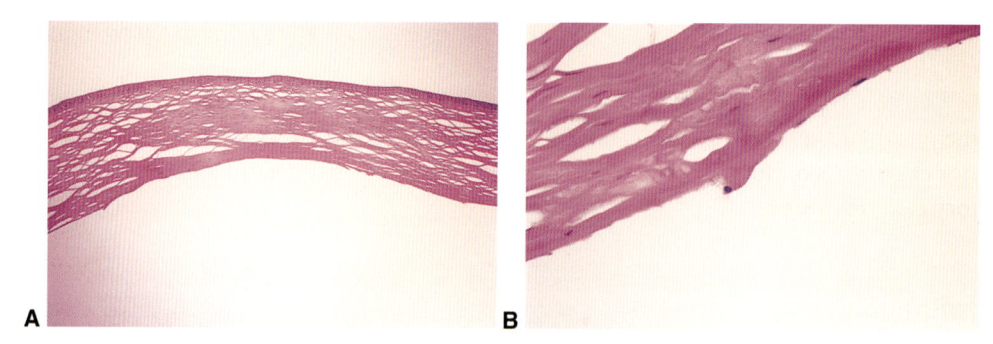

Figure 6-4 Posterior keratoconus. **A,** Anterior bowing of the posterior corneal surface accompanies corneal thinning. **B,** Descemet's membrane is thickened at the edge of the posterior concavity. *(Courtesy of Hans E. Grossniklaus, MD.)*

Posterior Keratoconus

A localized central or paracentral indentation of the posterior cornea without protrusion of the anterior surface is referred to as *posterior keratoconus,* also known as *internal ulcer of von Hippel.* The stroma may be thinned significantly, approaching one third normal corneal thickness, and often appears hazy. Descemet's membrane and endothelium are usually preserved in the area of the defect (Fig 6-4). Most cases occur in females and are unilateral, nonprogressive, and sporadic. Astigmatism and amblyopia may occur.

> Haney WP, Falls HF. The occurrence of congenital keratoconus posticus circumscriptus in two siblings presenting a previously unrecognized syndrome. *Am J Ophthalmol.* 1961;52:53–57.

Sclerocornea

Sclerocornea, a nonprogressive, noninflammatory scleralization of the cornea, may be limited to the corneal periphery or may involve the entire cornea. The limbus is usually poorly defined, and superficial vessels that are extensions of normal scleral, episcleral, and conjunctival vessels extend across the cornea. Both sexes are affected equally, and 90%

of cases are bilateral. Half of the cases are sporadic; the remainder are either autosomal dominant or recessive, the latter form being more severe. The most common ocular association is cornea plana, found in 80% of cases.

Histologically, the stromal lamellae of the cornea are irregularly thickened, without differentiation between sclera and cornea. The small- to medium-sized vessels observed clinically are present in the superficial stroma. No evidence of inflammation is present.

> Goldstein JE, Cogan DG. Sclerocornea and associated congenital anomalies. *Arch Ophthalmol.* 1962;67:761–768.

Congenital Corneal Staphyloma

Congenital corneal staphyloma is characterized by varying degrees of ectasia of the central, peripheral, or entire cornea. The posterior surface of the ectatic cornea is covered by remnants of anteriorly displaced iris. These findings may represent a severe expression of Peters anomaly or posterior keratoconus and may result from intrauterine trauma, maternal alcohol ingestion, or inflammation causing perforation.

Histologically, the scarred corneal and limbal tissues are thinned. Vascularization of the posterior aspect of the scar is often present in the area of the iris remnants. The anterior chamber is occluded by iris adhesions, and scattered collections of chronic inflammatory cells may be present.

Inflammations

Infectious

The cornea may be affected by infectious processes caused by a number of different microbial agents. Acute corneal inflammation is commonly characterized by edema and infiltration by inflammatory cells. Limbal hyperemia and iritis may be present. Severe inflammation can lead to corneal necrosis, ulceration, and perforation.

Bacterial infections

Corneal infections caused by bacterial agents often follow a disruption in the corneal epithelial integrity resulting from

- contact lens wear
- trauma
- contaminated ocular medications
- alteration in immunologic defenses (eg, use of topical or systemic immunosuppressives)
- antecedent corneal disease (eg, dry eye, corneal abrasion, bullous keratopathy, and so on)
- malposition of the eyelids

Some common bacterial organisms involved in corneal infections include *Staphylococcus aureus, Streptococcus pneumoniae, Pseudomonas aeruginosa,* and Enterobacteriaceae.

Scrapings obtained from infected corneas demonstrate collections of neutrophils admixed with necrotic debris. The presence of organisms may be demonstrated using tissue Gram stains such as Brown and Hopps (B&H) and Brown and Brenn (B&B). Growing the organism in culture remains the only method of obtaining accurate identification of specific organisms.

Herpes simplex virus keratitis

Usually a self-limited corneal epithelial disease, herpes simplex virus keratitis is characterized by a linear arborizing pattern of opacification and swelling of epithelial cells called a *dendrite*. Corneal scrapings obtained from a dendrite and prepared using the Giemsa stain reveal the presence of intranuclear viral inclusions. Infected epithelial cells may coalesce to form multinucleated giant cells. Chronic stromal keratitis may accompany or follow epithelial infection, leading to ulceration and scarring. With full-thickness stromal involvement, a granulomatous reaction can be seen, most often at the level of Descemet's membrane (Fig 6-5).

Fungal keratitis

Mycotic keratitis is often a complication of trauma or of corticosteroid use. Unlike most bacteria, fungi are able to penetrate the cornea and extend through Descemet's membrane into the anterior chamber. The most common organisms include *Aspergillus, Candida,* and *Fusarium.* Many fungi can be seen in tissue sections using special stains such as Grocott-Gomori methenamine–silver nitrate (GMS), PAS, or Giemsa (Fig 6-6). Other fungal organ-

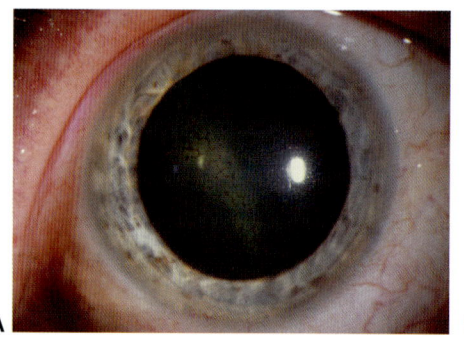

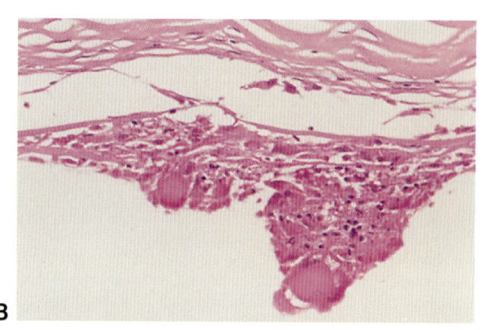

Figure 6-5 Herpes simplex virus keratitis. **A,** Clinical photograph depicting corneal dendrites. **B,** Note the granulomatous response to Descemet's membrane. Herpesvirus antigen has been detected in this area. *(Part A courtesy of Sander Dubovy, MD.)*

Figure 6-6 *Fusarium* keratitis. Grocott-Gomori methenamine–silver nitrate stain.

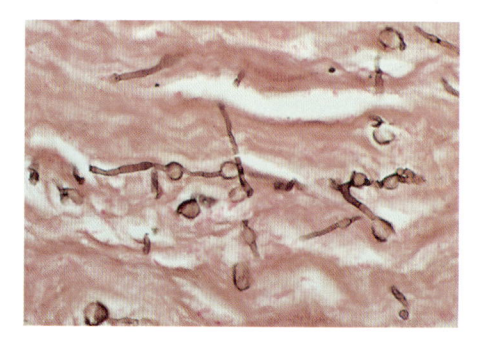

CHAPTER 6: Cornea • 79

isms, including *Candida* and organisms causing mucormycosis, are visible with routine hematoxylin and eosin (H&E) preparations.

Acanthamoeba *keratitis*

Acanthamoeba protozoa most commonly cause infection in soft contact lens wearers who do not take appropriate precautions in cleaning and sterilizing their lenses. The most frequently involved species are *A castellani* and *A polyphagia*. Patients presenting with *Acanthamoeba* keratitis usually have severe eye pain. Clinically, a ring infiltrate and radial keratoneuritis may be present. (See Section 8, *External Disease and Cornea*, Fig 7-29.)

Biopsy specimens or scrapings from infected areas may demonstrate cysts and trophozoites that may be visualized in H&E sections (Fig 6-7). Other techniques, such as the use of monoclonal antibodies, may enhance the recognition of cysts and trophozoites in tissue sections. Special culture techniques and media, including nonnutrient blood agar layered with *E coli*, are required to grow *Acanthamoeba*. The pathologic findings in corneal buttons removed because of this infection are quite variable, ranging from no inflammation to a marked granulomatous reaction.

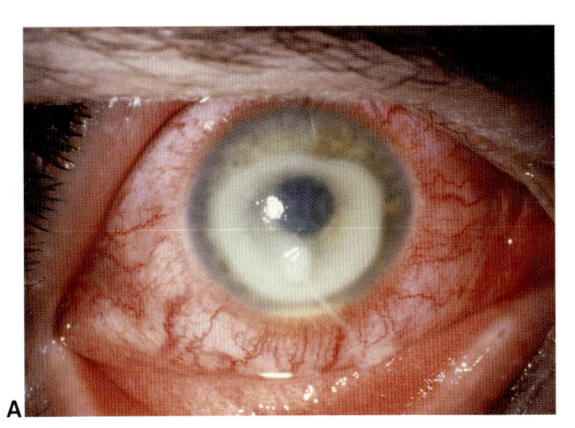

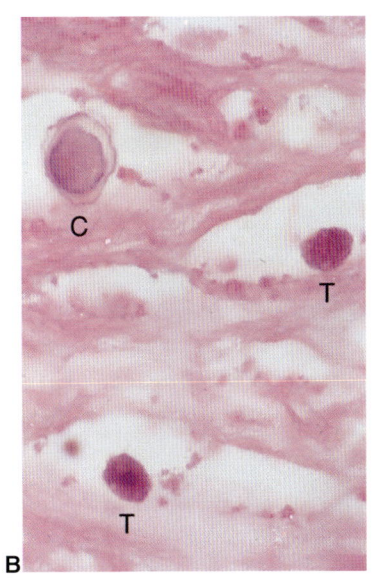

Figure 6-7 *Acanthamoeba* keratitis. **A,** Clinical photograph depicting ring infiltrate. **B,** Note the cyst *(C)* and trophozoite *(T)* forms. *(Part A courtesy of Sander Dubovy, MD.)*

Congenital syphilis

Transplacental infection of the fetus by *Treponema pallidum* may cause a nonsuppurative inflammation of the corneal stroma with relative sparing of the corneal epithelium and endothelium. Clinically, corneal stromal scarring at varying depths as well as deep stromal vascularization may be present. These changes are thought to result from an immunologic response to infectious microorganisms or their antigens in the corneal stroma. These clinical and histopathologic findings are frequently termed *interstitial keratitis*. Although congenital syphilis represents the classic cause of interstitial keratitis, other causative organisms include *Mycobacterium tuberculosis, M leprae, Borrelia burgdorferi,* and Epstein-Barr virus. (See also BCSC Section 8, *External Disease and Cornea.*)

Noninfectious

Corneal inflammation can also be caused by noninfectious agents. For example, foreign bodies may be retained in the cornea as a result of accidental or surgical trauma. Often, a localized granulomatous reaction may be present surrounding the foreign material. Foreign bodies are often birefringent and can be demonstrated on examination of tissue sections with polarized light.

Degenerations and Dystrophies

Degenerations

Corneal degenerations are secondary changes that occur in previously normal tissue. They are often associated with aging, are not inherited, and are not necessarily bilateral.

Salzmann nodular degeneration

Salzmann nodular degeneration is a noninflammatory corneal degeneration that may occur secondary to long-standing keratitis or may be idiopathic. It may be bilateral and is more commonly present in middle-aged and older women. Gray-white or blue-white raised lesions may be present, often in the central and paracentral cornea. Histopathologic examination discloses an absence of Bowman's layer and nodules composed of basement membrane–like material, hyaline material, cellular debris, and fibrocytes.

> Vannas A, Hogan MJ, Wood I. Salzmann's nodular degeneration of the cornea. *Am J Ophthalmol.* 1975;79:211–219.

Band keratopathy

Seen clinically as calcific plaques in the interpalpebral zone, band keratopathy is characterized by the deposition of calcium in the epithelial basement membrane, Bowman's layer, and anterior stroma (Fig 6-8). The calcium deposits appear as basophilic granules in H&E sections; the presence of calcium can be further confirmed by use of special stains such as alizarin red or the von Kossa stain. Band keratopathy may develop in any chronic local corneal disease, in association with systemic hypercalcemic states, and in eyes with prolonged chronic inflammation.

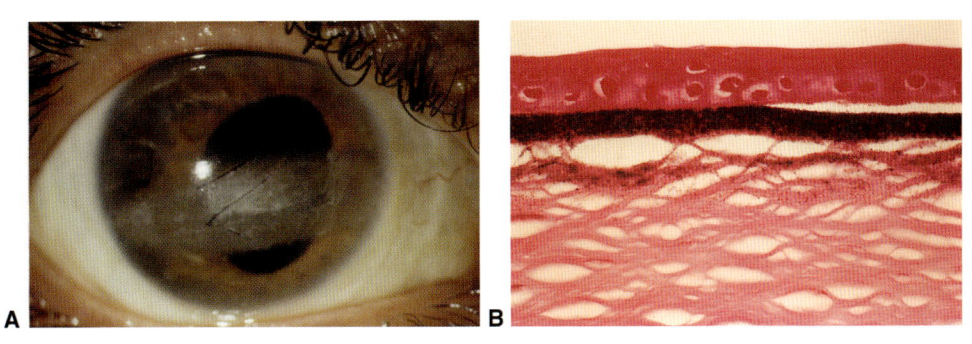

Figure 6-8 Band keratopathy. **A,** Clinical appearance shows white calcium deposition in the interpalpebral region of cornea. **B,** Calcium deposition in Bowman's layer appears black when stained with von Kossa stain. *(Part A courtesy of Sander Dubovy, MD; part B courtesy of Hans E. Grossniklaus, MD.)*

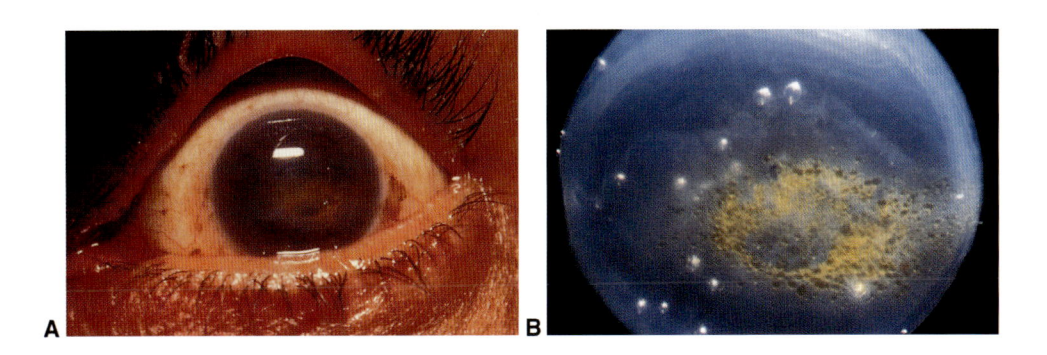

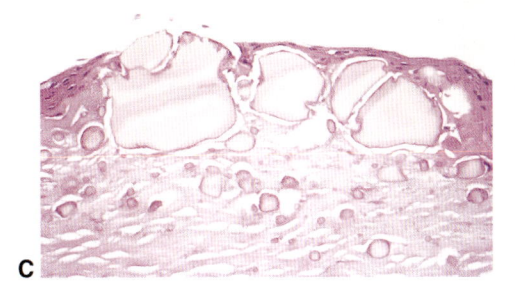

Figure 6-9 Actinic keratopathy (spheroidal degeneration). **A,** Clinical appearance shows golden-brown spheroidal deposits in the cornea. **B,** Gross appearance of corneal button. The air bubbles are artifacts. **C,** Histopathology shows lightly staining basophilic globules in the epithelium and superficial stroma. *(Courtesy of Hans E. Grossniklaus, MD.)*

Actinic keratopathy

Also known as *spheroidal degeneration* or *Labrador keratopathy,* actinic keratopathy involves damage to corneal collagen similar to that seen in pingueculae, pterygia, and solar elastosis of the skin. The actinic damage usually occurs within the palpebral fissure, similar to the pattern seen in band keratopathy. Clinical examination discloses translucent, golden-brown spheroidal deposits present in the superficial cornea. H&E-stained sections show basophilic globules in the superficial stroma, immediately subjacent to the epithelium. No associated inflammatory changes are present (Fig 6-9).

Pannus

Corneal pannus is the growth of tissue between the epithelium and Bowman's layer. This subepithelial fibrous tissue may have a significant vascular component, in which case the term *subepithelial fibrovascular pannus* is used. Bowman's layer may be disrupted (Fig 6-10). Pannus is frequently seen in cases of chronic corneal edema or prolonged corneal inflammation.

Bullous keratopathy

The end result of persistent stromal edema, bullous keratopathy is most frequently caused by the failure of the corneal endothelial cell layer to perform its normal pump function (Fig 6-11). The pump failure may occur either because the cells do not function normally or because there is a decrease in the number of endothelial cells below a critical level necessary to maintain corneal clarity. Although bullous keratopathy continues to be seen after

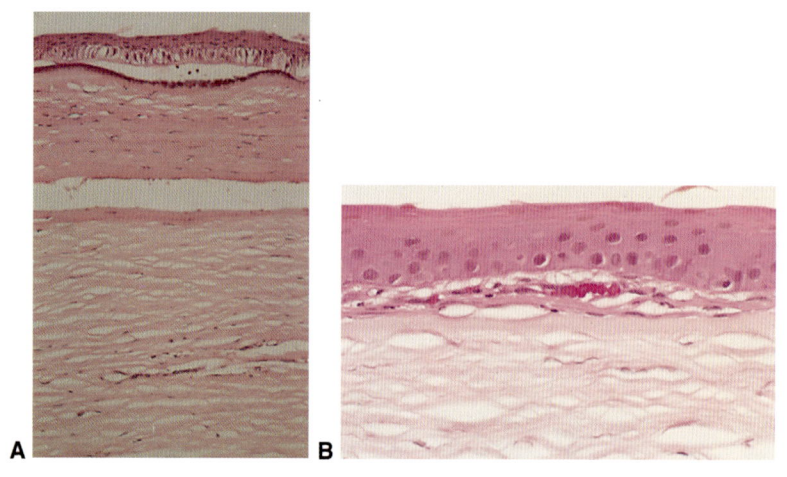

Figure 6-10 Pannus. **A,** This is degenerative pannus: fibrous connective tissue is interposed between the epithelium and Bowman's layer (note the basophilic stippling superficially in degenerative pannus, indicative of calcification). **B,** This is fibrovascular pannus, which may be accompanied by inflammatory cells and destruction of Bowman's layer (a condition sometimes called *inflammatory pannus*).

Figure 6-11 Bullous keratopathy. Note the swelling of the corneal epithelial cells (hydropic degeneration) and the subepithelial bulla *(arrow)*.

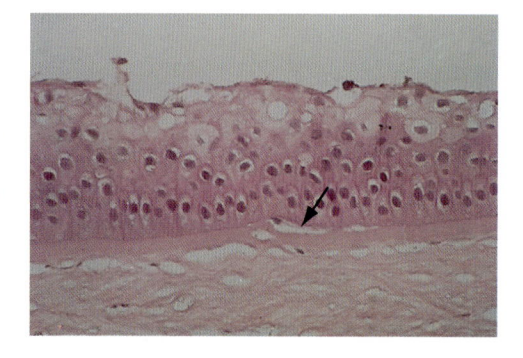

cataract surgery, its incidence has decreased since the advent of intraoperative viscoelastic agents that protect the corneal endothelium and the decreased use of iris plane and anterior chamber intraocular lenses.

In corneal buttons, varying degrees of diffuse corneal edema are present. The epithelium is separated from the underlying Bowman's layer, creating microcysts or coalescing to form bullae. The epithelial basement membrane may be thickened and redundant, and intraepithelial basement membrane material similar to that seen in map-dot-fingerprint dystrophy is often observed. There is a paucity of endothelial cells, and those cells remaining are flattened and attenuated. Descemet's membrane is preserved intact.

Keratoconus

Keratoconus, a noninflammatory condition, is characterized by a bilateral central ectasia of the cornea with anterior protrusion of the cornea. Although the condition is bilateral, 1 eye may be more severely affected. The alteration in the normal corneal contour produces myopia and irregular astigmatism. Keratoconus can occur as an isolated finding, or it may be associated with other ocular disorders or with systemic conditions, including atopy, Down syndrome, and Marfan syndrome.

The earliest histologic changes are focal discontinuities of the epithelial basement membrane and Bowman's layer. Central stromal thinning and anterior stromal scarring are usually present. Iron deposition in the basal epithelial layers *(Fleischer ring)* can often be demonstrated using the Prussian blue stain or Perls test. Spontaneous breaks in Descemet's membrane can lead to acute stromal edema, or *hydrops* (Fig 6-12). Other causes of spontaneous breaks in Descemet's membrane include obstetric forceps injury, congenital glaucoma *(Haab striae),* Terrien marginal degeneration, and pellucid marginal degeneration.

Drug-related alterations

Amiodarone, an oral anti-arrhythmic agent, may produce a whorl-like keratopathy similar to that observed in Fabry disease. This distinctive pattern is a result of lysosomal deposits within the basal layer of the corneal epithelium. Other drugs that may produce a whorl-like keratopathy include chloroquine, chlorpromazine, and indomethacin. These corneal changes usually do not produce symptoms, although patients may complain of halos or blurry vision.

Dystrophies

Dystrophies of the cornea are primary, inherited, bilateral disorders, categorized by the layer of the cornea most involved. Keratoconus (previously discussed) is often considered a dystrophy. Only the most common corneal dystrophies are discussed in the following sections.

Epithelial dystrophy

Also called *map-dot-fingerprint, Cogan microcystic,* or *anterior basement membrane dystrophy,* epithelial dystrophy may be the most common of the corneal dystrophies seen by the comprehensive ophthalmologist (Fig 6-13). In this condition, the basement membrane is thickened and may extend into the epithelium. In addition, abnormal epithelial cells with microcysts are present. A deposition of fibrillar material forms between the basement membrane and Bowman's layer. Patients with epithelial dystrophy often present with symptoms of recurrent erosion syndrome.

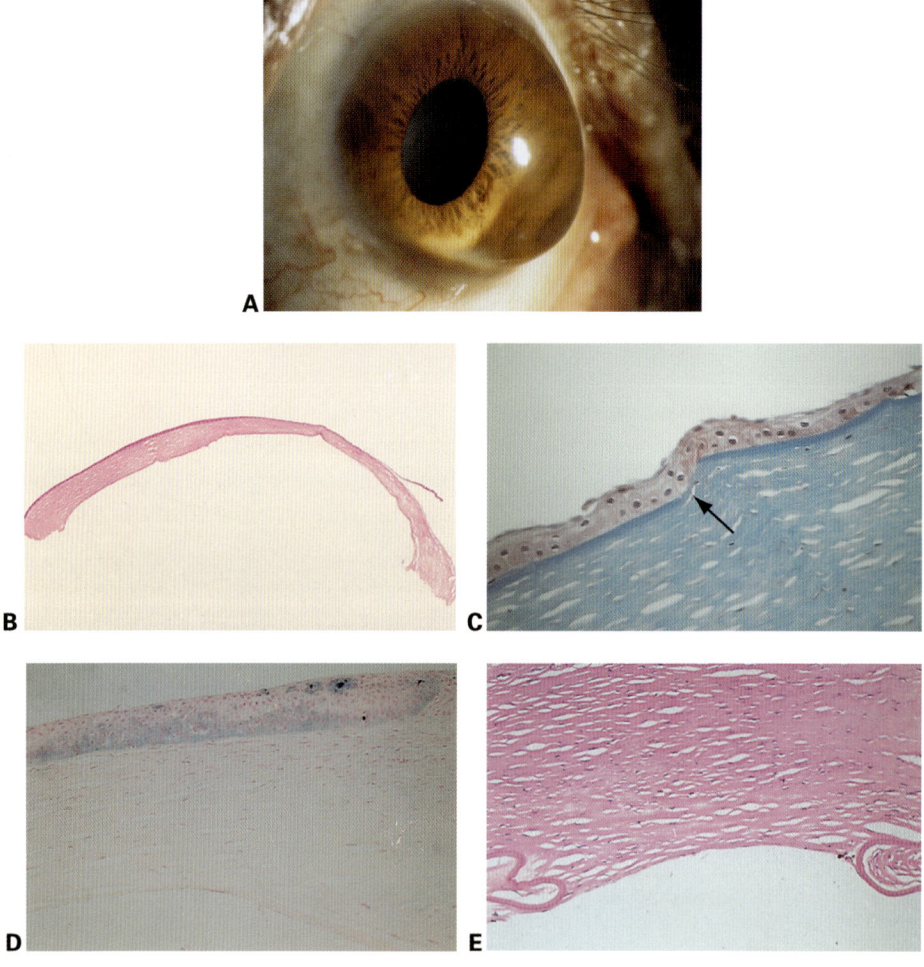

Figure 6-12 Keratoconus. **A,** Clinical appearance. **B,** Low-magnification view shows corneal stromal thinning. **C,** Masson trichrome stain demonstrates focal disruption of Bowman's layer *(arrow)*. **D,** Intraepithelial iron deposition (Fleischer ring). **E,** Rupture of Descemet's membrane, with rolled edges of Descemet's membrane at the edge of the rupture site. *(Part A courtesy of Sander Dubovy, MD; part C courtesy of Hans E. Grossniklaus, MD.)*

Macular dystrophy

Macular dystrophy, an autosomal recessive stromal dystrophy, involves the entire cornea to the limbus. Clinically, it is characterized by poorly defined stromal lesions with hazy intervening stroma. Mucopolysaccharide material is deposited both intracellularly and extracellularly in the corneal stroma. The material stains blue with the alcian blue and colloidal iron stains (Fig 6-14). Corneal thinning may occur as well. Two types of macular dystrophy have been described; these depend on the specific abnormality in the keratan sulfate and dermatan sulfate–proteoglycan metabolism. The genes for macular dystrophy have been identified on chromosome 16q.

CHAPTER 6: Cornea • 85

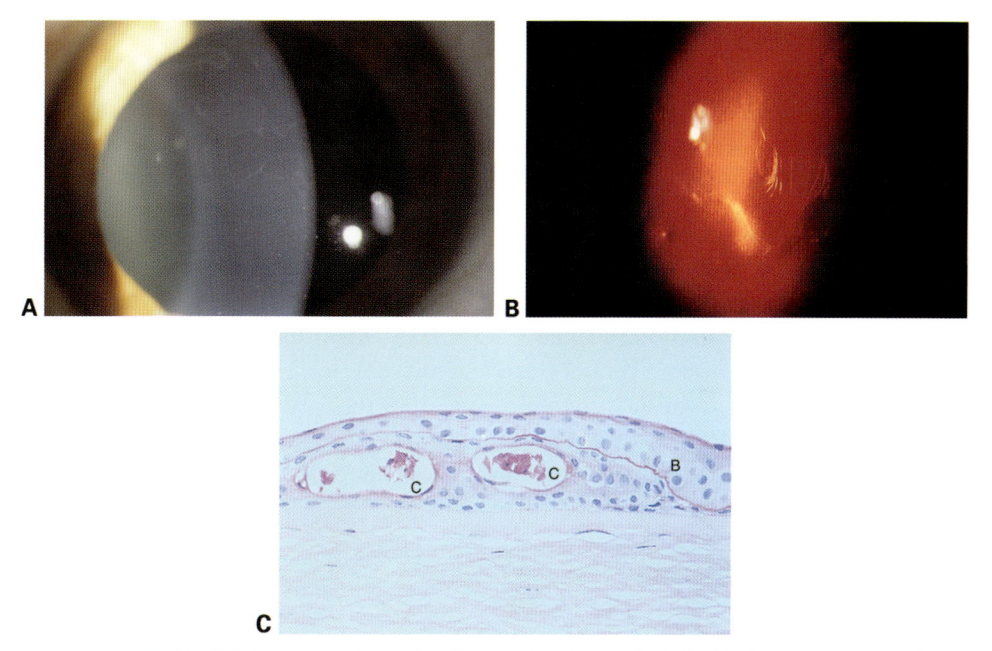

Figure 6-13 Epithelial dystrophy (map-dot-fingerprint dystrophy). **A,** Clinical appearance depicting fine, lacy opacities. **B,** Clinical appearance of cornea using retroillumination to demonstrate numerous wavy lines and dotlike lesions. **C,** The changes in primary map-dot-fingerprint dystrophy are almost identical to those seen in cases of chronic corneal epithelial edema. Note the intraepithelial basement membrane *(B)* and the degenerating intraepithelial cells trapped within cystic spaces *(C)*. *(Part A courtesy of Sander Dubovy, MD.)*

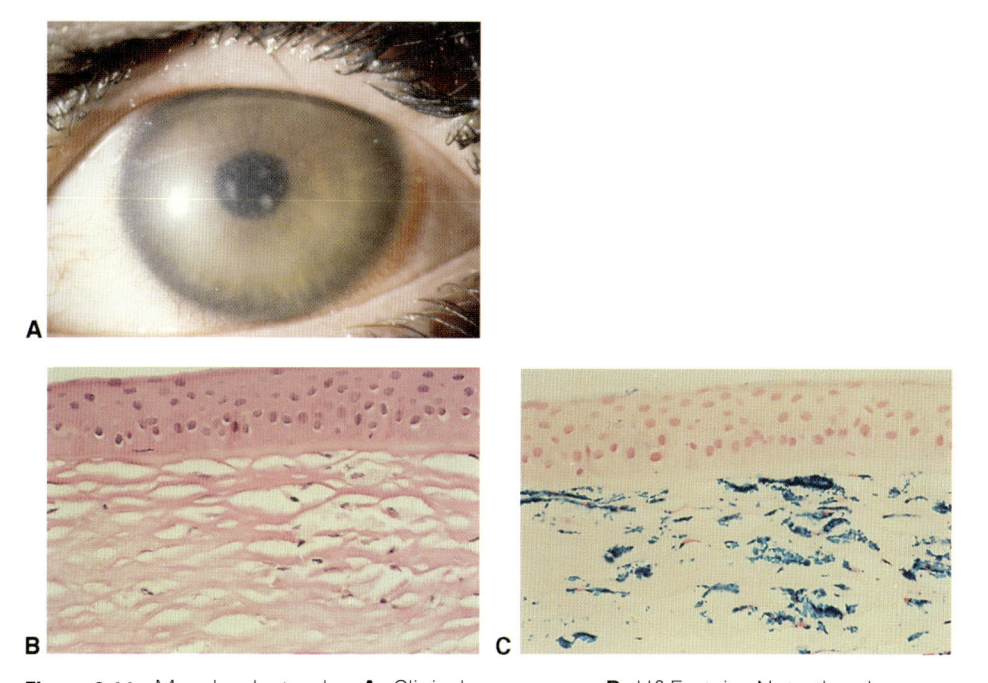

Figure 6-14 Macular dystrophy. **A,** Clinical appearance. **B,** H&E stain. Note the clear spaces surrounding the keratocytes and in the stroma. **C,** Colloidal iron stain for mucopolysaccharides. *(Part A courtesy of Sander Dubovy, MD.)*

86 • Ophthalmic Pathology and Intraocular Tumors

Granular dystrophy

Granular dystrophy is an autosomal dominant stromal dystrophy that involves the central cornea and has sharply defined lesions with clear intervening stroma (Fig 6-15). Histologically, irregularly shaped, well-circumscribed depositions of hyaline material are visible in the stroma. This material stains bright red with the Masson trichrome stain.

Lattice dystrophy

Lattice dystrophy is an autosomal dominant condition that involves the central cornea and is characterized by refractile lines with hazy intervening stroma (Fig 6-16). The disorder is a primary localized corneal amyloidosis, in which the amyloid deposits may result from epithelial cells and keratocytes. Histologically, the amyloid deposits are concentrated most heavily in the anterior stroma, but they may also occur in the subepithelial area. The amyloid material stains positive with the Congo red stain and demonstrates metachromasia with crystal violet stain. The amyloid material is birefringent, appearing

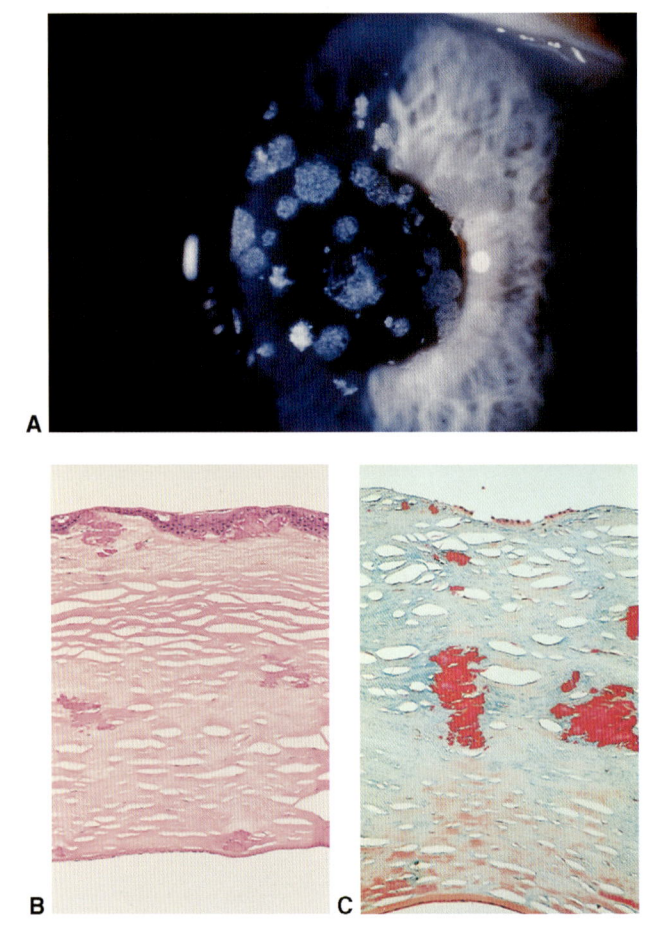

Figure 6-15 Granular dystrophy. **A,** Clinical appearance; note the clear intervening stroma. **B,** H&E stain. Note the chunky stromal deposits at all levels of the cornea. **C,** Masson trichrome stain. The corneal stroma stains blue, and the granular deposits stain brilliant red.

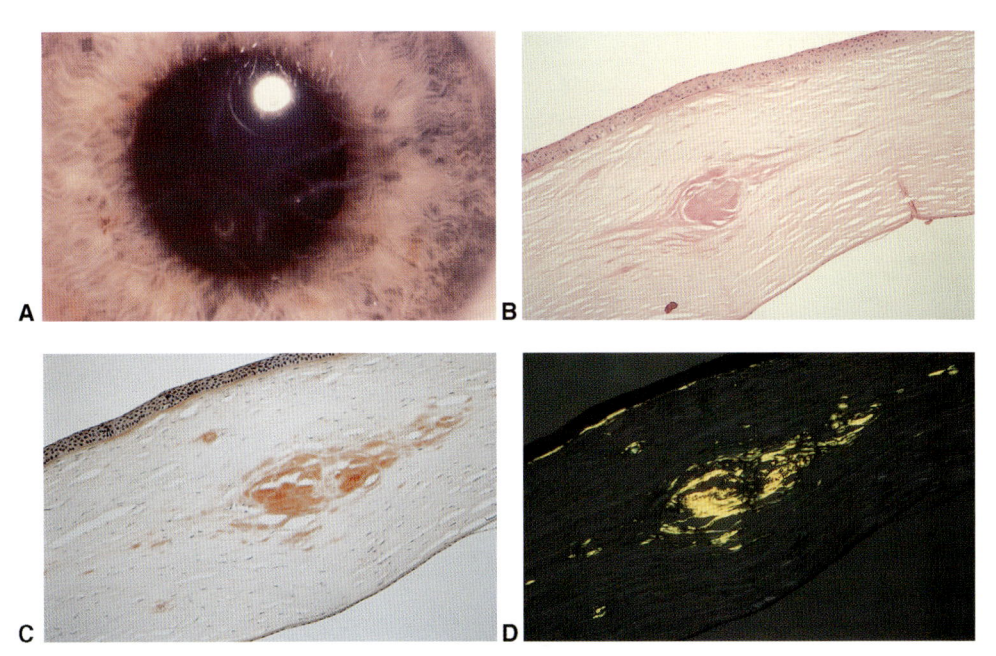

Figure 6-16 Lattice dystrophy. **A,** Clinical appearance. **B,** H&E stain shows scattered fusiform, eosinophilic material deposited at all levels of the stroma. **C,** Congo red stain demonstrates that the fusiform deposits are amyloid. **D,** Examination of Congo red stain with polarized light shows birefringence of amyloid deposits. *(Parts B, C, D, courtesy of Hans E. Grossniklaus, MD.)*

Table 6-1 Histopathologic Differentiation of Macular, Granular, and Lattice Dystrophies

Dystrophy	Masson	Alcian Blue	PAS	Congo Red	Birefringence
Macular	−	+	−	−	−
Granular	+	−	−	−	−
Lattice	+	−	+	+	+

apple green under polarized light. Recurrence of amyloid deposits in the corneal graft following penetrating keratoplasty occurs more frequently in lattice dystrophy than in granular or macular dystrophy.

See Table 6-1 for a histopathologic comparison of the macular, granular, and lattice dystrophies.

Avellino dystrophy

Features of both granular and lattice dystrophy appear in Avellino dystrophy, first described in patients tracing their ancestry to Avellino, Italy. Histologically, both hyaline deposits (typical of granular dystrophy) and amyloid deposits (characteristic of lattice dystrophy) are present within the corneal stroma. This dystrophy, like granular and lattice dystrophy, has been mapped to chromosome 5q.

Fuchs dystrophy

Fuchs dystrophy has a variable inheritance pattern and occurs more commonly in women. It is one of the leading causes of bullous keratopathy. This condition can be recognized clinically before corneal decompensation occurs by the appearance of guttae in Descemet's membrane. In corneal buttons, Descemet's membrane appears diffusely thickened. Focal, anvil-shaped excrescences of basement membrane material are seen protruding into the anterior chamber or buried within the thickened Descemet's membrane. The endothelial cells are usually sparse to absent. As in bullous keratopathy from other causes, there are varying degrees of secondary epithelial basement membrane changes and subepithelial fibrosis (Fig 6-17).

Pigment Deposits

Krukenberg spindle occurs in the pigment dispersion syndrome. The melanin pigment is primarily located within the endothelial cells but is also free on the posterior corneal surface (Fig 6-18).

Blood staining of the cornea may complicate hyphema when the intraocular pressure (IOP) is very high; however, if the endothelium is compromised, blood staining can occur

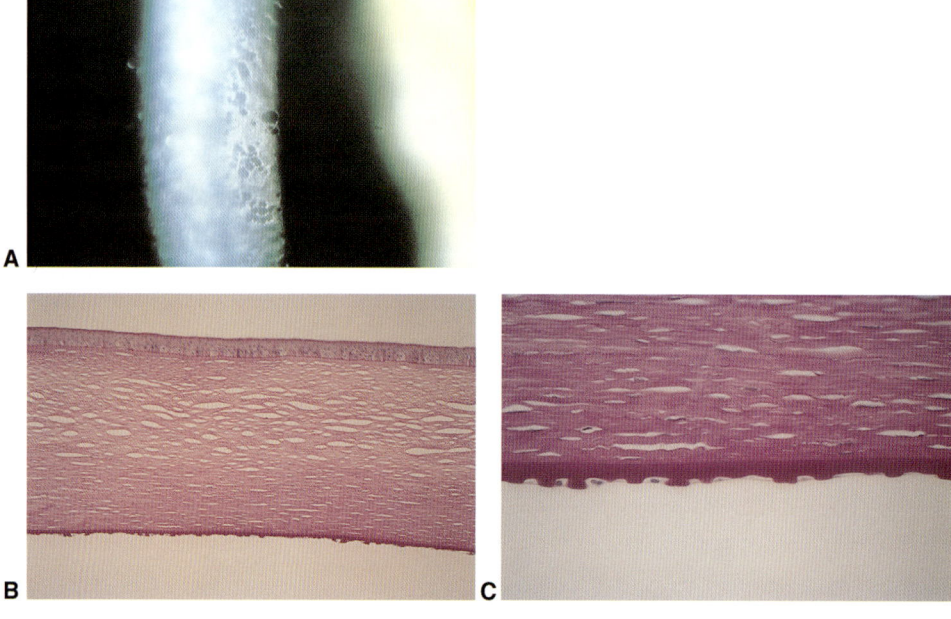

Figure 6-17 Fuchs dystrophy. **A,** Retroillumination of cornea shows "beaten bronze" appearance. **B,** Histology shows diffuse edema of corneal epithelium and stroma. **C,** Higher magnification of Descemet's membrane and posterior corneal stroma using PAS stain shows numerous focal areas of thickening of Descemet's membrane (guttae). *(Part A reproduced from* External Disease and Cornea: A Multimedia Collection. *San Francisco: American Academy of Ophthalmology; 2000. Parts B and C courtesy of Hans E. Grossniklaus, MD.)*

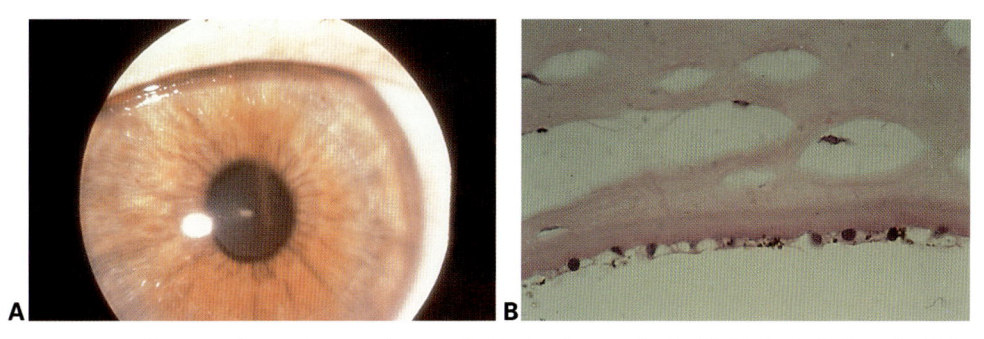

Figure 6-18 Pigment dispersion syndrome. **A,** Krukenberg spindle. **B,** Melanin is found within the endothelial cells. (See also Figure 7-13.) *(Part A courtesy of L.J. Katz, MD; part B courtesy of Debra J. Shetlar, MD.)*

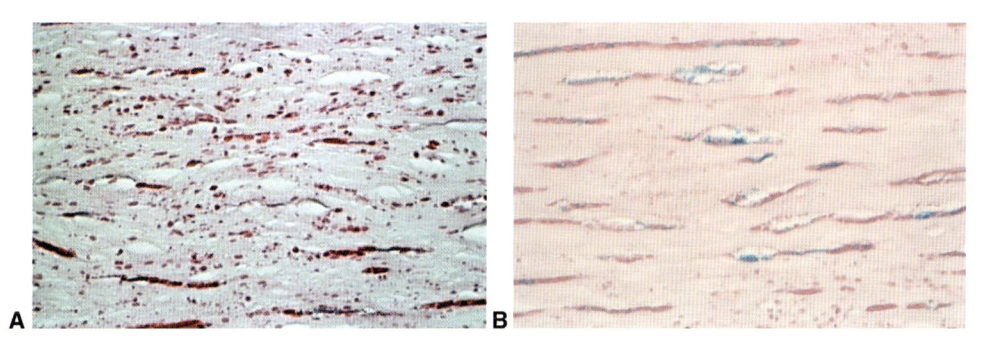

Figure 6-19 A, Corneal blood staining, H&E stain. The orange particles represent hemoglobin in the corneal stroma. **B,** An iron stain demonstrates iron confined to the stromal keratocytes. *(Courtesy of Hans E. Grossniklaus, MD.)*

even at normal or low IOP. In acute blood staining, hemoglobin is demonstrated in the corneal stroma. Later, iron may be demonstrated in the keratocytes (Fig 6-19).

Iron lines result from pooling of tears in areas where the corneal surface is irregular. Histologically, iron is found within the basal epithelial cells and can be demonstrated using the Prussian blue stain or Perls test. Some of the named iron lines include the following:

- Hudson-Stähli (junction of upper two thirds and lower one third of aging cornea)
- Fleischer (in keratoconus)
- Stocker (at the advancing edge of a pterygium)
- Ferry (anterior to a filtering bleb)

The *Kayser-Fleischer ring* is a brown ring seen in the periphery of the cornea in Wilson disease. It corresponds to copper deposition in Descemet's membrane.

Neoplasia

Primary conjunctival intraepithelial neoplasia may extend from the limbus and involve the corneal epithelium. *Dysplasia* of the corneal epithelium refers to abnormal maturation

Figure 6-20 Clinical appearance of corneal epithelial dysplasia. Note the multiple, poorly demarcated superficial opacities. *(Courtesy of Sander Dubovy, MD.)*

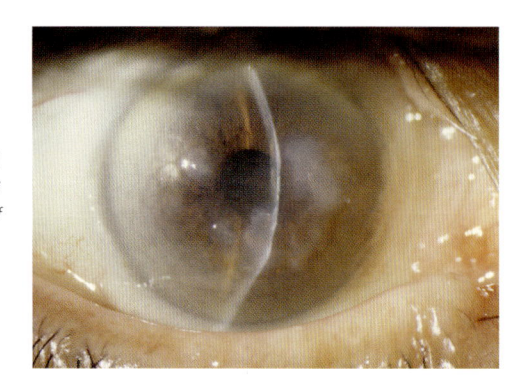

of the epithelium as it differentiates from the basal layer to the superficial layers (Fig 6-20). This condition has been described further in Chapter 5, Conjunctiva. Rarely, primary intraepithelial neoplasia may arise in the clear cornea.

Carcinoma in situ describes full-thickness dysplastic involvement of the epithelium. Bowman's layer normally acts as a natural barrier against invasion by neoplasia; therefore, invasive squamous cell carcinoma involving the corneal stroma is seen only if the disease is very advanced or if Bowman's layer is compromised.

CHAPTER 7

Anterior Chamber and Trabecular Meshwork

Topography

The anterior chamber is bounded anteriorly by the corneal endothelium, posteriorly by the anterior surface of the iris–ciliary body and pupillary portion of the lens, and peripherally by the trabecular meshwork (Fig 7-1). The depth of the anterior chamber is about 3.4–3.7 mm. The trabecular meshwork is derived from the neural crest.

Trabecular Beams and Endothelium

The outermost corneoscleral meshwork is composed of multiple layers of collagenous sheets that are lined by very thin endothelium. This endothelium forms bridges between the sheets. The uveal meshwork, the innermost portion of the trabecular meshwork, is composed of 2 to 3 layers of intersecting trabecular beams that course meridionally from the ciliary body and iris root to the zone between the corneoscleral and trabecular endothelium. These beams, or cords, are covered by a slightly thicker layer of endothelium. Trabecular beams are thicker in individuals with primary infantile glaucoma than in normal individuals. Schlemm's canal encircles the trabecular meshwork and is joined to the corneoscleral meshwork by the internal collector channel. External collector veins channel aqueous back into the vascular system (Fig 7-2).

Congenital Anomalies

Schwalbe's line varies in prominence depending on the number and thickness of inserted cords at the zone of transition between the corneal and trabecular endothelium. Thickening of Schwalbe's line is known as *posterior embryotoxon* (Fig 7-3) and has been associated with open-angle glaucoma, sclerocornea, and other ocular and systemic anomalies related to maldevelopment of neural crest cells.

Axenfeld-Rieger syndrome represents a group of congenital anterior segment defects previously called *mesodermal dysgenesis* and a variety of eponyms. The single most important clinical feature of these phenotypes is that they confer at least a 50% risk of developing glaucoma. The syndrome is often hereditary with an autosomal dominant inheritance

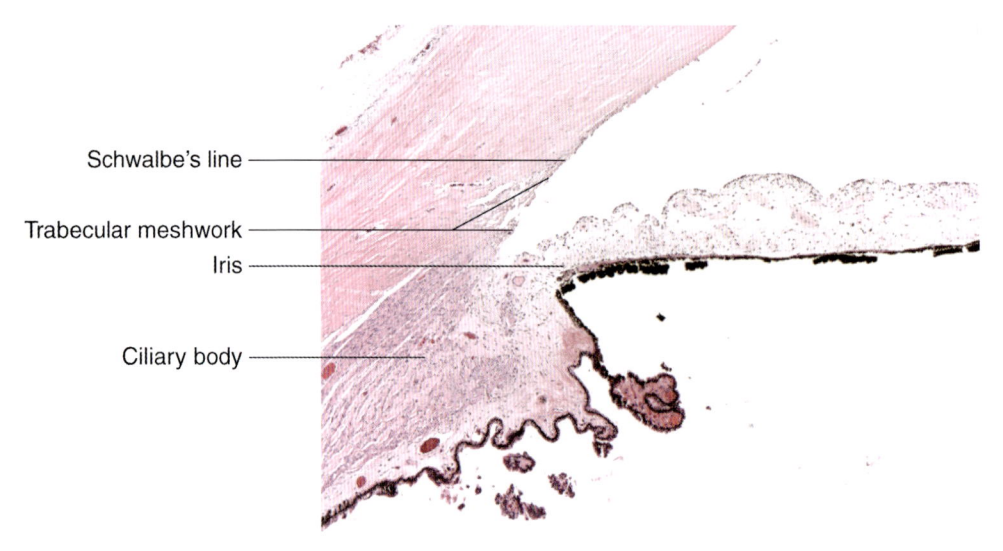

Figure 7-1 The normal anterior chamber angle, the site of drainage for the major portion of the aqueous humor flow, is defined by the anterior border of the iris, the face of the ciliary body, the internal surface of the trabecular meshwork, and the posterior surface of the cornea. *(Courtesy of Nasreen A. Syed, MD.)*

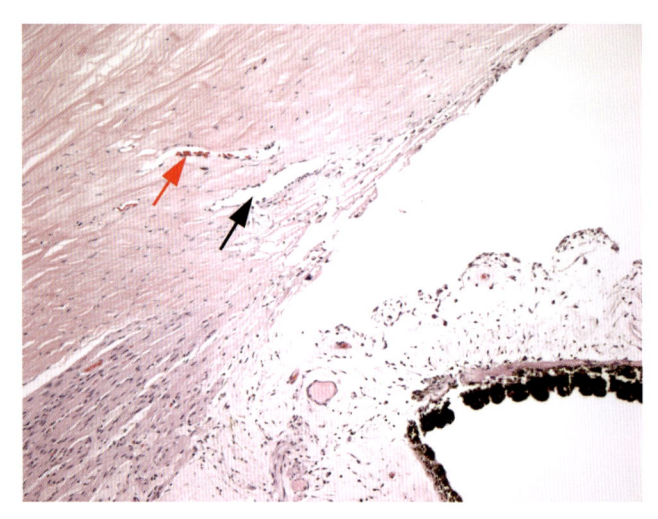

Figure 7-2 Light micrograph of the anterior chamber angle demonstrates Schlemm's canal *(black arrow)* to the trabecular meshwork in the sclera. One of the external collector vessels can be seen adjacent to Schlemm's canal *(red arrow)*. *(Courtesy of Nasreen A. Syed, MD.)*

pattern. Mutations in the homeodomain transcription factor gene *PITX2* (chromosome 4q25) have been found in some patients with this syndrome. Other chromosomal loci, namely 6p25 and 13q14, have been linked to the related phenotypes. The following conditions are included under the name *Axenfeld-Rieger syndrome*.

Axenfeld anomaly is a congenital anomaly in which Schwalbe's line is anteriorly displaced and iris bands extend to the cornea (Fig 7-4). If the development of the meshwork is defective and glaucoma is present, the condition is called *Axenfeld syndrome*.

CHAPTER 7: Anterior Chamber and Trabecular Meshwork • 93

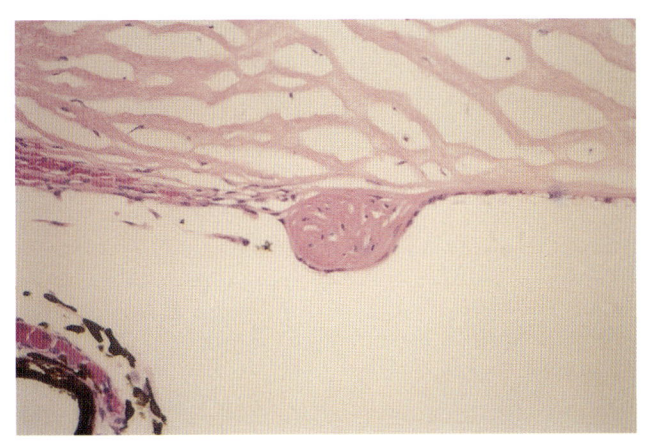

Figure 7-3 Posterior embryotoxon. Light micrograph shows a nodular prominence at the termination of Descemet's membrane. *(Courtesy of Hans E. Grossniklaus, MD.)*

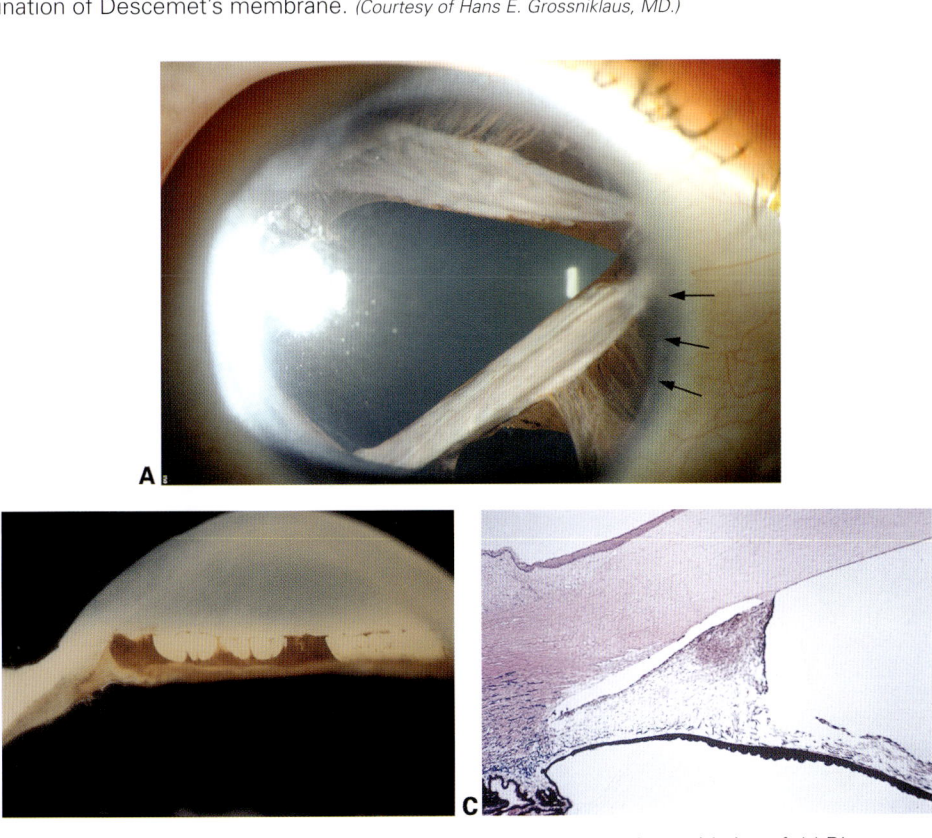

Figure 7-4 A, Clinical photograph of the anterior segment in a patient with Axenfeld-Rieger syndrome. Iris atrophy, polycoria, and iris strands in the periphery are present. Posterior embryotoxon can be seen laterally *(arrows)*. **B,** Gross photograph shows a prominent Schwalbe's line and the anterior insertion of iris strands (Axenfeld anomaly). **C,** Light micrograph shows iris strands that insert anteriorly on Schwalbe's line. *(Part A courtesy of Wallace L.M. Alward, MD. Copyright University of Iowa; part B courtesy of Robert Y. Foos, MD; part C reproduced from Yanoff M, Fine BS. Ocular Pathology: A Color Atlas. New York: Gower; 1988.)*

Rieger anomaly is the term used to describe iris and pupillary abnormalities in combination with the findings of Axenfeld anomaly. Rieger anomaly is associated with the later onset of glaucoma. If Rieger anomaly is associated with dental and skeletal abnormalities, the condition is called *Rieger syndrome*.

> Alward WL. Axenfeld-Rieger syndrome in the age of molecular genetics. *Am J Ophthalmol.* 2000;130:107–115.
>
> Espinoza HM, Cox CJ, Semina EV, Amendt BA. A molecular basis for differential developmental anomalies in Axenfeld-Rieger syndrome. *Hum Mol Genet.* 2002;11:743–753.
>
> Maclean K, Smith J, St. Heaps L, et al. Axenfeld-Rieger malformation and distinctive facial features: clues to a recognizable 6p25 microdeletion syndrome. *Am J Med Genet.* 2005;132:381–385.

Degenerations

Iridocorneal Endothelial Syndrome

The iridocorneal endothelial (ICE) syndrome refers to a spectrum of acquired abnormalities affecting the cornea, anterior chamber angle, and iris. Abnormal proliferation of corneal endothelium is a constant feature of all forms of the ICE syndrome. When these cells cover the angle, secondary angle-closure glaucoma develops. Over time, peripheral anterior synechiae may form, closing the angle (Fig 7-5). Three different clinical presentations are known:

- iris nevus (Cogan-Reese) syndrome
- Chandler syndrome
- essential iris atrophy

Figure 7-5 ICE syndrome. Descemet's membrane lines the anterior surface of the iris *(arrows)*. The iris is apposed to the cornea (peripheral anterior synechiae, *asterisk*).

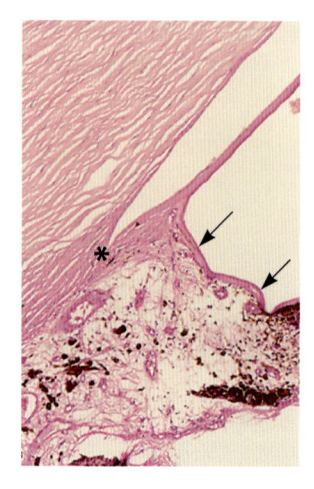

The first letter for each type forms the mnemonic *ICE*. Most patients are young to middle-aged adults who are affected unilaterally. See also BCSC Section 10, *Glaucoma*, which discusses secondary angle-closure glaucoma and covers in depth the issues discussed throughout this chapter.

> Albert DM, Jakobiec FA, eds. *Principles and Practice of Ophthalmology: Basic Sciences.* Philadelphia: Saunders; 1994:1448–1454.

Secondary Glaucoma With Material in the Trabecular Meshwork

Exfoliation syndrome

Sometimes known as *pseudoexfoliation,* exfoliation syndrome is a systemic condition, usually identified in people over 50 years of age and characterized by deposits of PAS-positive fibrils on the lens capsule, zonular fibers, iris, ciliary body, trabecular meshwork, cornea, conjunctiva, and orbital soft tissues. These deposits distinguish exfoliation syndrome from the rare *true exfoliation,* which is the splitting of the lens capsule induced by infrared radiation. Ocular involvement in exfoliation syndrome may be asymmetric. The deposits take the form of distinct fibrils that contain elements of elastic fibers such as fibrillin and α-elastin, as well as noncollagenous basement membrane material such as laminin. The fibrils are coated with the glycosaminoglycan hyaluronic acid (Figs 7-6, 7-7).

The trabecular meshwork in exfoliation syndrome also contains an excessive amount of pigment, but its distribution is more uneven than in pigmentary glaucoma (see "Pigment dispersion associations" later in the chapter). Transillumination defects and circumferential ridges are prominent in the posterior iris. About 10%–23% of patients with exfoliation syndrome have glaucoma: exfoliative glaucoma is the most common identifiable type of glaucoma. Exfoliation syndrome has been associated with systemic hypertension, cerebrovascular events, and myocardial infarction. There is increased risk of zonular dehiscence and capsular rupture during cataract extraction in patients with exfoliation syndrome.

> Ritch R, Schlötzer-Schrehardt U. Exfoliation syndrome. *Surv Ophthalmol.* 2001;45:265–315.

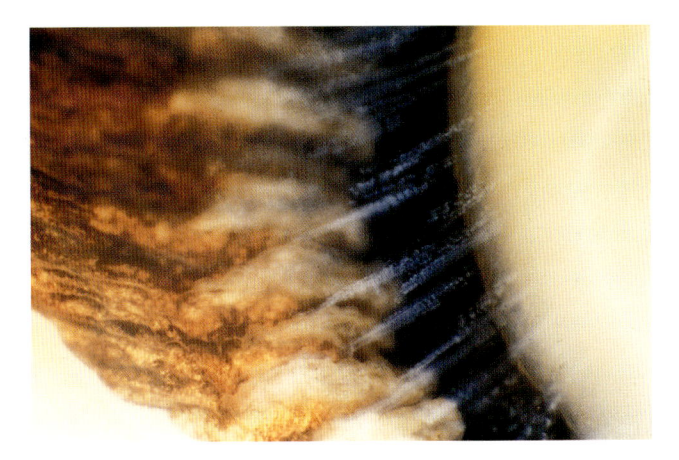

Figure 7-6 Gross photograph shows fibrillar deposits on the lens zonule in pseudoexfoliation. *(Courtesy of Hans E. Grossniklaus, MD.)*

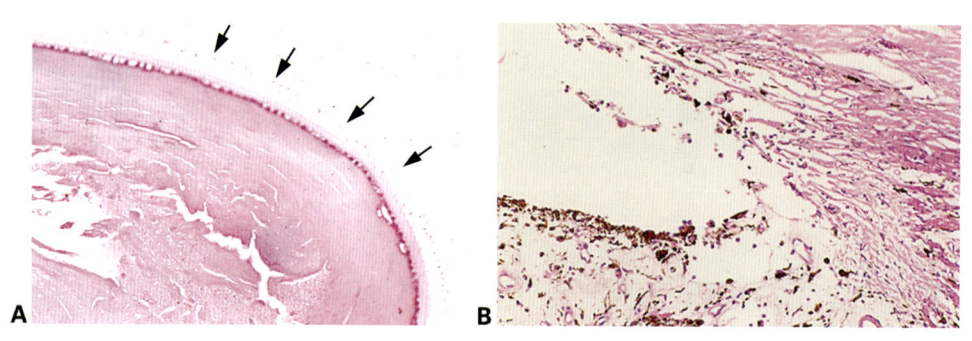

Figure 7-7 A, Abnormal material that resembles iron filings on the edge of a magnet *(arrows)* appears on the lens capsule. **B,** Note the intense pigmentation in the angle. *(Part A courtesy of Nasreen A. Syed, MD.)*

Phacolytic glaucoma

The condition known as *phacolytic glaucoma* occurs when denatured lens protein leaks from a hypermature cataract and occludes the trabecular meshwork. Although some controversy persists regarding the pathogenesis of phacolytic glaucoma, evidence suggests that the abnormal lens protein leaking into the anterior chamber may be directly responsible for the increased resistance to outflow. Macrophages, containing numerous vacuoles, may be present (Fig 7-8). BCSC Section 9, *Intraocular Inflammation and Uveitis,* discusses lens-induced uveitis in more detail.

Trauma

Following an intraocular hemorrhage, blood breakdown products may accumulate in the trabecular meshwork. Hemolyzed erythrocytes may obstruct aqueous outflow and lead to a secondary open-angle glaucoma known as *ghost cell glaucoma.* These ghost erythrocytes are tan in color, spherical in shape, and rigid. Their rigidity makes it difficult for the cells to escape through the trabecular meshwork (Fig 7-9).

In some cases of secondary open-angle glaucoma associated with chronic intraocular hemorrhage, histologic examination has revealed hemosiderin within endothelial cells of the trabecular meshwork and within macrophages. The effect of hemosiderin on the trabecular meshwork and on the pathogenesis of glaucoma is not known. The iron stored in the cells may be an enzyme toxin that damages trabecular function in hemosiderosis oculi. Alternatively, the hemosiderin may be a sign of damage that has occurred during oxidation of hemoglobin. Iron deposition in hemosiderosis oculi can be demonstrated within many ocular epithelial structures by means of the Prussian blue reaction.

In other cases of hemorrhage-associated glaucoma, macrophages in the anterior chamber are noted to contain phagocytosed erythrocytes. In *hemolytic glaucoma,* hemoglobin-laden macrophages block the trabecular outflow channels. It is possible that macrophages are a sign of trabecular obstruction rather than the actual cause.

Blunt injury to the globe may be associated with traumatic hyphema and with recession of the angle, the most common manifestation of this type of trauma. The probability that glaucoma will develop as a late sequela of hyphema depends, in part, on the amount

CHAPTER 7: Anterior Chamber and Trabecular Meshwork • 97

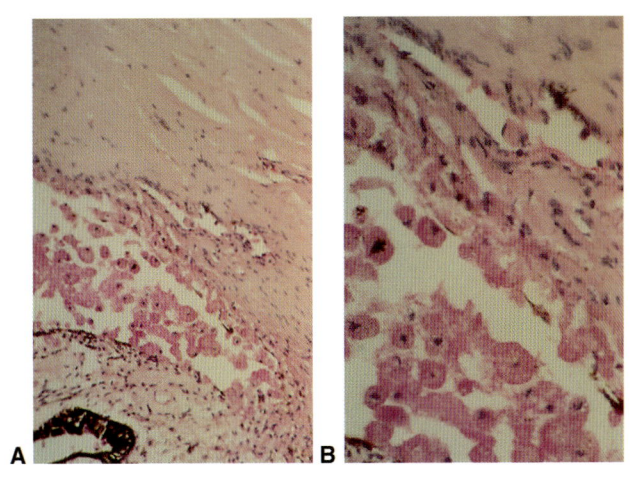

Figure 7-8 Phacolytic glaucoma. **A,** Low magnification of macrophages filled with degenerated lens cortical material in the angle. **B,** Higher magnification.

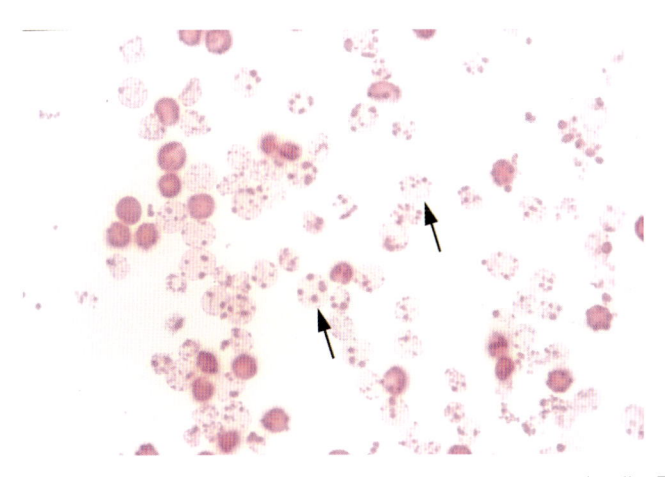

Figure 7-9 Aqueous aspirate demonstrating numerous ghost red blood cells. The degenerating hemoglobin is present as small globules known as Heinz bodies *(arrows)*. *(Courtesy of Nasreen A. Syed, MD.)*

of angle recession. Between 5% and 10% of patients having greater than 180° of angle recession eventually develop chronic glaucoma.

Histologically, angle recession represents a tear in the ciliary body between the longitudinal and circular muscles (Fig 7-10). If the longitudinal muscle is detached from the scleral spur, the tear is referred to as a *cyclodialysis.* Tears in the root of the iris *(iridodialysis)* may also occur with blunt trauma (Fig 7-11; see also Fig 2-7).

Although recession of the angle provides evidence of past blunt trauma, it does not necessarily mean that the trauma is the direct cause of glaucoma. Because glaucoma usually takes years to develop following angle recession, progressive degenerative changes in the remaining trabecular meshwork may be an important factor in the pathogenesis of postcontusion glaucoma.

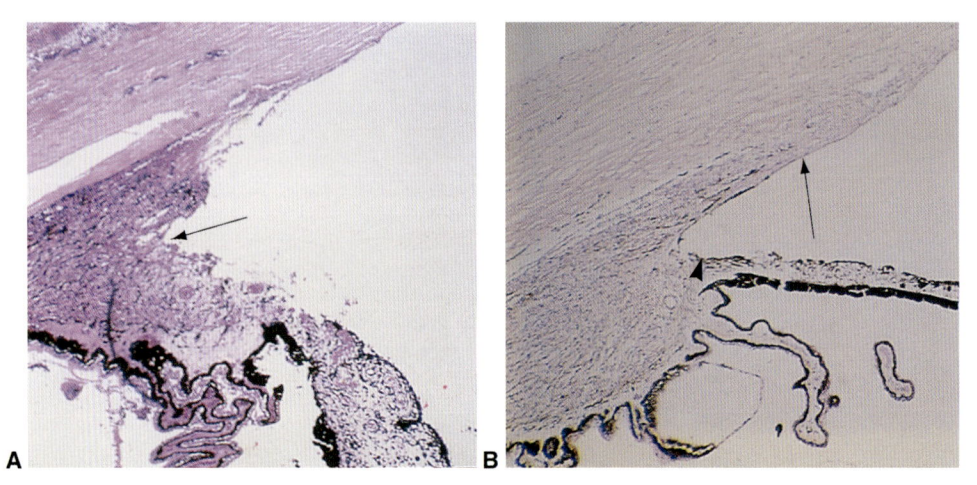

98 • Ophthalmic Pathology and Intraocular Tumors

Figure 7-10 **A,** Contusion injury to the ciliary body. There is a rupture in the face of the ciliary body in the plane between the external longitudinal muscle fibers of the ciliary body and the internal circular and oblique fibers *(arrow)*. Concurrent injury to the trabecular meshwork often occurs. **B,** Contusion angle deformity. The iris root *(arrowhead)* is displaced posteriorly in relation to the longitudinal muscle bundle and its insertion into the scleral spur *(arrow)*. In the region of the injury, the anterior chamber may be deep. Although clinically and histologically unapparent, injury to the drainage structures can be significant.

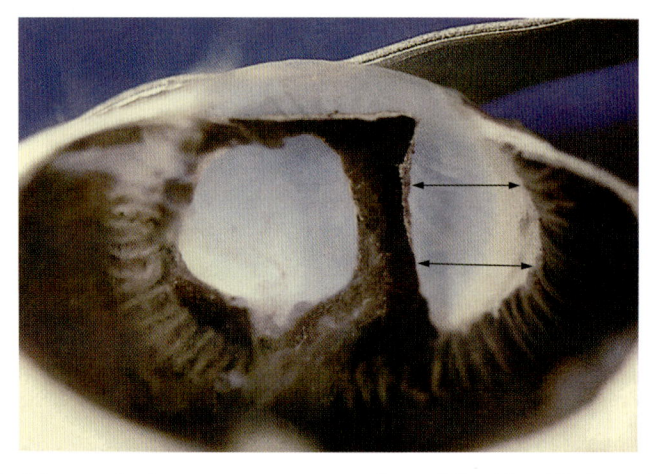

Figure 7-11 Blunt trauma to the eye may cause rupture of the iris at its base *(arrows)*, a point of relative weakness, resulting in iridodialysis.

Pigment dispersion associations

Pigment dispersion may be associated with a variety of other conditions in which pigment epithelium or uveal melanocytes are injured, such as uveitis (uveitic glaucoma) or uveal melanoma. These conditions are characterized by pigment within the trabecular meshwork and in macrophages littering the angle (Fig 7-12).

Secondary open-angle glaucoma can occur as a result of the *pigment dispersion syndrome* (Fig 7-13). This type of glaucoma is characterized by radially oriented defects in the midperipheral iris and pigment in the trabecular meshwork, the corneal endothelium

CHAPTER 7: Anterior Chamber and Trabecular Meshwork • 99

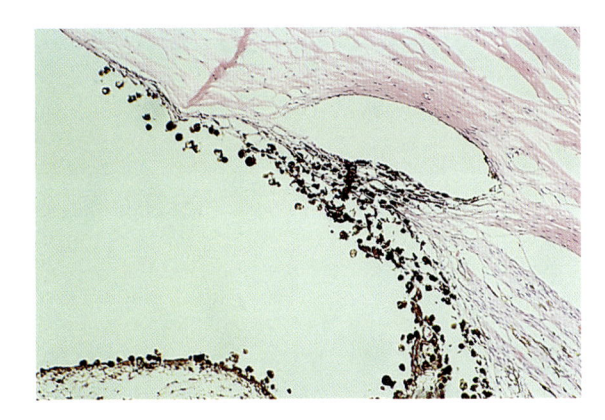

Figure 7-12 Secondary open-angle glaucoma. The trabecular meshwork is obstructed by macrophages that have ingested pigment from a necrotic intraocular melanoma *(melanomalytic glaucoma)*.

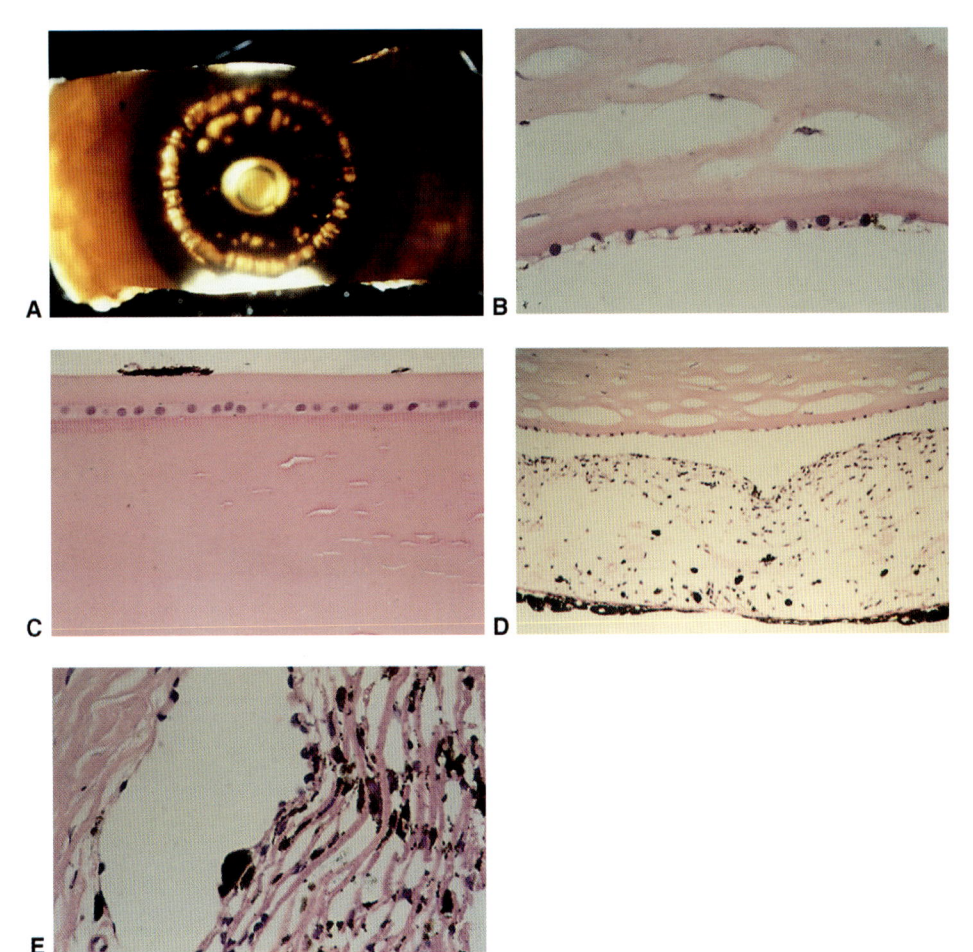

Figure 7-13 Pigment dispersion syndrome. **A,** Gross photograph demonstrating radially oriented transillumination defects in the iris. **B,** Krukenberg spindle. Melanin is present within the corneal endothelial cells. **C,** Scheie stripe. Melanin is present on the anterior surface of the lens. **D,** Note the focal loss of iris pigment epithelium. Chafing of the zonules against the epithelium may release the pigment that is dispersed in this condition. **E,** Note the accumulation of pigment in the trabecular meshwork.

(Krukenberg spindle), and other anterior segment structures such as the lens capsule. See Figure 6-18 for a clinical photograph of a Krukenberg spindle. The dispersed pigment is presumed to be iris pigment epithelium mechanically rubbed off by contact with lens zonular fibers. Histologic studies of eyes with pigmentary glaucoma show large accumulations of pigment granules and cellular debris in the trabecular meshwork and phagocytosed pigment in and on endothelial cells of the cornea. Pigment is present both intracellularly and extracellularly in the trabecular meshwork.

Neoplasia

Melanocytic nevi and melanomas that arise in the iris or extend to the iris from the ciliary body may obstruct the trabecular meshwork (Fig 7-14). See also Chapter 17, Melanocytic Tumors. In addition, pigment elaborated from the melanomas may be shed into the trabecular meshwork and produce secondary glaucoma.

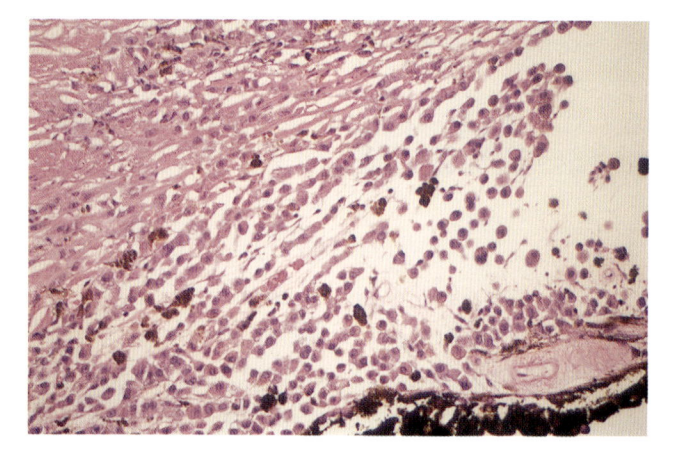

Figure 7-14 Photomicrograph shows malignant melanoma cells filling the anterior chamber angle and obstructing the trabecular meshwork. *(Courtesy of Hans E. Grossniklaus, MD.)*

CHAPTER 8

Sclera

Topography

The sclera is the white, nearly opaque portion of the outer wall of the eye, covering from four fifths to five sixths of the eye's circumference. It is continuous anteriorly at the limbus with the corneal stroma. Posteriorly, the outer two thirds of the sclera merges with the dura of the optic nerve sheath; the inner one third continues as the lamina cribrosa, through which pass the axonal fibers of the optic nerve. The diameter of the scleral shell averages 22.0 mm, and its thickness varies from 1.0 mm posteriorly to 0.3 mm just posterior to the insertions of the 4 rectus muscles. Histologically, the sclera is divided into 3 layers (from outermost inward): episclera, stroma, and lamina fusca (Fig 8-1). The sclera is derived from the neural crest.

Episclera

The episclera is a thin fibrovascular layer that covers the outer surface of the scleral stroma. It is thickest anterior to the rectus muscle insertions and immediately surrounding the optic nerve and thinnest at the limbus and posterior to the rectus muscle insertions at the equator of the eye. The episclera is composed of loosely arranged collagen fibers and a vascular plexus.

Stroma

The bulk of the sclera is made up of sparsely vascularized, dense, type I collagen fibers whose diameters range from 28 nm to more than 300 nm; the thicker fibers are more centrifugally arranged. In general, collagen fibers in the stroma course parallel to the external surface of the scleral shell, but individual fibers are randomly arranged and may branch and curl. In comparison to the corneal stroma, scleral collagen fibers are thicker and more variable in thickness and orientation. Transmural emissarial channels provide outlets within the stroma as follows (Fig 8-2):

- in the posterior region, for posterior ciliary arteries and nerves
- in the equatorial region, for vortex veins
- in the anterior regions, for anterior ciliary arteries, veins, and nerves

Ciliary nerves may have pigmented melanocytes along their nerve sheaths that appear as pigmentation on the epibulbar surface (eg, Axenfeld nerve loop).

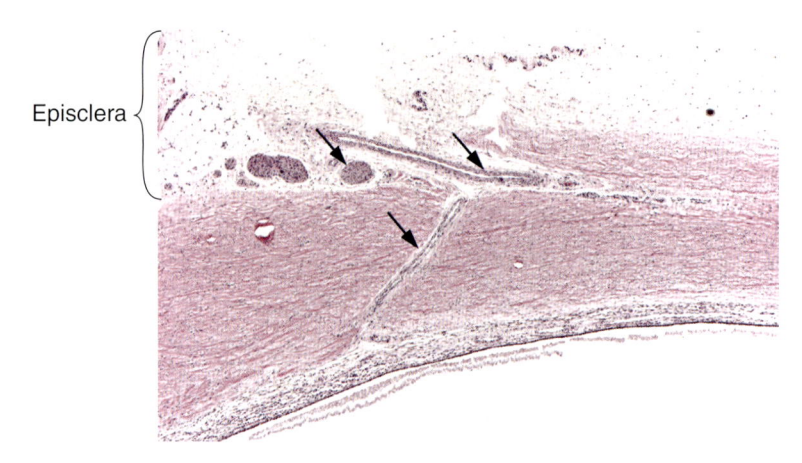

102 • Ophthalmic Pathology and Intraocular Tumors

Figure 8-1 Normal sclera demonstrating emissary structures, including ciliary arteries and nerves entering and traversing the sclera *(arrows)*. *(Courtesy of Nasreen A. Syed, MD.)*

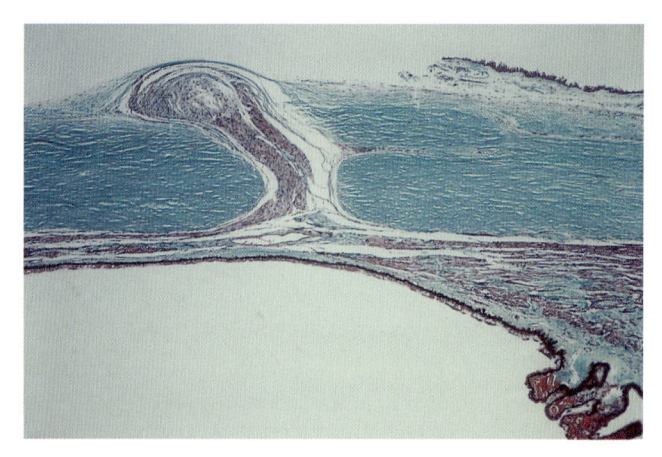

Figure 8-2 An emissarial channel through the sclera for the Axenfeld nerve loop is present overlying the pars plana (trichrome stain). *(Courtesy of Harry H. Brown, MD.)*

Lamina Fusca

The lamina fusca is a thin network of bridging collagen fibers that loosely binds the uvea to the sclera. Sclerouveal attachments are strongest along major emissarial canals and the anterior base of the ciliary body. The lamina fusca contains variable numbers of melanocytes.

Congenital Anomalies

Choristoma

Limbal dermoids are discussed in Chapter 5, Conjunctiva, and an example is shown in Figure 6-3.

Episcleral osseous choristomas are found most commonly in the superotemporal quadrant of the epibulbar surface, 0.5–1.0 cm posterior to the limbus. The clinical appearance is that of a single stationary hard white plaque, round to oval in shape, and measuring up to 1.0 cm in diameter, beneath the conjunctiva. No other congenital anomalies are associated. The histopathologic appearance demonstrates mature lamellar bony trabeculae; rarely, hematopoietic elements occupy the marrow space.

Nanophthalmos

An eye that is uniformly reduced in size except for the lens, which is normal or slightly enlarged, results in severe hyperopia. Nanophthalmos is usually bilateral. The sclera is abnormally thick, which is thought to predispose to uveal effusion because of reduced protein permeability and impaired venous outflow through the vortex veins. Glaucoma, which is common in nanophthalmic eyes, may be caused by a variety of mechanisms, including angle closure, pupillary block, and open angle with elevated episcleral venous pressure.

Inflammations

Episcleritis

Simple episcleritis most commonly presents as a slightly tender, movable, sectorial red area involving the anterior episclera. It affects males and females equally, most commonly in the third to fifth decades, and usually has no association with antecedent injury or systemic illness. Histopathologic examination shows vascular congestion and stromal edema associated with a chronic inflammatory infiltrate, composed primarily of lymphocytes, in a perivascular distribution. Granulomatous inflammation and necrosis are not present. The diagnosis is made on clinical findings, and complete resolution is the rule, with or without topical corticosteroid therapy. The condition may be recurrent, however, and can ultimately cause fibrosis and scar formation.

In contrast to simple episcleritis, *nodular episcleritis* more often affects females and those with rheumatoid arthritis. It is characterized by tender, elevated, rounded, pink-red nodules on the anterior episclera. Histopathologically, the nodules are composed of necrobiotic granulomatous inflammation, a palisading arrangement of epithelioid histiocytes around a central core of necrotic collagen. This light microscopic pattern is the same as that seen in rheumatoid nodules in subcutaneous tissue. Spontaneous resolution is the expected outcome, and topical corticosteroids or nonsteroidal anti-inflammatory drugs (NSAIDs) may reduce symptoms. See BCSC Section 8, *External Disease and Cornea,* for further discussion of this condition and of those covered in the following sections.

Scleritis

Scleritis is a painful, often progressive ocular disease with potentially serious sequelae. There is a high association with systemic autoimmune vasculitic connective tissue diseases.

104 • Ophthalmic Pathology and Intraocular Tumors

Such diseases include

- rheumatoid arthritis
- systemic lupus erythematosus
- polyarteritis nodosa
- Wegener granulomatosis
- relapsing polychondritis
- Reiter syndrome

The inflammation may be localized to the anterior or the posterior sclera, or it may affect other ocular tissues, particularly the cornea and uvea. *Anterior scleritis* is usually a severely painful sectoral inflammation of episclera and sclera with intense photophobia (Fig 8-3). The disease is bilateral in approximately 50% of cases. *Posterior scleritis* is marked by a different constellation of signs and symptoms: patients present with unilateral proptosis, retrobulbar pain, gaze restriction, and visual field loss. Contiguous spread of inflammation may result in optic neuritis or retinal and choroidal detachments; it may even give the mistaken impression of an intraocular neoplasm.

Histopathologic examination of scleritis reveals 2 main categories: necrotizing and nonnecrotizing inflammation. Either type may occur anteriorly or posteriorly. *Necrotizing inflammation* may be nodular or diffuse (so-called *brawny scleritis,* Fig 8-4). Both patterns demonstrate a palisading arrangement of epithelioid histiocytes and multinucleated giant cells surrounding sequestered areas of necrosis (Fig 8-5). Peripheral to the histiocytes is a rim of lymphocytes and plasma cells. Multiple foci may show different stages of evolution. In the course of healing, the necrotic stroma is resorbed, leaving in its wake a thinned scleral remnant prone to staphyloma formation (Fig 8-6). Severe ectasia of the scleral shell

Figure 8-3 This patient has a sectoral nodular anterior scleritis that causes severe ocular pain and photophobia. *(Courtesy of Harry H. Brown, MD.)*

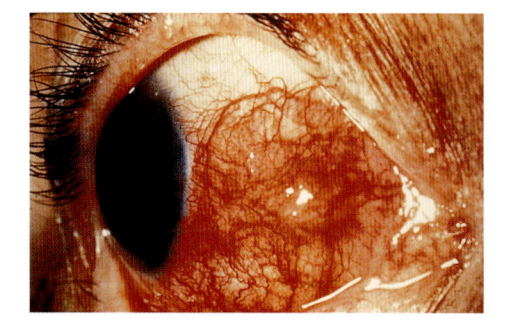

Figure 8-4 Diffuse posterior scleritis (brawny scleritis) demonstrates marked thickening of the posterior sclera. *(Courtesy of Harry H. Brown, MD.)*

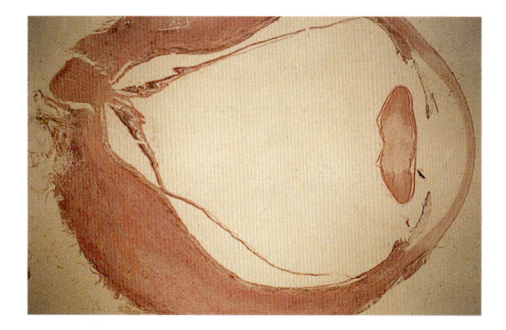

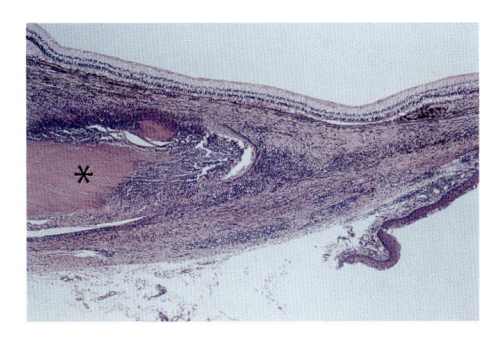

Figure 8-5 An area of necrosis *(asterisk)* is sequestered by a zonal inflammatory reaction of histiocytes, lymphocytes, and plasma cells in this necrotizing granulomatous scleritis. *(Courtesy of Harry H. Brown, MD.)*

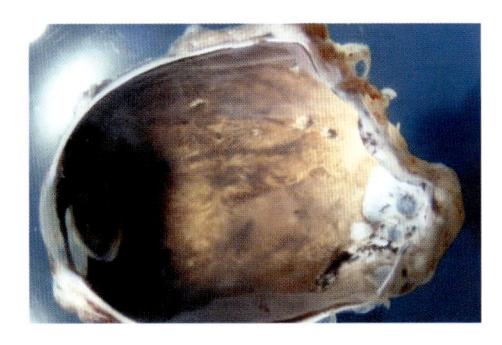

Figure 8-6 A posterior staphyloma is present in this eye as a sequela of scleritis. *(Courtesy of Hans E. Grossniklaus, MD.)*

predisposes to herniation of uveal tissue through the defect, a condition known as *scleromalacia perforans*.

Nonnecrotizing inflammation is characterized by a perivascular lymphocytic and plasma cell infiltrate without a granulomatous inflammatory component. Vasculitis may be present in the form of fibrinoid necrosis of vessel walls. Treatment with NSAIDs usually leads to resolution without significant weakening of the scleral shell.

> Dubord PJ, Chambers A. Scleritis and episcleritis: diagnosis and management. *Focal Points: Clinical Modules for Ophthalmologists.* San Francisco: American Academy of Ophthalmology; 1995, module 9.

Degenerations

Senile calcific plaques occur commonly in elderly persons as flat, firm, gray rectangular to oval patches that appear bilaterally and measure less than 1.0 cm in greatest dimension. They are located anterior to the insertions of the medial and lateral rectus muscles (Fig 8-7). On histologic sections, the calcium appears within the midportion of the scleral stroma. It initially occurs as a finely granular deposition but may progress to involve both superficial and deep layers as a confluent plaque. Senile calcific plaques may be highlighted by special stains such as the von Kossa stain. The etiology is unknown; dehydration and actinic damage have been proposed but not proven.

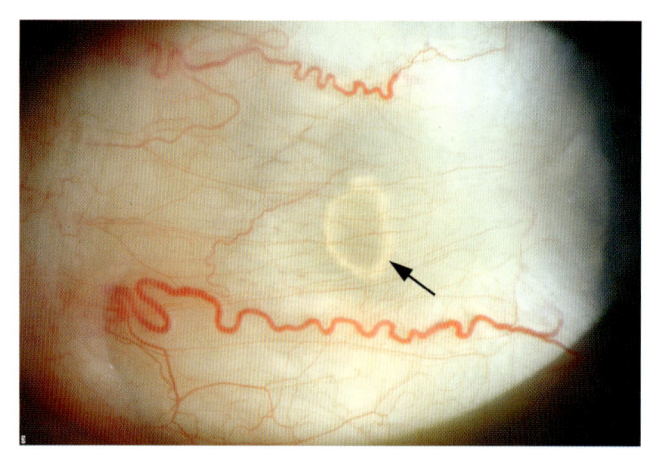

106 • Ophthalmic Pathology and Intraocular Tumors

Figure 8-7 A calcific plaque of the sclera *(arrow)*. Such plaques are typically located just anterior to the insertion of the medial or lateral rectus muscles. *(Courtesy of Vinay A. Shah, MBBS.)*

Corneal staphylomas are discussed in Chapter 6, Cornea. *Scleral staphylomas* are ectasias lined by uveal tissue that may occur at points of weakness in the scleral shell, either in inherently thin areas (such as posterior to the rectus muscle insertions) or in areas weakened by tissue destruction (as in scleritis associated with rheumatoid arthritis; see Fig 8-6). In children, staphylomas may occur as a result of long-standing increased IOP or axial myopia, owing to the relative distensibility of the sclera in younger, as compared with older, individuals. Age at onset and location, therefore, vary according to the underlying etiology. Staphylomas appear as variably sized and shaped patches of blue-purple discoloration of the sclera caused by increased visibility of the underlying uveal pigment and vasculature. Histopathologic examination invariably reveals thinned sclera, with or without fibrosis and scarring, again depending on the cause.

Neoplasia

Neoplasms of the sclera are exceedingly rare. Tumors most likely originate in the episclera or Tenon's capsule rather than in the sclera proper. Reported examples include fibrous histiocytoma and melanocytoma. Nodular fasciitis is included in this discussion, although it is a reactive proliferative process.

Fibrous histiocytoma is a benign neoplasm formed by a proliferation of spindle cells, characteristically in a matlike *(storiform)* pattern. Although more common in the orbit, it may occasionally involve the sclera. For more information on this neoplasm, see Chapter 14, Orbit.

Nodular fasciitis is a reactive process that may, rarely, cause a tumor in the episclera. Antecedent trauma has been implicated as an etiologic factor for the development of nodular fasciitis in other body sites, but no such association has been identified in the sclera. The disease usually affects young adults as a rapidly growing, round to oval, firm white-gray nodule measuring 0.5–1.5 cm and appearing at the limbus or anterior to a rectus muscle insertion. Although self-limited, it is usually excised because of its rapid growth. Histopathologic examination reveals a circumscribed spindle cell proliferation in which individual cells are likened to the appearance of fibroblasts growing in tissue culture. These spindle cells aggregate in whorling fascicles, admixed with a chronic inflammatory infiltrate and lipid-laden histiocytes, in a myxoid background. Older lesions may show foci of dense collagen deposition. Although mitotic figures may be present, atypical (eg, tripolar) mitotic figures are absent. The cellular nature of these proliferations and the presence of mitotic figures may lead to the histologic misinterpretation as sarcoma (soft tissue malignancy), a pitfall to avoid.

CHAPTER 9

Lens

Topography

The crystalline lens is a soft, elastic, avascular, biconvex structure that in the adult measures 9–10 mm in diameter and 3.5 mm in anteroposterior thickness (Fig 9-1). The lens is derived from surface ectoderm. BCSC Section 11, *Lens and Cataract*, discusses in depth the structure, embryology, and pathology of the lens.

Capsule

The lens capsule is composed of a thick basement membrane that surrounds the entire lens and is elaborated by the lens epithelial cells. It is thickest anteriorly (12–21 μm) and peripherally near the equator and thinnest posteriorly (2–9 μm). The capsule provides insertions for the zonular fibers and plays an important part in molding the lens shape in accommodation.

Epithelium

The lens epithelium is derived from the cells of the original lens vesicle that did not differentiate into primary fibers. Although epithelial cells located centrally do not usually undergo mitosis, those located peripherally in the equatorial zone actively divide. The anterior or axial cells form a single layer of cuboidal cells with their basilar surface toward the anterior lens capsule, whereas the cells nearer the equator appear more elongated as they differentiate into lens fibers.

Cortex and Nucleus

New lens fibers are continuously laid down from the outside as the lens epithelial cells differentiate. The oldest fibers, the embryonic and fetal lens nucleus, were produced in embryonic life, have lost their nuclei, and persist in the center of the lens. The outermost fibers, which are the most recently formed, make up the cortex of the lens and are composed of fibers derived from the differentiated lens epithelial cells.

Zonular Fibers

The lens is supported by the zonular fibers that attach to the anterior and posterior lens capsule in the midperiphery (Fig 9-2). These fibers hold the lens in place through their attachments to the ciliary body processes.

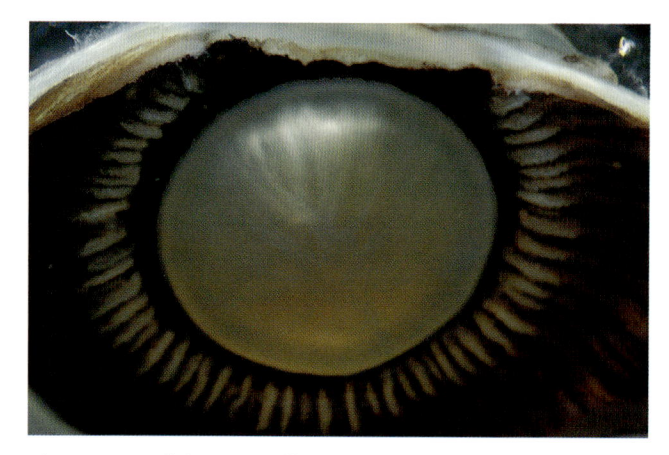

110 • Ophthalmic Pathology and Intraocular Tumors

Figure 9-1 Posterior aspect of the crystalline lens, depicting its relationship to the peripheral iris and ciliary body. *(Courtesy of Hans E. Grossniklaus, MD.)*

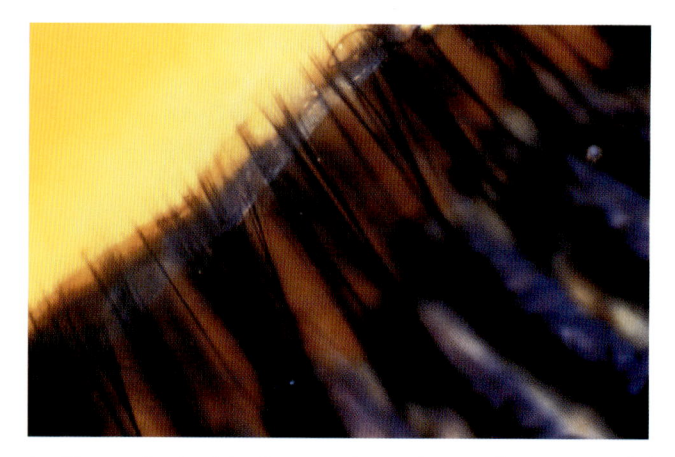

Figure 9-2 Zonular fibers attached to the anterior and posterior aspect of the lens capsule. *(Reproduced with permission from Wilson DJ, Jaeger MJ, Green WR. Effects of extracapsular cataract extraction on the lens zonules. Ophthalmology. 1987;94:467–470.)*

Congenital Anomalies

Ectopia Lentis

With ectopia lentis, the lens may be partially dislocated *(subluxation)* or totally dislocated *(luxation)* (Fig 9-3). Congenital ectopia lentis may occur as an isolated phenomenon *(simple ectopia lentis)* or as part of an inherited syndrome that has systemic manifestations.

Marfan syndrome is a disorder of connective tissue with ocular, musculoskeletal, and cardiovascular manifestations. The lens is usually displaced upward or in a superotemporal

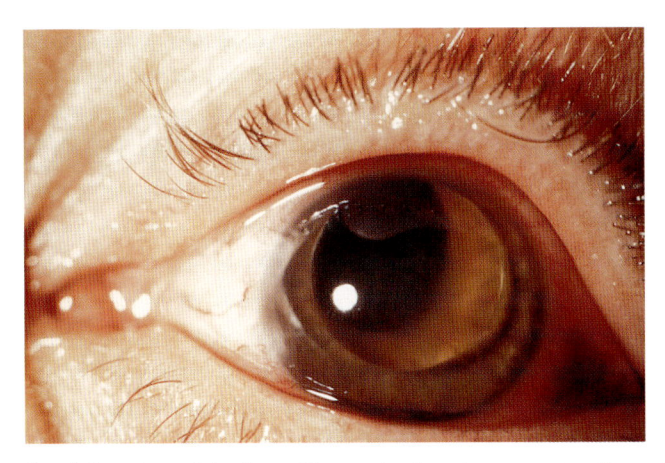

Figure 9-3 Anterior dislocation of the lens. The entire lens is present in the anterior chamber. *(Courtesy of Debra J. Shetlar, MD.)*

Table 9-1 Conditions Associated With Ectopia Lentis

With systemic abnormalities
 Marfan syndrome: lens dislocated up
 Homocystinuria: lens dislocated down
 Weill-Marchesani syndrome: superotemporal or temporal displacement of spherophakic lens
 Others: hyperlysinemia, Ehlers-Danlos syndrome, Crouzon disease, and oxycephaly

With other congenital ocular abnormalities
 Aniridia
 Uveal coloboma
 Buphthalmos
 Megalocornea
 High myopia
 Corectopia
 Peters anomaly

direction, and axial myopia is often present. Marfan syndrome is caused by mutations in the fibrillin gene on chromosome 15.

In patients with *homocystinuria,* the lens is displaced inferonasally, or it may luxate into the anterior chamber or posterior segment. This autosomal recessive trait is caused by a defect in cystathionine β–synthase. Other conditions associated with ectopia lentis are listed in Table 9-1.

Congenital Cataract

Lens opacities present at birth or developing during the first year of life are called *congenital cataracts.* The term *infantile cataracts* is also used for those not seen at birth. Congenital cataracts may be unilateral or bilateral. In general, about one third of these cataracts are associated with other disease syndromes, one third occur as an inherited trait, and one third result from undetermined causes. See also BCSC Section 6, *Pediatric Ophthalmology and Strabismus.*

Posterior polar cataracts are congenital opacities that may range from the small white spot of a Mittendorf dot to a larger, plaque-shaped opacity that is due to persistence of the retrolental vascular tissue (persistent fetal vasculature [PFV]). The posterior capsule may rupture and lead to lens-induced inflammation and/or extension of vessels and fibroblasts into the lens. Removing these cataracts is difficult, as the lens capsule may be thinned or absent, leading to a high rate of posterior capsule rupture.

Rubella cataract

Rubella cataract occurs in the fetus if the mother is exposed to the rubella virus during the first or second trimester of pregnancy. The lens opacity is only one of several birth anomalies associated with in utero rubella exposure. Histologically, the lens is microspherophakic, and retained lens fiber nuclei are present. Rubella virus may be cultured from surgically removed lenses.

Inflammations

Phacoantigenic Endophthalmitis

Also known as *lens-induced granulomatous endophthalmitis* or *phacoanaphylactic endophthalmitis,* this type of lens-induced intraocular inflammation is mediated by IgG immunoglobulins directed against lens protein. The inflammation may follow accidental or surgical trauma to the lens. Histologically, lens-induced granulomatous endophthalmitis consists of a central nidus of degenerating lens material surrounded by concentric layers of inflammatory cells (zonal granuloma). Multinucleated giant cells and neutrophils are present within the inner layer adjacent to the degenerating lens material. Lymphocytes and histiocytes make up the intermediate mantle of cells. These cells may be surrounded by fibrous connective tissue and collagen, depending on the duration of the inflammatory response (Figs 9-4, 9-5). See also BCSC Section 9, *Intraocular Inflammation and Uveitis.*

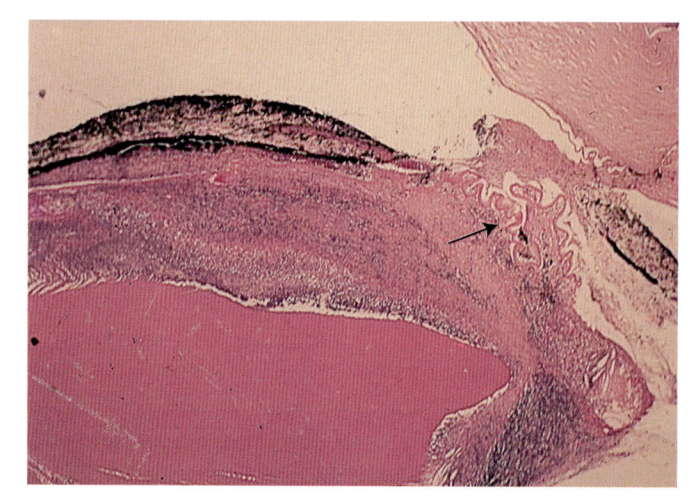

Figure 9-4 Phacoantigenic endophthalmitis, in which inflammatory reaction surrounds the lens *(lower left).* The torn capsule can be observed in the pupillary region *(arrow).* Also note corneal scar *(upper right),* representing the site of ocular penetration.

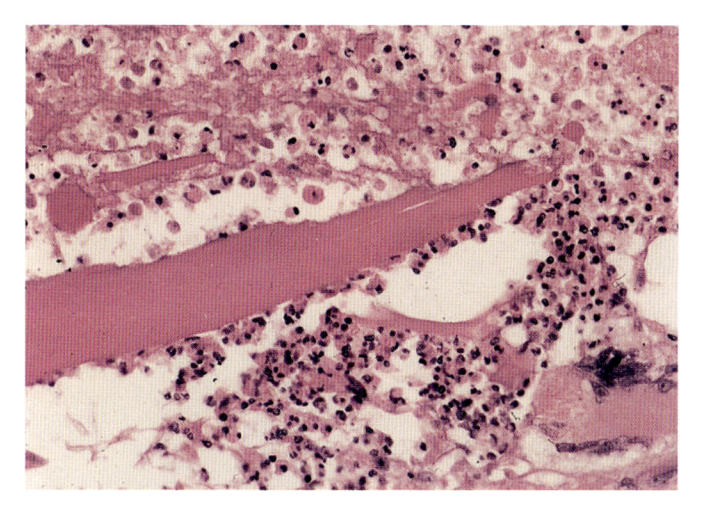

Figure 9-5 Phacoantigenic endophthalmitis. Granulomatous inflammation, including giant cells *(lower right)*, surrounds inciting lens fibers.

Phacolytic Glaucoma

In a hypermature cataract, the liquefied cortical material may leak through the capsule and gain access to the anterior chamber. This material incites a marked nongranulomatous inflammatory response in which numerous macrophages phagocytize the lens protein material. Collections of these protein-laden macrophages, as well as extracellular lens protein, may obstruct the trabecular meshwork and thereby cause a type of secondary glaucoma known as *phacolytic glaucoma,* which was also discussed in Chapter 7. Cytologic examination of aqueous humor from patients with phacolytic glaucoma reveals collections of macrophages containing eosinophilic lens protein and extracellular proteinaceous material (see Fig 7-8). The treatment for phacolytic glaucoma is surgical removal of the lens and irrigation of the anterior chamber.

Propionibacterium acnes Endophthalmitis

Chronic postoperative endophthalmitis secondary to *P acnes* may develop following cataract surgery, usually 2 months to 2 years later. It may be characterized by granulomatous keratic precipitates, a small hypopyon, vitritis, and a white plaque containing *P acnes* and residual lens material sequestered within the capsular bag (Figs 9-6, 9-7). Onset of the inflammation may follow Nd:YAG laser capsulotomy that allows release of the sequestered organisms.

Degenerations

Cataract and Other Abnormalities

Capsule

Mild thickening of the lens capsule can be associated with pathologic proliferation of lens epithelium or with chronic inflammation of the anterior segment. Focal, internally directed

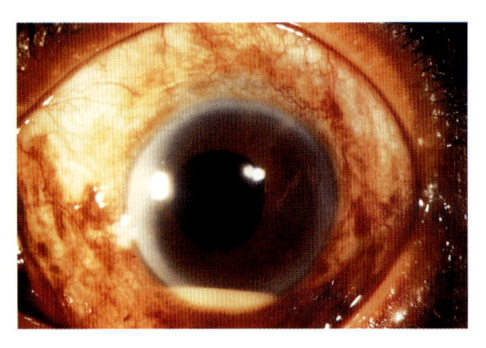

114 • Ophthalmic Pathology and Intraocular Tumors

Figure 9-6 Clinical photograph of eye with *P acnes* endophthalmitis. Note injection of the conjunctiva and small hypopyon. *(Courtesy of William C. Lloyd III, MD, and Ralph C. Eagle, Jr, MD.)*

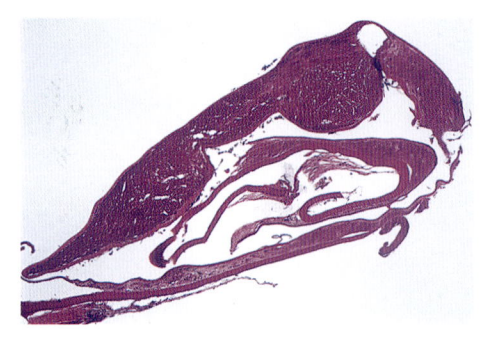

Figure 9-7 Histopathology of a lens capsule from a case of *P acnes* endophthalmitis. *(Courtesy of William C. Lloyd III, MD, and Ralph C. Eagle Jr, MD.)*

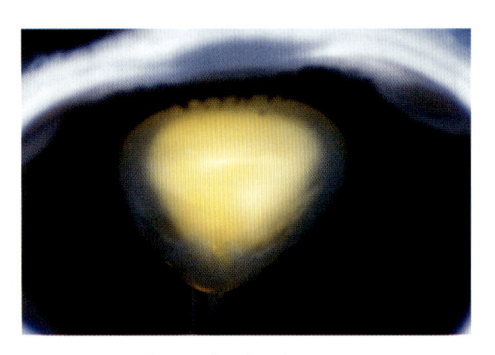

Figure 9-8 Posterior lenticonus. *(Courtesy of Hans E. Grossniklaus, MD.)*

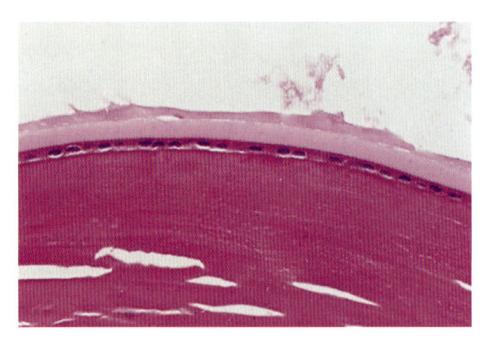

Figure 9-9 Exfoliation syndrome (pseudoexfoliation). Abnormal material appears on the anterior lens capsule like iron filings on the edge of a magnet.

excrescences of the lens capsule are seen in several conditions, including aniridia and Lowe syndrome.

Coronary, or *cerulean, cataracts* consist of wartlike excrescences on the capsule. With time, these excrescences are replaced by clumps of epithelium, resulting in granular debris in the peripheral cortex.

In *posterior lenticonus,* the lens capsule is abnormally thin, and the lens bulges into the anterior aspect of the vitreous (Fig 9-8). The outermost layers of the adult nucleus and cortex in the region of the bulge become opacified. *Anterior lenticonus* is much rarer and shows more extensive cytoarchitectural abnormalities.

Exfoliation syndrome, also known as *pseudoexfoliation,* is not an abnormality of the lens capsule per se but is the result of the deposition of a fibrillary proteinlike material on the anterior lens capsule. The material is also deposited on other intraocular structures. Histologically, the eosinophilic deposits appear sprinkled on the surface of the capsule like iron filings standing upright on the surface of a magnet (Fig 9-9). See also Chapter 7, Anterior Chamber and Trabecular Meshwork.

Epithelium

A severe elevation of IOP causes injury to the lens epithelial cells, leading to degeneration of the cells. Clinically, patches of white flecks *(glaukomflecken)* are seen beneath the lens capsule. Histology shows focal areas of necrotic lens epithelial cells beneath the anterior lens capsule. Associated degenerated subepithelial cortical material is also present. See also BCSC Section 10, *Glaucoma*.

Chronic iritis may cause degeneration and necrosis, as well as proliferation of anterior lens epithelium. Epithelial hyperplasia may be associated with the formation of subcapsular fibrous plaques (Fig 9-10). In this situation, the epithelial cells have undergone metaplastic transformation into cells capable of producing collagen. These functionally transformed epithelial cells arise in response to a variety of stimuli, including chronic inflammation or trauma. Following resolution of the inciting stimulus, the lens epithelium may produce another capsule, thereby totally surrounding the fibrous plaque and producing a duplication cataract.

Retention of iron-containing metallic foreign bodies in the lens may lead to lens epithelial degeneration and necrosis secondary to *siderosis*. The presence of iron within the epithelial cells can be nicely demonstrated by the use of the Prussian blue stain or Perls test.

Posterior subcapsular cataract may be the most common abnormality involving the lens epithelium. This condition is often associated with cortical degeneration and nuclear sclerosis. The process begins with epithelial disarray at the equator, followed by posterior migration of the lens epithelium. As the cells migrate posteriorly, they enlarge and swell to 5–6 times their normal size. These swollen cells, referred to as *bladder cells* or *Wedl cells*, can cause significant visual impairment if they involve the axial portion of the lens (Fig 9-11). Conditions often associated with posterior subcapsular cataracts include chronic vitreal inflammation, ionizing radiation, and prolonged use of corticosteroids.

Disruption of the lens capsule often results in proliferation of the lens epithelial cells. Following extracapsular cataract extraction, for example, remaining epithelial cells can

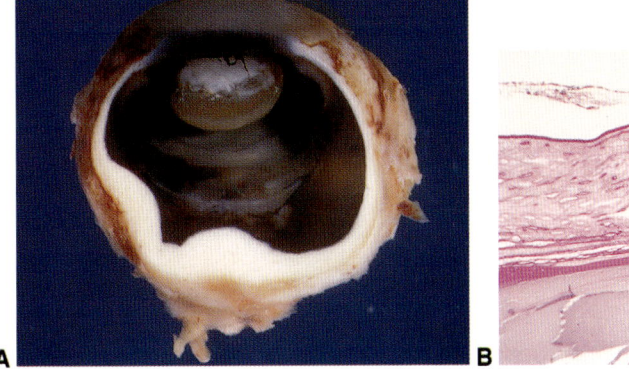

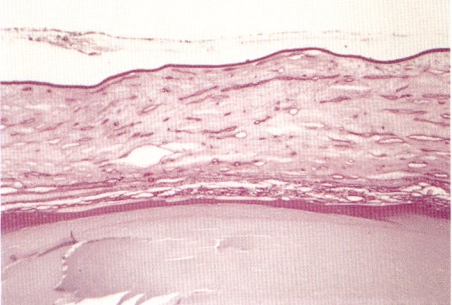

Figure 9-10 Anterior subcapsular cataract in a phthisical globe. **A,** Gross appearance. **B,** Fibrous plaque is present anterior to the original anterior capsule. *(Courtesy of Hans E. Grossniklaus, MD.)*

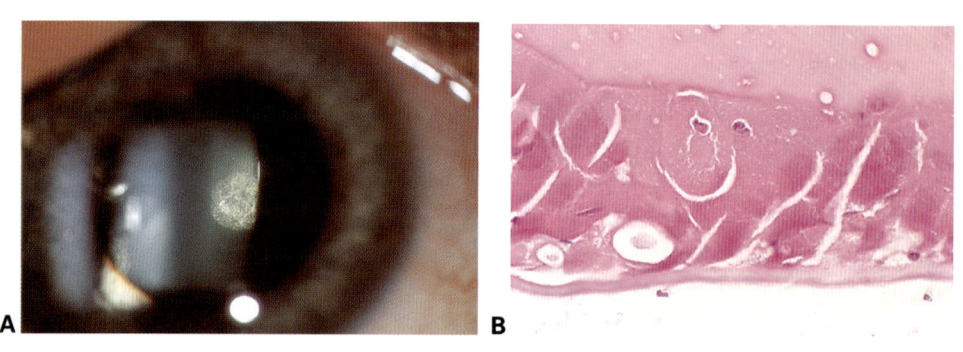

116 • Ophthalmic Pathology and Intraocular Tumors

Figure 9-11 Posterior subcapsular cataract. **A,** Viewed at the slit lamp. **B,** With bladder cells (Wedl cells). *(Part A courtesy of CIBA Pharmaceutical Co., division of CIBA-GEIGY Corp. Reproduced with permission from* Clinical Symposia. *Illustration by John A. Craig; part B courtesy of Debra J. Shetlar, MD.)*

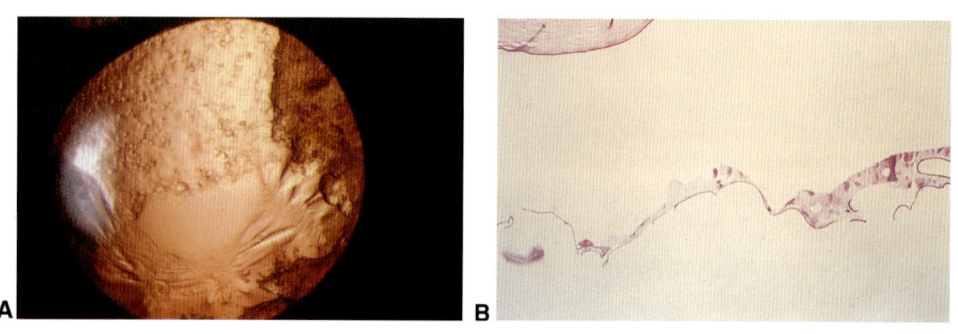

Figure 9-12 Elschnig pearls. **A,** Clinical appearance using retroillumination to demonstrate posterior capsule opacities. **B,** Histology depicting proliferating lens epithelium on posterior capsule. *(Part A courtesy of Sander Dubovy, MD; part B courtesy of Debra J. Shetlar, MD.)*

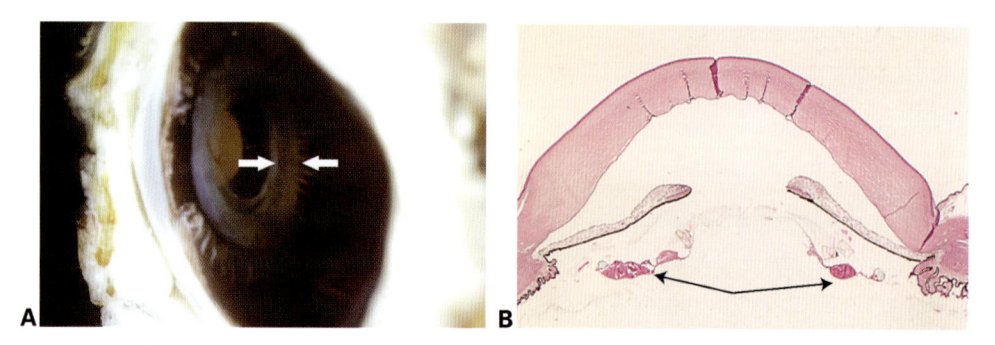

Figure 9-13 Soemmerring ring cataract. **A,** A ring cataract found adjacent to a posterior chamber intraocular lens *(arrows)*. **B,** Ring cataract, photomicrograph *(arrows)*. *(Part A courtesy of Sander Dubovy, MD.)*

proliferate and cover the inner surface of the posterior capsule. These collections of proliferating epithelial cells may form partially transparent globular masses called *Elschnig pearls* (Fig 9-12). Sequestration of proliferating lens fibers in the equatorial region, often as a result of incomplete cortical removal during cataract surgery, may create a doughnut-shaped configuration referred to as a *Soemmerring ring* (Fig 9-13).

Cortex

Opacities of the cortical lens fibers are most often associated with nuclear sclerosis or posterior subcapsular cataracts. Clinically, cortical degenerative changes fall into 2 broad categories:

1. generalized discolorations with loss of transparency
2. focal opacifications

Generalized loss of transparency cannot be diagnosed histologically with reliability, as histologic stains that are used to colorize the lens after it is processed prevent the assessment of lens clarity. The earliest sign of focal cortical degeneration is hydropic swelling of the lens fibers with decreased intensity of the eosinophilic staining. Focal cortical opacities become more apparent when fiber degeneration is advanced enough to cause liquefactive change. Light microscopy shows the accumulation of eosinophilic globules *(morgagnian globules)* in slitlike spaces between the lens fibers, which is a reliable histologic sign of cortical degeneration (Fig 9-14). As focal cortical lesions progress, the slitlike spaces become confluent, forming globular collections of lens protein. Ultimately, the entire cortex can become liquefied, allowing the nucleus to sink downward and the capsule to wrinkle *(morgagnian cataract)* (Fig 9-15).

Denatured lens protein can escape through an intact capsule and provoke an anterior chamber inflammatory reaction composed predominantly of macrophages. This condition, sometimes known as *phacolytic glaucoma,* was discussed earlier in this chapter and in Chapter 7.

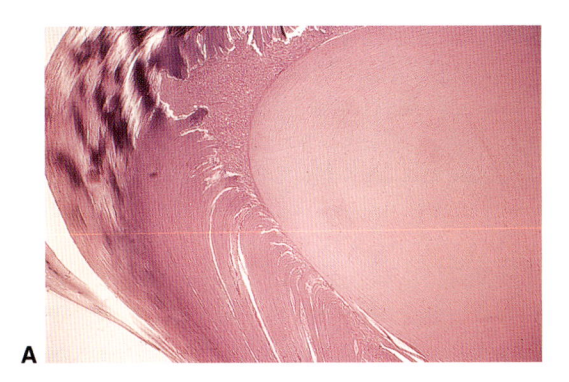

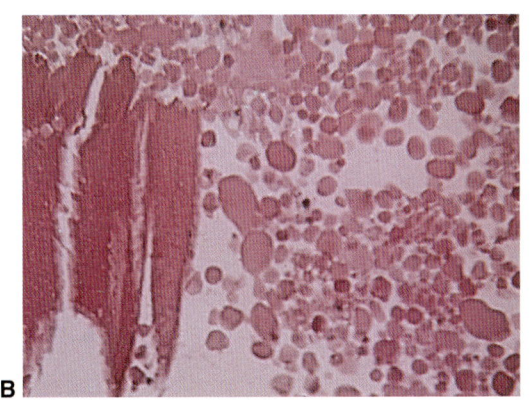

Figure 9-14 Cataract. **A,** Extensive cortical changes are present. **B,** Cortical degeneration. Lens cells (fibers) have swollen and fragmented to form morgagnian globules. The lenticular fragments are opaque and will increase osmotic pressure within the capsule. *(Courtesy of Hans E. Grossniklaus, MD.)*

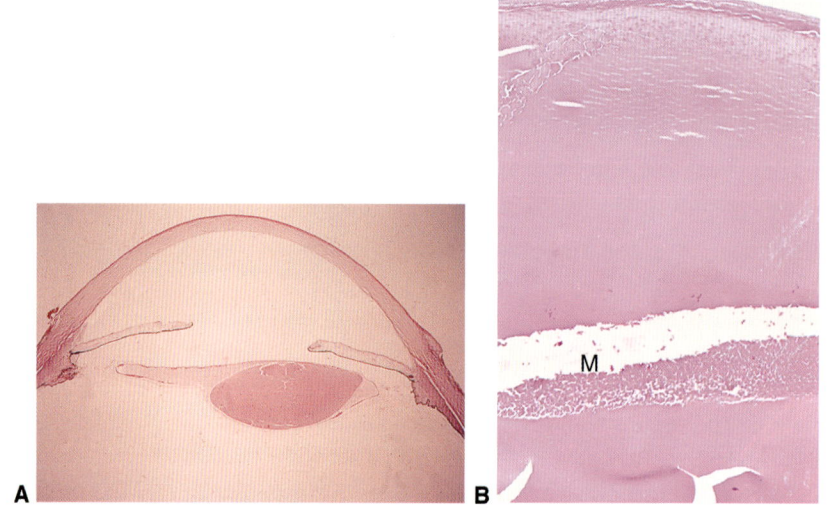

Figure 9-15 Morgagnian cataract. **A,** The lens cortex is liquefied, leaving the lens nucleus floating free within the capsular bag. **B,** Note the artifactitious (sharply angulated) clefts in this nuclear sclerotic cataract. A zone of morgagnian globules *(M)* is identified. *(Part A courtesy of Debra J. Shetlar, MD.)*

Nucleus

The continued production of lens fibers subjects the nucleus in the adult lens to the lifelong stress of mechanical compression. This compression causes hardening of the lens nucleus. Aging is also associated with alterations in the chemical composition of the nuclear fibers that may cause them to accumulate urochrome pigment. These changes in the nucleus increase the index of refraction, inducing a myopic shift of the refractive error.

The pathogenesis of nuclear discoloration is poorly understood and probably involves more than 1 mechanism. Clinically, the lens nucleus may appear yellow, brunescent, or deep brown. The histologic appearance, however, will not necessarily correlate to the clinical appearance because of the absorption of eosin dye (Fig 9-16).

Nuclear cataracts are difficult to assess histologically because they take on a subtle homogeneous eosinophilic appearance. The loss of cellular laminations probably correlates better with nucleus firmness than it does with optical opacification clinically. The more homogeneous the nucleus becomes, the less likely it is to artifactitiously fracture during sectioning.

Occasionally, crystalline deposits identified as calcium oxalate crystals may be identified within a nuclear cataract. The examiner can identify these crystals by viewing sections under polarized light.

Neoplasia and Associations With Systemic Disorders

There are no reported examples of neoplasms arising in the human lens. Premature opacification of the lens has been noted in many clinical situations, including the following:

- diabetes mellitus
- galactosemia

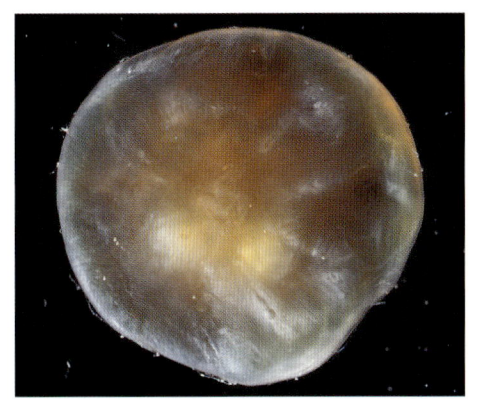

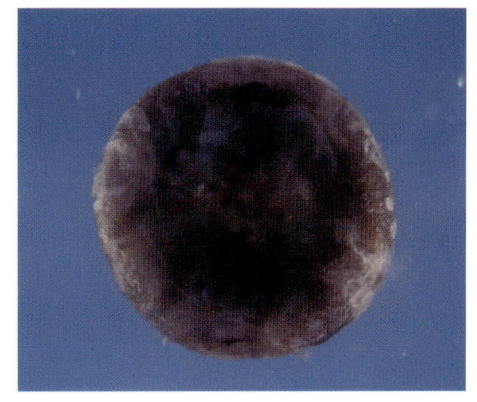

Figure 9-16 Surgically extracted lens nuclei showing varying degrees of brunescence and opacification. *(Courtesy of Hans E. Grossniklaus, MD.)*

- hypercupremia
- Fabry disease
- Down syndrome
- corticosteroid use

Exogenous agents, such as electric shock and radiation, may also play causative roles in the formation of cataracts. Retained intralenticular foreign bodies, especially those containing iron, may lead to cataract formation.

Pathology of Intraocular Lenses

Placement of an intraocular lens (IOL) following the removal of a cataract has become standard in most cases of cataract surgery. The selection of the type of IOL and the location of placement depends on a host of factors and may lead to a number of pathologic situations.

Decentration

Lens malpositions are almost certain to occur with asymmetric fixation of haptics. Placement of both haptics within the capsular bag is most likely to present with a well-centered optic (Fig 9-17). In the early 1980s, when posterior chamber IOLs were first introduced, the most likely etiology of decentration was surgical inexperience, with the haptics extending out of the capsular bag through tears in the anterior lens capsule after can-opener capsulotomy. With improvement of surgical techniques and the use of continuous curvilinear capsulorrhexis, the anterior capsule was made more stable and able to support a permanent in-the-bag fixation. Currently, the majority of IOLs are placed in the posterior chamber. However, IOLs may occasionally be placed in the anterior chamber, particularly if there is insufficient zonule support of the lens capsule (Fig 9-18).

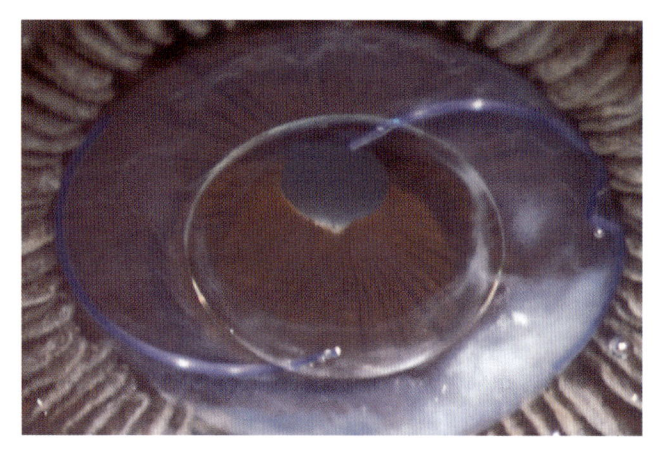

120 • Ophthalmic Pathology and Intraocular Tumors

Figure 9-17 Posterior view of posterior chamber intraocular lens that is positioned within the capsular bag. *(Courtesy of Hans E. Grossniklaus, MD.)*

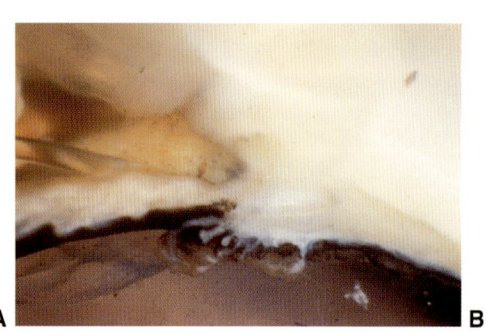

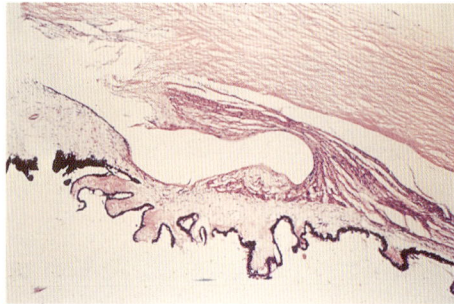

Figure 9-18 Anterior chamber IOL. **A,** Gross appearance of iris root and ciliary body with lens haptic. **B,** Microscopic appearance of anterior chamber. The IOL has been removed during tissue processing; the site where the haptic has partially eroded through the iris root can be seen. *(Reproduced with permission from Champion R, McDonnell PJ, Green WR. Intraocular lenses: histopathologic characteristics of a large series of autopsy eyes. Surv Ophthalmol. 1985;30:1–32. Photographs courtesy of W. Richard Green, MD.)*

Inflammation

Noninfectious causes

Inflammation following the implantation of an IOL may be caused by the lens itself through contact and chafing of the lens against the surrounding ciliary epithelium. This may lead to anterior segment inflammation and/or uveitis-glaucoma-hyphema (UGH) syndrome.

Infectious causes

Infectious generalized endophthalmitis may occur secondary to any intraocular procedure, including cataract extraction with IOL placement. Localized endophthalmitis may occur secondary to a focal sequestered infection that is present within the lens capsule and cataractous lens remnants (eg, *P acnes*, described earlier).

Corneal Complications

Corneal decompensation, including pseudophakic corneal edema and pseudophakic bullous keratopathy, may occur secondary to endothelial cell damage.

Retinal Complications

Cystoid macular edema may occur after cataract surgery, with fluid collecting within the inner and outer plexiform layers of the neural retina. See BCSC Section 12, *Retina and Vitreous*. Retinal detachment occurs in 2%–3% of eyes following intracapsular cataract extraction and in 0.5%–2.0% of eyes following extracapsular cataract extraction. The incidence following phacoemulsification is felt to be smaller. See BCSC Section 11, *Lens and Cataract*.

>   Apple DJ, Raab MF. *Ocular Pathology Clinical Applications and Self-Assessment.* 5th ed. St. Louis: Mosby-Year Book; 1998:161–179.

CHAPTER 10

Vitreous

Topography

The vitreous humor makes up most of the volume of the globe and is important in many diseases that affect the eye. BCSC Section 12, *Retina and Vitreous,* discusses the vitreous in detail.

The average volume of the adult vitreous is 4 cc. The vitreous is composed of 99% water and several macromolecules, including

- types II and IX collagen
- glycosaminoglycans
- soluble proteins
- glycoproteins

The outer portion of the vitreous has a greater number of collagen fibrils and is termed the *vitreous cortex.* The outer surface of the cortex is known as the *hyaloid face.*

The vitreous is bordered anteriorly by the lens, where its attachment to the lens capsule is called the *hyaloideocapsular ligament.* This attachment is firm in young patients and becomes increasingly tenuous with age. The vitreous is attached to the internal limiting membrane (ILM) of the retina by the insertion of the cortical collagen into the basement membrane structure that comprises the basal lamina of the ciliary epithelium and the ILM.

The vitreous attaches most firmly to the vitreous base, a 360° band that straddles the ora serrata and varies in width from 2 to 6 mm. The vitreous base extends more posteriorly with advancing age. Other relatively firm attachments of the vitreous are

- at the margins of the optic nerve head
- along the course of major retinal vessels
- in a circular area around the fovea
- at the edges of areas of vitreoretinal degeneration such as lattice degeneration

The strength of the vitreoretinal attachment is important in the pathogenesis of retinal tears and detachment, macular hole formation, and vitreous hemorrhage from neovascularization.

The embryologic development of the vitreous is generally divided into 3 stages:

1. primary vitreous
2. secondary vitreous
3. tertiary vitreous

The *primary vitreous* consists of fibrillar material; mesenchymal cells; and vascular components: the hyaloid artery, vasa hyaloidea propria, and tunica vasculosa lentis. The *secondary vitreous* begins to form at approximately the ninth week of gestation and is destined to become the main portion of the vitreous in the postnatal and adult eye. The primary vitreous atrophies with formation of the secondary vitreous, leaving only Cloquet's canal and, occasionally, the Bergmeister papilla and Mittendorf dot as vestigial remnants. The secondary vitreous is relatively acellular and completely avascular. The cells present in the secondary vitreous are called *hyalocytes,* and they exhibit features distinguishing them from macrophages and glial cells. The zonular fibers represent the *tertiary vitreous*.

Congenital Anomalies

Persistent Fetal Vasculature

Persistent fetal vasculature (PFV; also known as *persistent hyperplastic primary vitreous,* or *PHPV*) is characterized by the persistence of variable components of the primary vitreous and is most often unilateral. In most cases of clinically significant PFV, a fibrovascular plaque in the retrolental space extends laterally to involve the ciliary processes, which may be pulled centripetally by traction from the fibrovascular tissue. The clinical and gross appearance of elongated ciliary processes results. The anterior fibrovascular plaque is generally contiguous posteriorly with a remnant of the hyaloid artery that may attach to the optic nerve head (Fig 10-1). Involvement of the posterior structures may be more extensive, with tractional detachment of the peripapillary retina resulting from traction from preretinal membranes. The lens is often cataractous, and nonocular tissues such as adipose tissue and cartilage may be present in the retrolental mass. Eyes affected by PFV are often microphthalmic.

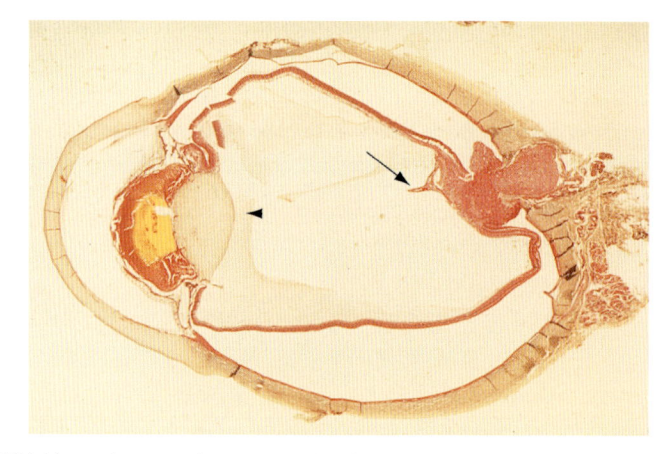

Figure 10-1 PFV. Note the prominent anterior fibrovascular plaque *(arrowhead)*. The posterior remnant of the persistent hyaloid is evident at the optic nerve head *(arrow)*. *(Courtesy of Hans E. Grossniklaus, MD.)*

Bergmeister Papilla

Persistence of a small part of the posterior portion of the hyaloid artery is referred to as a *Bergmeister papilla*. This anomaly generally takes the form of a veil-like structure overlying the optic nerve head or a finger-like projection extending from the surface of the optic nerve head.

Mittendorf Dot

The hyaloid artery attaches to the tunica vasculosa lentis just inferior and nasal to the center of the lens. With regression of these vascular structures, it is not uncommon to see a focal lens opacity at this site, which is referred to as a *Mittendorf dot* (see Fig 2-47 in BCSC Section 2, *Fundamentals and Principles of Ophthalmology*).

Peripapillary Vascular Loops

Retinal vessels may grow into a Bergmeister papilla and then return to the optic nerve head, creating the appearance of a vascular loop. These loops should not be mistaken for neovascularization of the optic nerve head.

Vitreous Cysts

Vitreous cysts generally occur in eyes with no other pathologic findings, but they have been seen in eyes with retinitis pigmentosa, with uveitis, and with remnants of the hyaloid system. Histologic studies have suggested the presence of hyaloid remnants in the vitreous cysts. The exact origin of the cysts is not known.

Inflammations

As a relatively acellular and completely avascular structure, the vitreous is not an active participant in inflammatory disorders. It does become involved secondarily in inflammatory conditions of adjacent tissues, however. The most notable involvement of the vitreous is in infectious endophthalmitis secondary to bacterial or fungal agents. The vitreous may also become involved secondarily with the inflammatory response associated with the following:

- toxocariasis
- toxoplasmosis
- acute retinal necrosis (ARN)
- cytomegalovirus (CMV) retinitis
- sarcoidosis
- pars planitis
- other forms of noninfectious retinitis

See also BCSC Section 9, *Intraocular Inflammation and Uveitis*.

Inflammatory conditions cause predictable changes in the vitreous. Marked neutrophilic infiltration of the vitreous occurs in acute inflammatory conditions such as bacterial endophthalmitis (Fig 10-2). This infiltration leads to liquefaction of the vitreous, with

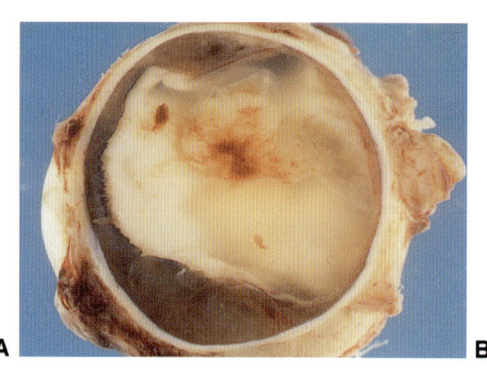

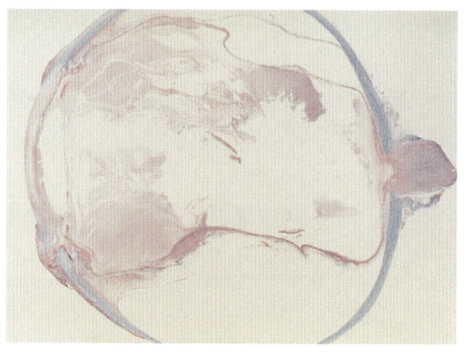

Figure 10-2 A, Gross photograph of opacification and infiltration of the vitreous as a result of bacterial endophthalmitis. **B,** Section shows cellular infiltration of vitreous in endophthalmitis (retinal detachment is artifactitious). *(Courtesy of Hans E. Grossniklaus, MD.)*

subsequent detachment of the posterior vitreous. Severe cases may be accompanied by formation of fibrocellular membranes, which typically form in the retrolental space and may exert traction on the peripheral retina. Chronic inflammatory conditions such as pars planitis (intermediate uveitis) and sarcoidosis may lead to infiltration of the vitreous with chronic inflammatory cells as well as to neovascularization of the anterior or posterior vitreous.

Degenerations

Syneresis and Aging

Syneresis of the vitreous is defined as liquefaction of the gel. Syneresis of the central vitreous is an almost universal consequence of aging. It also occurs as a consequence of vitreous inflammation and hemorrhage and in the setting of pathologic myopia. The prominent lamellae and strands that develop in aging and following inflammation or hemorrhage are the result of abnormally aggregated vitreous fibers around syneretic areas (Fig 10-3). Syneresis is one of the contributing factors leading to vitreous detachment.

Hemorrhage

A constellation of histopathologic findings may develop in the vitreous following vitreous hemorrhage. After 3–10 days, red blood cell clots undergo fibrinolysis and red blood cells may diffuse throughout the vitreous cavity. At this time, breakdown of the red blood cells also occurs. Loss of hemoglobin from the red blood cells produces ghost cells (Fig 10-4) and hemoglobin spherules (Fig 10-5). Obstruction of the trabecular meshwork by these cells may lead to *ghost cell glaucoma*. (See Fig 7-9 and BCSC Section 10, *Glaucoma.*)

The process of red blood cell dissolution attracts macrophages, which phagocytose the effete red blood cells. The hemoglobin is broken down to hemosiderin, then removed from the eye. In massive hemorrhages, cholesterol crystals caused by the breakdown of red blood cell membranes may be present, often surrounded by a foreign body giant cell reaction. Cholesterol

CHAPTER 10: Vitreous • 127

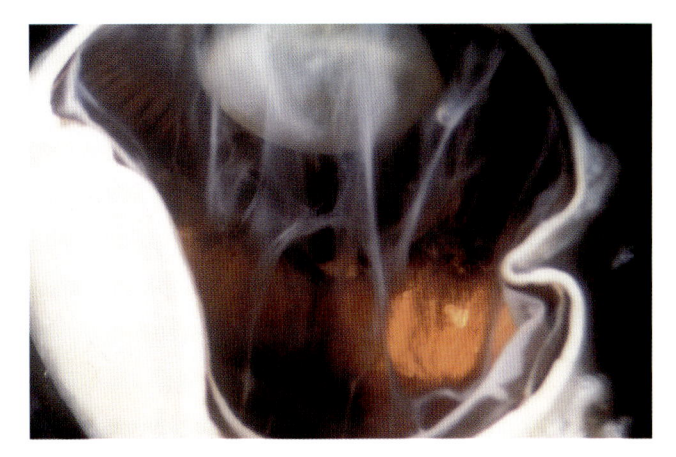

Figure 10-3 Gross photograph of vitreous condensations outlining syneretic cavities. *(Courtesy of Hans E. Grossniklaus, MD.)*

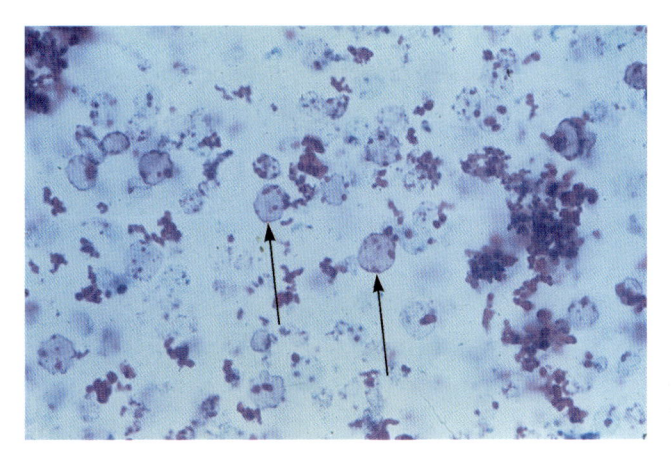

Figure 10-4 Ghost cells *(arrows)* represent red blood cells that have lost much of their intracellular hemoglobin. *(Courtesy of Hans E. Grossniklaus, MD.)*

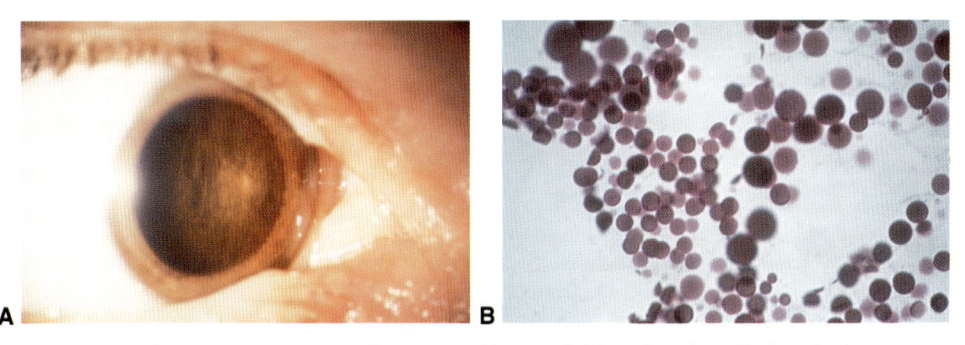

Figure 10-5 A, Clinical photograph of retrolental hemoglobin spherules. **B,** Cytologic preparation of hemoglobin spherules removed from the vitreous cavity. *(Reproduced with permission from Spraul CW, Grossniklaus HE. Vitreous hemorrhage.* Surv Ophthalmol. *1997;42:3–39.)*

appears clinically as refractile intravitreal crystals. As mentioned previously, syneresis of the vitreous and posterior vitreous detachment are common after vitreous hemorrhage.

Asteroid Hyalosis

Asteroid hyalosis is a condition with a spectacular clinical appearance (see Fig 12-6, BCSC Section 12, *Retina and Vitreous*) but little clinical significance. Asteroid bodies are rounded structures measuring 10–100 nm that stain positively with alcian blue and positively with stains for neutral fats, phospholipids, and calcium (Fig 10-6). The bodies stain metachromatically and exhibit birefringence. Occasionally, asteroid bodies will be surrounded by a foreign body giant cell, but the condition is not generally associated with an inflammatory reaction.

The exact mechanism of formation of asteroid bodies is not known; however, element mapping by electron spectroscopic imaging has revealed a homogeneous distribution of calcium, phosphorus, and oxygen. The electron energy loss spectra of these elements show details similar to those found for hydroxyapatite. In addition, high contrast and sensitivity against a calcium-specific chelator highlights the crystalline, apatite-like nature of asteroid bodies. Immunofluorescence microscopy has revealed the presence of chondroitin-6-sulfate at the periphery of asteroid bodies; and carbohydrates specific for hyaluronic acid were observed by lectin-gold labeling to be part of the inner matrix of asteroid bodies. Thus, asteroid bodies exhibit structural and elemental similarity to hydroxyapatite, and proteoglycans and their glycosaminoglycan side chains appear to play a role in regulating the biomineralization process.

> Winkler J, Lunsdorf H. Ultrastructure and composition of asteroid bodies. *Invest Ophthalmol Vis Sci.* 2001;42:902–907.

Vitreous Amyloidosis

The term *amyloidosis* refers to a group of diseases that lead to extracellular deposition of amyloid. Amyloid is composed of various proteins that have a characteristic ultrastructural appearance of nonbranching fibrils with variable length and a diameter of 75–100 Å (Fig 10-7). The proteins forming amyloid also have in common the ability to form a tertiary structure characterized as a β-pleated sheet, which then enables the proteins to bind Congo red stain and show birefringence in polarized light (Fig 10-8).

Amyloid may be derived from various types of protein, and the protein of origin is characteristic for different forms of amyloidosis. Amyloid deposits occur in the vitreous when

Figure 10-6 Asteroid bodies surrounded by a foreign-body reaction. *(Courtesy of Hans E. Grossniklaus, MD.)*

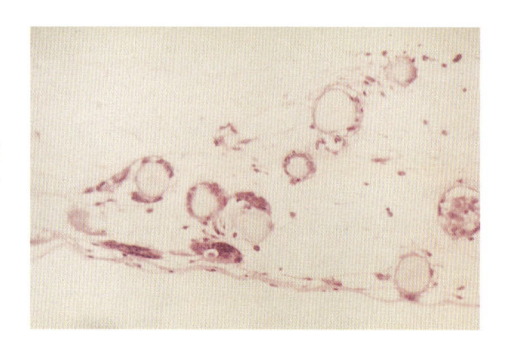

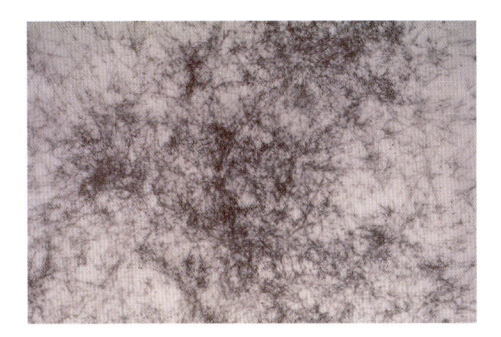

Figure 10-7 Electron photomicrograph shows characteristic amyloid fibrils. *(Courtesy of David J. Wilson, MD.)*

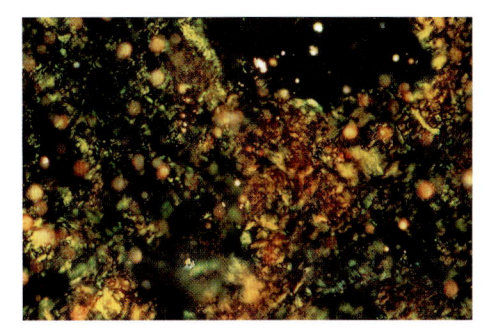

Figure 10-8 Polarized light photomicrograph of the Congo red–stained vitreous from a patient with familial amyloid polyneuropathy. *(Courtesy of David J. Wilson, MD.)*

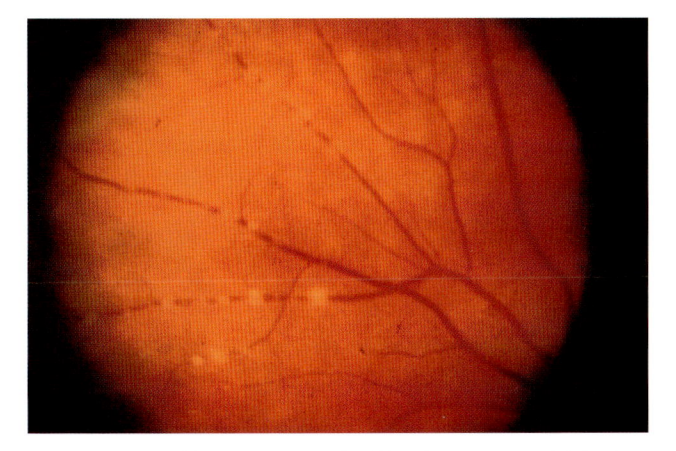

Figure 10-9 Perivascular sheathing associated with vitreous amyloidosis. *(Courtesy of Hans E. Grossniklaus, MD.)*

the protein forming the amyloid is *transthyretin,* previously known as *prealbumin.* Multiple genetic mutations have been described that result in various amino acid substitutions in the transthyretin protein. The most common mutations were originally described based on their clinical findings as *familial amyloid polyneuropathy (FAP)* types I and II. Systemic manifestations in patients with this type of amyloidosis include vitreous opacities and perivascular infiltrates (Fig 10-9), peripheral neuropathy, cardiomyopathy, and carpal tunnel syndrome.

The mechanism by which the vitreous becomes involved is not known with certainty. Because amyloid deposits are found within the walls of retinal vessels and in the retinal pigment epithelium (RPE), amyloid may gain access to the vitreous through these tissues. In addition, because transthyretin is a blood protein, it may gain access to the vitreous by crossing the blood–aqueous barrier at the ciliary body.

Posterior Vitreous Detachment

Posterior vitreous detachment (PVD) occurs when a dehiscence in the vitreous cortex allows fluid from a syneretic cavity to gain access to the potential subhyaloid space, causing the remaining cortex to be stripped from the ILM (Fig 10-10). As fluid drains out of the syneretic cavities under the newly formed posterior hyaloid, the vitreous body collapses anteriorly. Vitreous detachment generally occurs rapidly, so that over the course of a few hours to days the vitreous collapses anteriorly and remains attached only at its base.

A weakening of the adherence of the cortical vitreous to the ILM with age also plays a role in PVDs. The reported incidence of PVD varies between 31% and 65% at age 65 and is increased by intraocular inflammation, aphakia or pseudophakia, trauma, and vitreoretinal disease. PVD is important in the pathogenesis of many conditions, including retinal tears and detachment, vitreous hemorrhage, and macular hole formation.

Rhegmatogenous Retinal Detachment and Proliferative Vitreoretinopathy

Retinal tears form from vitreous traction on the retina during or after PVD or secondary to ocular trauma. Tears are most likely to occur at sites of greatest vitreoretinal adhesion, such as the vitreous base or the margin of lattice degeneration (Fig 10-11). The histopathology of retinal tears reveals that the vitreous is adherent to the retina along the flap of the tear. In the area of retina separated from the underlying RPE, there is loss of photoreceptors.

Retinal detachment occurs when vitreous traction and fluid currents resulting from eye movements combine to overcome the forces maintaining retinal adhesion to the RPE. The principal histopathologic findings in retinal detachment consist of the following:

- degeneration of the outer segments of the photoreceptors
- eventual loss of photoreceptor cells as a result of apoptosis, or programmed cell death
- migration of Müller cells
- proliferation and migration of RPE cells

Small cystic spaces develop in the detached retina, and in chronic detachment, these cysts may coalesce into large macrocysts (Fig 10-12).

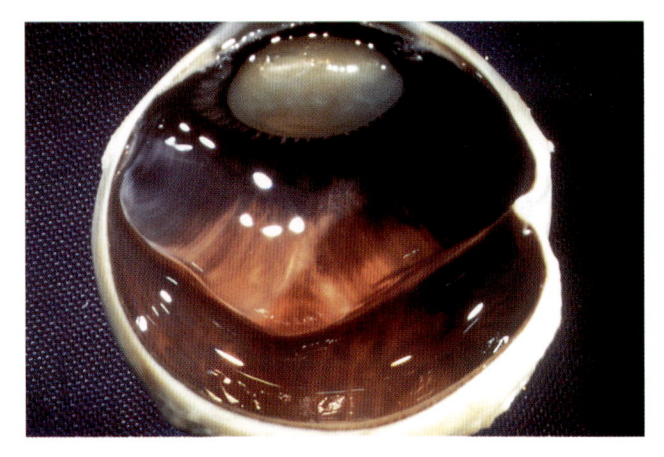

Figure 10-10 Gross photograph of posterior vitreous detachment. *(Courtesy of Hans E. Grossniklaus, MD.)*

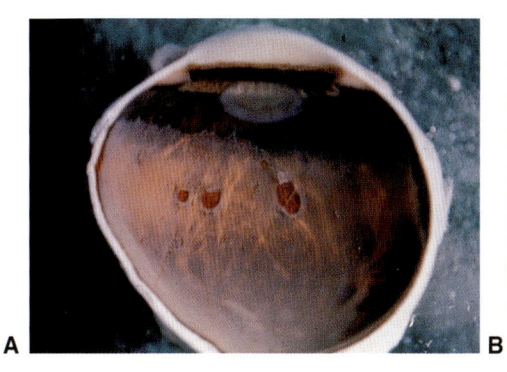

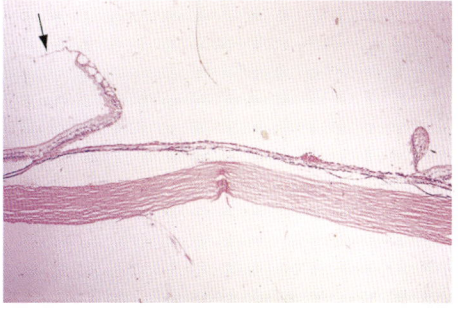

Figure 10-11 A, Gross photograph of retinal tears at vitreous base. **B,** Photomicrograph shows condensed vitreous *(arrow)* attached to anterior flap of retinal tear. *(Courtesy of W. Richard Green, MD.)*

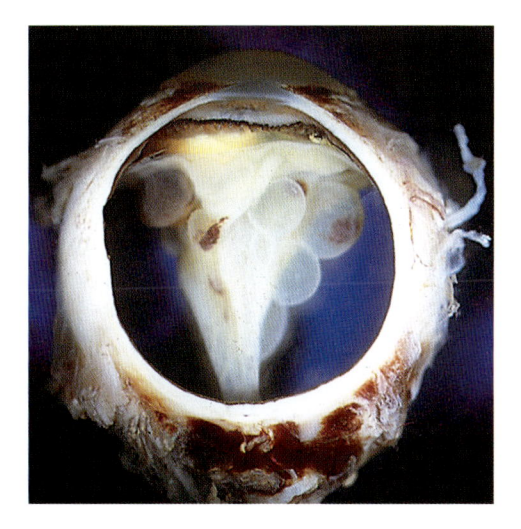

Figure 10-12 Long-standing total retinal detachment with macrocystic degeneration of the retina.

With rhegmatogenous retinal detachment, cellular membranes may form on either surface (anterior or posterior) of the retina (Fig 10-13). Clinically, this process is referred to as *proliferative vitreoretinopathy (PVR)*. Membranes form as a result of proliferation of RPE cells and contain other cellular elements, including glial cells (Müller cells, fibrous astrocytes), macrophages, fibroblasts, myofibroblasts, and possibly hyalocytes. The cell biology of membrane formation in the vitreous is complex and involves the interaction of various growth factors, integrins, and cellular proliferation. Recent studies have shown a significant association between clinical grades of PVR and the expression levels of specific cytokines and/or growth factors in the vitreous fluid.

> Harada C, Mitamura Y, Harada T. The role of cytokines and trophic factors in epiretinal membranes: involvement of signal transduction in glial cells. *Prog Retin Eye Res.* 2005;25:149–164; Dec 27 [Epub].

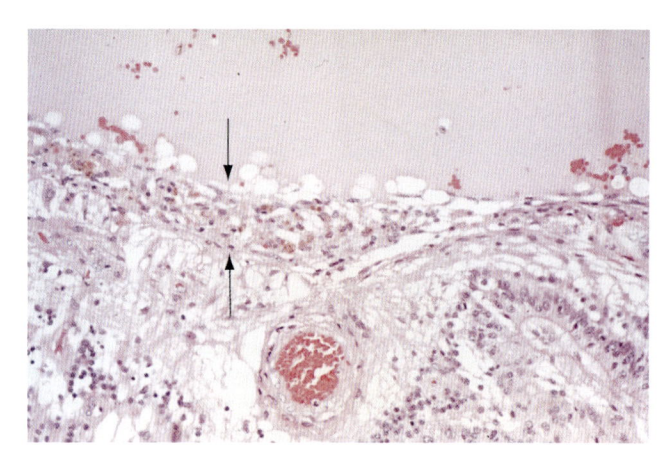

Figure 10-13 Preretinal membrane *(between arrows)* on the surface of the retina, secondary to proliferative vitreoretinopathy. *(Courtesy of David J. Wilson, MD.)*

Macular Holes

Idiopathic macular holes most likely form as the result of degenerative changes in the vitreous. Current imaging studies such as optical coherence tomography (OCT) have greatly advanced our understanding of the anatomical features of full-thickness macular holes and early macular hole formation. These studies are most consistent with a focal anteroposterior traction mechanism, but some inconsistencies in clinical cases suggest a role for degeneration of the inner retinal layers. Localized perifoveal vitreous detachment (an early stage of age-related PVD) appears to be the primary pathogenetic event in idiopathic macular hole formation (Fig 10-14). Detachment of the posterior hyaloid from the pericentral retina exerts anterior traction on the foveola and localizes the dynamic vitreous traction associated with ocular rotations into the perifoveolar region.

OCT has clarified the pathoanatomy of early macular hole stages, beginning with a foveal pseudocyst (stage 1a), typically followed by disruption of the outer retina (stage 1b), before progressing to a full-thickness dehiscence (stage 2). Histologically, full-thickness macular holes are similar to holes in other locations. A full-thickness retinal defect with rounded tissue margins (stage 3) is accompanied by loss of the photoreceptor outer segments in adjacent retina that is separated from the RPE by subretinal fluid (Fig 10-14D). An epiretinal membrane composed of Müller cells, fibrous astrocytes, and fibroblasts with myoblastic differentiation is often present on the surface of the retina adjacent to the macular hole. Cystoid macular edema in the parafoveal retina adjacent to the full-thickness macular hole is relatively common. Following surgical repair of macular holes, closer apposition of the remaining photoreceptors and variable glial scarring close the macular defect.

> Gass JD. Reappraisal of biomicroscopic classification of stages of development of a macular hole. *Am J Ophthalmol.* 1995;119:752–759.
> Johnson MW. Improvements in the understanding and treatment of macular hole. *Curr Opin Ophthalmol.* 2002;13:152–160.
> Smiddy WE, Flynn HW Jr. Pathogenesis of macular holes and therapeutic implications. *Am J Ophthalmol.* 2004;137:525–537.

CHAPTER 10: Vitreous • 133

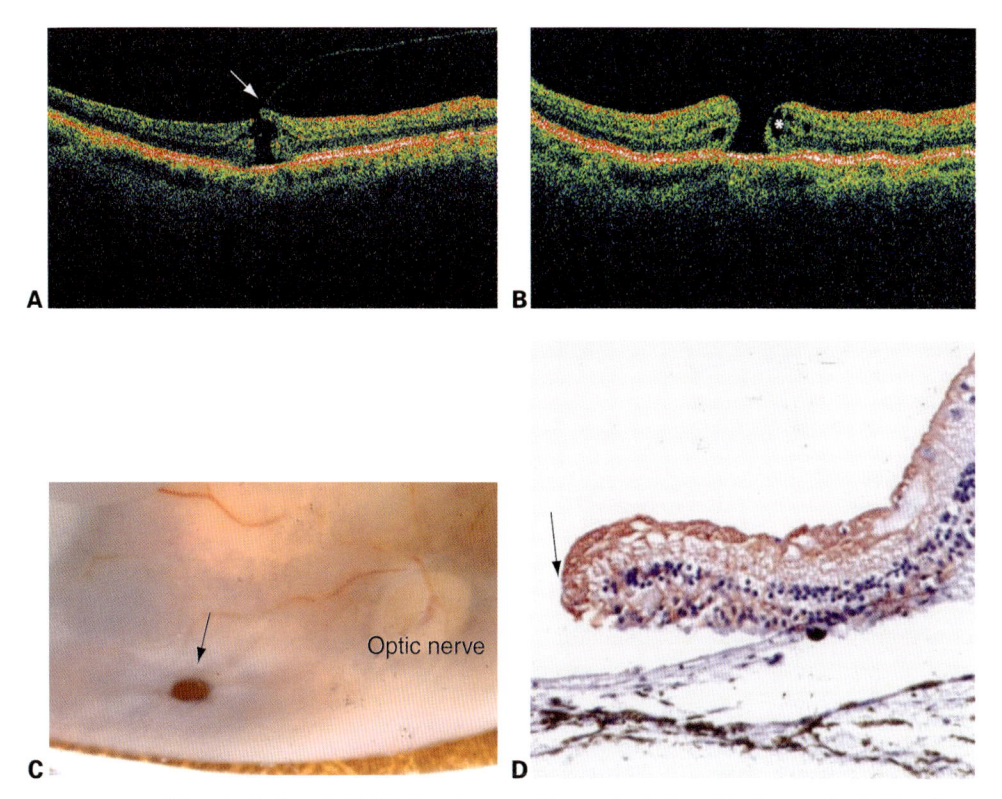

Figure 10-14 Macular holes. **A,** OCT of early stage 2 macular hole with vitreoretinal adhesion to lamellar flap *(arrow)*. **B,** OCT of stage 3 macular hole with full-thickness retinal defect, rounded margins, and CME *(asterisk)*. **C,** Gross photograph of full-thickness macular hole *(arrow)*. **D,** Histopathology of full-thickness macular hole showing rounded gliotic margin *(arrow)* with positive staining for glial fibrillary acidic protein (GFAP), highlighting the Müller cells and fibrous astrocytes. *(Parts A and B courtesy of Robert H. Rosa, Jr, MD, and Terry Hanke, CRA; parts C and D courtesy of Patricia Chévez-Barrios, MD.)*

Neoplasia

Intraocular Lymphoma

Primary neoplastic involvement of the vitreous is uncommon because of the relatively acellular nature of the vitreous. However, the vitreous can be the site of primary involvement in cases of B-cell lymphoma. This type of lymphoma has been referred to as *primary intraocular/central nervous system lymphoma, large cell lymphoma,* and *reticulum cell sarcoma.* Immunohistochemical and molecular genetic studies have confirmed that this entity is a B-cell lymphoma. In rare cases, vitreous involvement may occur in T-cell lymphomas.

The most common presentation of *primary intraocular lymphoma (PIOL)* is as a posterior uveitis. Some patients have sub-RPE infiltrates (Fig 10-15) with a very characteristic speckled pigmentation overlying tumor detachments of the RPE. The sub-RPE infiltrates are present in a minority of patients with intraocular lymphoma. Approximately 50% of

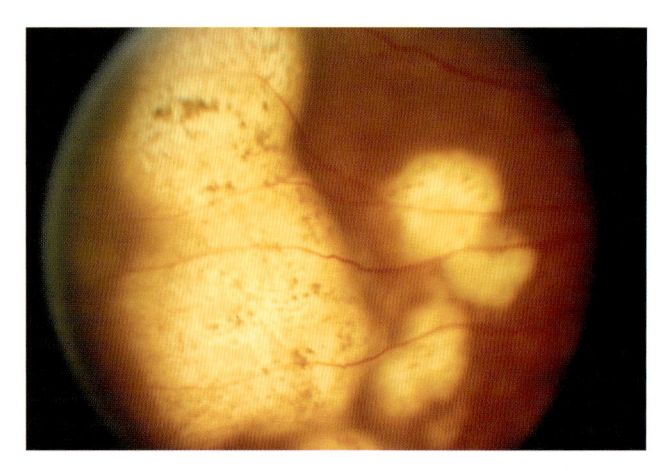

Figure 10-15 Sub-RPE infiltrates in a patient with primary intraocular lymphoma. Note the characteristic speckled pigmentation over the tumor detachments of the RPE. *(Courtesy of Robert H. Rosa, Jr, MD.)*

Figure 10-16 Cytologic preparation of vitreous lymphoma. Note the atypical cells *(arrowheads)* with large nuclei and multiple nucleoli. Cell ghosts *(arrows)* are also present. *(Courtesy of David J. Wilson, MD.)*

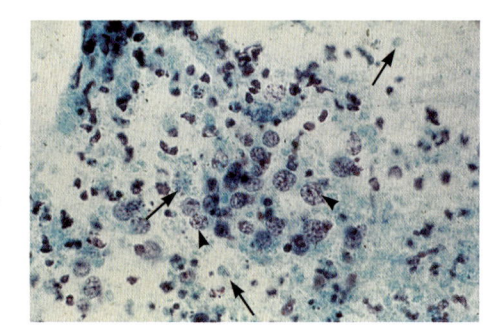

patients presenting with ocular findings have concomitant involvement of the central nervous system.

The diagnosis of intraocular lymphoma is made by cytologic analysis of vitrectomy specimens. Immunohistochemical study of cell markers, flow cytometry, or gene amplification studies can be performed on vitreous specimens, although the standard method of diagnosis is cytology.

Cytologically, the vitreous infiltrate in intraocular lymphoma is heterogeneous. The atypical cells are large lymphoid cells, frequently with a convoluted nuclear membrane and multiple, conspicuous nucleoli. An accompanying infiltrate of small lymphocytes almost always appears, and the normal cells may obscure the neoplastic cell population. These small round lymphocytes are largely reactive T cells. Numerous cell ghosts are usually present, and this feature is very suggestive of a diagnosis of intraocular lymphoma (Fig 10-16). Immunohistochemically, the viable tumor cells can be labeled as a monoclonal population of B cells. Demonstration of a monoclonal population is helped by the use of flow cytometry. Other laboratory tests that may be useful in the diagnosis and follow-up of patients with intraocular lymphoma are determination of the interleukin-10 to

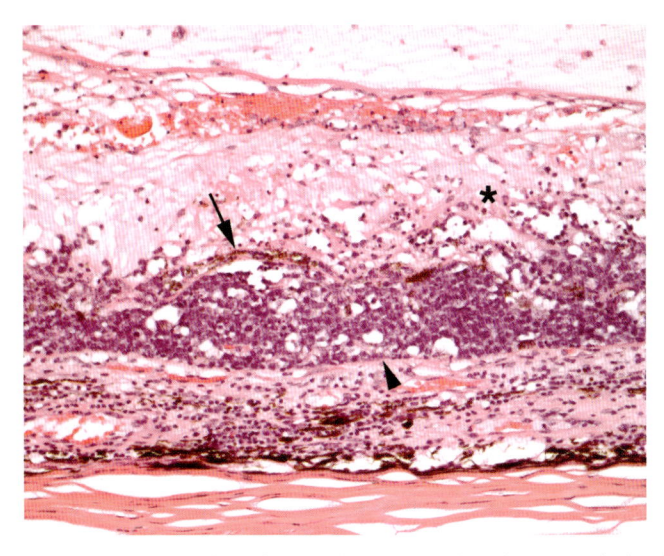

Figure 10-17 Primary intraocular lymphoma. Note the detachment of the RPE by tumor *(arrow)* overlying retinal gliosis *(asterisk)*, and intact Bruch's membrane *(arrowhead)*. Secondary chronic inflammation is present in the choroid. *(Courtesy of Robert H. Rosa, Jr, MD.)*

interleukin-6 ratio and the use of microdissection and polymerase chain reaction (PCR) for the detection of immunoglobulin gene rearrangement and translocation.

The subretinal/sub-RPE infiltrates are composed of atypical lymphoid cells (Fig 10-17). With or without treatment, the subretinal infiltrates tend to resolve, leaving a focal area of RPE atrophy. Optic nerve and retinal infiltration may also be present. Infiltrates in these locations tend to be perivascular and may lead to ischemic retinal or optic nerve damage. The choroid is most often free of atypical cells; however, secondary chronic inflammation may be present in the choroid. In the setting of systemic lymphoma with ocular involvement, the choroid (rather than the vitreous, retina, or subretinal space) is the primary site of involvement.

> Coupland SE, Hummel M, Muller HH, Stein H. Molecular analysis of immunoglobulin genes in primary intraocular lymphoma. *Invest Ophthalmol Vis Sci.* 2005;46:3507–3514.
> Levy-Clarke GA, Chan CC, Nussenblatt RB. Diagnosis and management of primary intraocular lymphoma. *Hematol Oncol Clin North Am.* 2005;19:739–749.
> Read RW, Zamir E, Rao NA. Neoplastic masquerade syndromes. *Surv Ophthalmol.* 2002;47: 81–124.

CHAPTER 11

Retina and Retinal Pigment Epithelium

Topography

The retina and the retinal pigment epithelium (RPE) make up 2 distinct layers that together line the inner two thirds of the globe:

1. The RPE is a pigmented layer derived from the outer layer of the optic cup.
2. The neurosensory retina is a delicate, transparent layer derived from the inner layer of the optic cup.

Anteriorly, the RPE becomes continuous with the pigmented epithelium of the ciliary body, and the retina becomes continuous with the nonpigmented ciliary body epithelium. Posteriorly, the RPE terminates at the optic nerve, just prior to the termination of Bruch's membrane. The nuclear, photoreceptor, and synaptic layers of the retina gradually taper at the optic nerve head, and only the nerve fiber layer (NFL) continues on to form the optic nerve. BCSC Section 12, *Retina and Vitreous*, discusses in depth the anatomy of the retina, as well as other topics covered in this chapter.

Retina

The topographic variation in the structures of the retina is striking, with regional variation in the neural structures as well as the retinal vasculature. The neurosensory retina has 9 layers (Fig 11-1). Beginning on the vitreous side and progressing to the choroidal side, they are

1. internal limiting membrane (ILM; a true basement membrane synthesized by Müller cells)
2. nerve fiber layer
3. ganglion cell layer
4. inner plexiform layer
5. inner nuclear layer
6. outer plexiform layer

7. outer nuclear layer (nuclei of the photoreceptors)
8. external limiting membrane (ELM; not a true membrane but rather an apparent membrane formed by a series of desmosomes between Müller cells and photoreceptors)
9. photoreceptors (inner and outer segments) of the rods and cones

The arrangement of the retina (in tissue sections oriented perpendicular to the retinal surface) is vertical from outer to inner layers, except for the NFL, where the axons run horizontally toward the optic nerve head. Consequently, deposits and hemorrhages in the deep retinal layers have a round appearance clinically when viewed on edge, whereas those in the NFL have a feathery appearance.

The blood supply of the retina comes from 2 sources, with a watershed zone inside the inner nuclear layer. The *retinal blood vessels* supply the NFL, ganglion cell layer, inner plexiform layer, and inner two thirds of the inner nuclear layer. The *choroidal vasculature* supplies the outer one third of the inner nuclear layer, outer plexiform layer, outer nuclear layer, photoreceptors, and RPE. Because of this division of the blood supply to the retina, ischemic choroidal vascular lesions and ischemic lesions attributed to the retinal vasculature produce different histologic pictures. Ischemic retinal injury produces inner ischemic atrophy of the retina, and choroidal ischemia produces outer ischemic retinal atrophy.

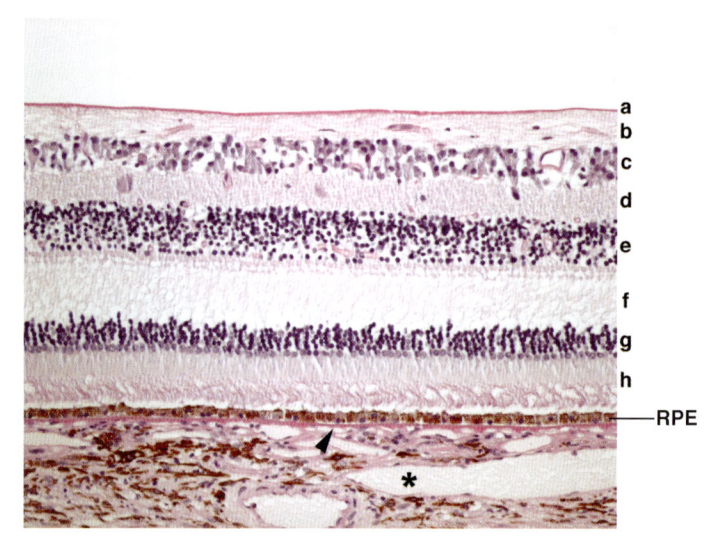

Figure 11-1 Normal retinal layers. From vitreous to choroid: **a,** internal limiting membrane; **b,** nerve fiber layer; **c,** ganglion cell layer; **d,** inner plexiform layer; **e,** inner nuclear layer; **f,** outer plexiform layer; **g,** outer nuclear layer; **h,** photoreceptors (inner/outer segments) for rods and cones. RPE = retinal pigment epithelium. Bruch's membrane, *arrowhead;* choroid, *asterisk.* The external limiting membrane (ELM) is not shown in this figure. *(Courtesy of Robert H. Rosa, Jr, MD.)*

Retinal Pigment Epithelium

The RPE consists of a monolayer of hexagonal cells with apical microvilli and a basement membrane at the base of the cells. This monolayer has the following specialized functions:

- vitamin A metabolism
- maintenance of the outer blood–retina barrier
- phagocytosis of the photoreceptor outer segments
- absorption of light
- heat exchange
- formation of the basal lamina of the inner portion of Bruch's membrane
- production of the mucopolysaccharide matrix that surrounds the photoreceptor outer segments
- active transport of materials into and out of the subretinal space

Compared with that of the retina, the topographic variation of the RPE is subtle. In the macula, the RPE is taller, narrower, and more heavily pigmented, and it forms a regular hexagonal array. In the equatorial and midperipheral area, the RPE cells are larger in diameter and thinner. Variability in the diameter of the RPE cells increases in the peripheral retina. The amount of cytoplasmic pigment, primarily lipofuscin, increases with age, particularly within the RPE in the macular region.

Macula

Histologically, the term *macula* refers to that area of the retina where the ganglion cell layer is thicker than a single cell (Fig 11-2). Clinically, this area corresponds approximately with the area of the retina bound by the inferior and superior vascular arcades. The macula is subdivided into the *foveola,* the *fovea,* the *parafovea,* and the *perifovea.* Only photoreceptor cells appear in the central foveola; the ganglion cells, other nucleated cells (including Müller cells), and blood vessels are not present. The concentration of cones is greater in the macula than in the peripheral retina, and only cones are present in the fovea.

Nerve fibers in the outer plexiform layer (nerve fiber layer of Henle) of the macula run obliquely (see Fig 11-2). This morphologic feature results in the flower-petal appearance of cystoid macular edema (CME) seen on fluorescein angiography and the star-shaped configuration of hard exudates seen ophthalmoscopically in conditions that cause macular edema. Xanthophyll pigment gives the macula its yellow appearance clinically and grossly (macula lutea), but the xanthophyll dissolves during tissue processing and is not present in histologic sections.

Congenital Anomalies

Albinism

Albinism is a general term that refers to a congenital dilution of the pigment of the skin, the eyes and the skin, or just the eyes. True albinism has been subdivided into *oculocutaneous*

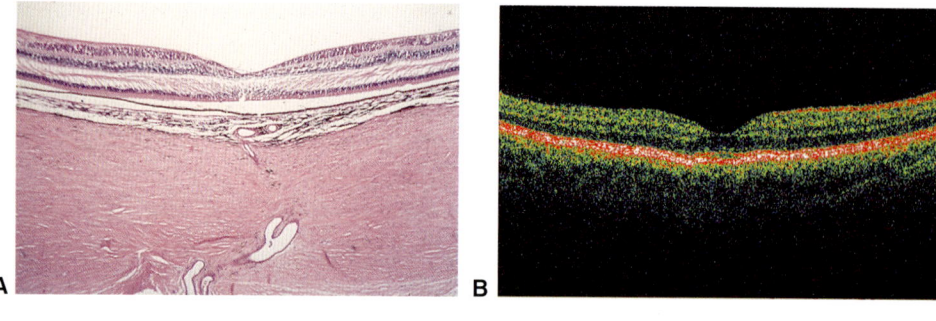

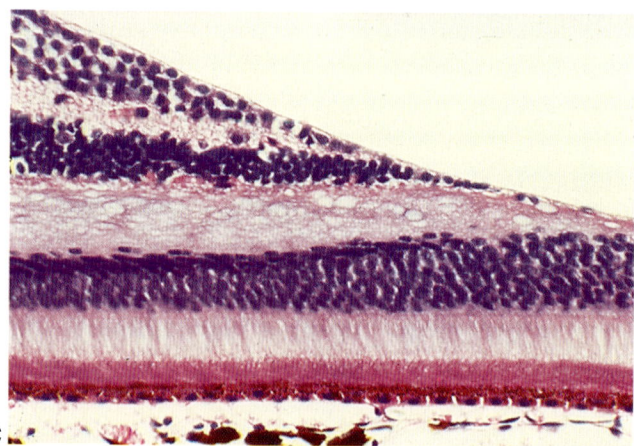

140 • Ophthalmic Pathology and Intraocular Tumors

Figure 11-2 A, The normal macula is identified histologically by a multicellular, thick ganglion cell layer and an area of focal thinning, the foveola. Clinically, the macula lies between the inferior and superior vascular arcades. **B,** Optical coherence tomography (OCT) of the macula showing in vivo histologic assessment with tremendous details of the lamellar architecture of the retina. **C,** In the region of the foveola, the inner cellular layers are absent, with an increased density of pigment in the RPE. The incident light falls directly on the photoreceptor outer segments, reducing the potential for distortion of light by overlying tissue elements. *(Part B courtesy of Robert H. Rosa, Jr, MD, and Terry Hanke, CRA.)*

and *ocular albinism*. This distinction is somewhat helpful clinically, but in reality all cases of ocular albinism have some degree of mild cutaneous involvement. There is a pathophysiologic difference between the 2 types of albinism: in oculocutaneous albinism the amount of melanin in each melanosome is reduced, whereas in ocular albinism the number of melanosomes is reduced.

Many different types of oculocutaneous and ocular albinism have been described, but the ocular involvement always conforms to 1 of 2 clinical patterns:

1. congenitally subnormal visual acuity and nystagmus
2. normal or minimally reduced visual acuity and no nystagmus, a clinical pattern termed *albinoidism* because the visual consequences are much milder

CHAPTER 11: Retina and Retinal Pigment Epithelium • 141

Albinism and albinoidism share clinical features such as photophobia, iris transillumination, and hypopigmented fundi (Fig 11-3) as a result of the reduction in melanin content of the RPE and choroid. These 2 patterns also differ: albinism is accompanied by foveal hypoplasia, whereas albinoidism shows normal or nearly normal foveal architecture.

Two types of ocular albinism have important systemic associations:

1. *Hermansky-Pudlak syndrome:* albinism associated with a hemorrhagic disorder characterized by easy bruising
2. *Chédiak-Higashi syndrome:* an abnormality of neutrophils resulting in an increased susceptibility for infection

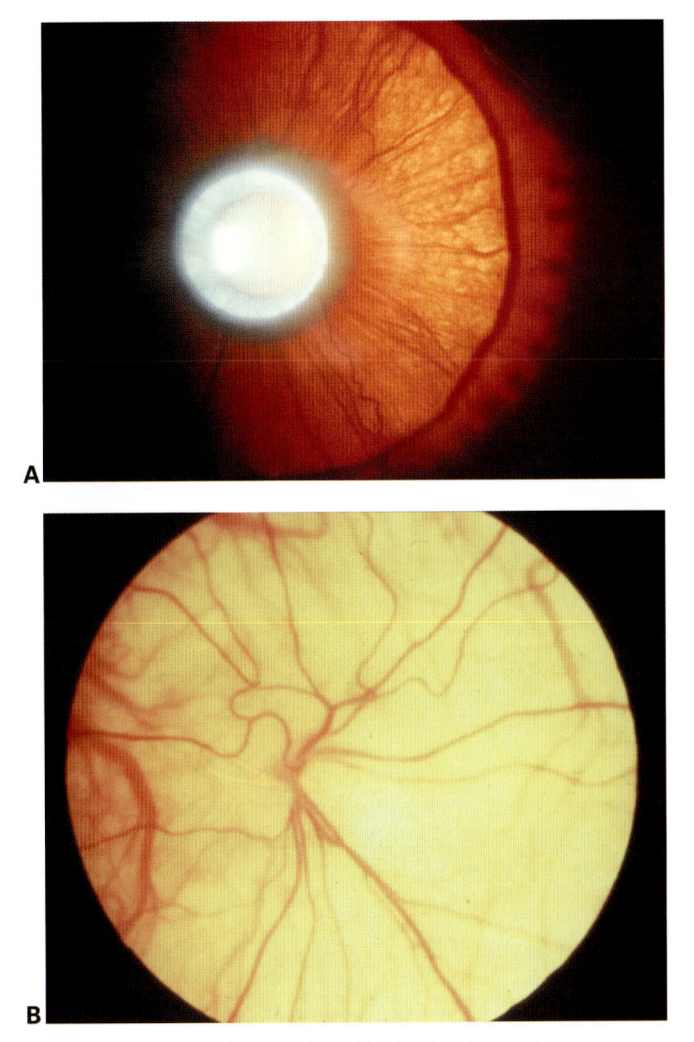

Figure 11-3 Albinisim. **A,** Iris transillumination. **B,** Fundus hypopigmentation. *(Courtesy of Robert H. Rosa, Jr., MD.)*

BCSC Section 6, *Pediatric Ophthalmology and Strabismus,* discusses albinism in greater detail.

Myelinated (Medullated) Nerve Fibers

Generally, myelination of the optic pathways terminates at the lamina cribrosa. However, myelination of the nerve fibers in the NFL can occur and produce a striking clinical appearance (see Fig 25-3, BCSC Section 6, *Pediatric Ophthalmology and Strabismus*). Areas of myelination are usually contiguous with the optic nerve head, but myelination may occur in isolation from the optic nerve head as well. The area of myelination is typically small, but large areas can produce a clinically significant scotoma. The myelin is produced by oligodendroglial cells within the NFL. Myelinated nerve fibers have been associated with myopia, amblyopia, strabismus, and nystagmus.

Vascular Anomalies

The numerous congenital anomalies of the retinal vasculature include

- capillary hemangioma (hemangioblastoma) and cavernous hemangioma
- proliferative retinopathy associated with anencephaly
- parafoveal telangiectasia
- Leber miliary aneurysm
- Coats disease
- familial exudative retinopathy
- racemose angioma (Wyburn-Mason syndrome)
- vascular loop

One histopathologic study of parafoveal telangiectasia revealed focal endothelial degeneration, accumulation of lipid within the walls of vessels, and extensive degeneration of pericytes. These findings were more pronounced in the area of clinically abnormal vessels but were also present diffusely in the retinal vasculature. In that study, no dilated or telangiectatic vessels were present.

Leber miliary aneurysm shows varying degrees of retinal capillary nonperfusion and aneurysmal dilation of retinal vessels. The changes in Leber miliary aneurysm are similar to those present to a greater degree in Coats disease. In Coats disease, exudative retinal detachment occurs as a result of leakage from abnormalities in the peripheral retina, including telangiectatic vessels, microaneurysms, and saccular dilations of retinal vessels (Fig 11-4). These changes are most often unilateral but may be bilateral. Histologically, retinal detachments secondary to Coats disease are characterized by the presence of "foamy" macrophages in the subretinal space.

Congenital Hypertrophy of the RPE

Congenital hypertrophy of the RPE (CHRPE), a relatively common congenital lesion, is characterized clinically by a flat, dark black lesion varying in size from a few to 10 mm in diameter (see Fig 17-10 in Chapter 17). Frequently, central lacunae and a peripheral zone of less dense pigmentation appear within the lesion. This lesion is histopathologically characterized by enlarged RPE cells with densely packed and larger-than-normal, spherical melanin granules (Fig 11-5). This benign congenital condition can generally be distinguished from choroidal nevi and malignant melanoma on the basis of ophthalmoscopic features. Adenocarcinoma of the RPE may develop, rarely, in an area of CHRPE.

In addition, CHRPE may be present in Gardner syndrome, or familial adenomatous polyposis. In this syndrome, bilateral or multiple (greater than 4) areas of RPE hypertrophy are a marker for the presence of the phenotype in members of pedigrees affected with the syndrome and indicate a significant risk for colorectal carcinoma. Four different types of RPE hypertrophy have been described in Gardner syndrome, and 1 of these types is similar to that present in CHRPE. Histopathologic study of the RPE changes in Gardner syndrome is more consistent with hyperplasia of the RPE than with hypertrophy. The RPE changes in Gardner syndrome are probably more appropriately termed *hamartomas*,

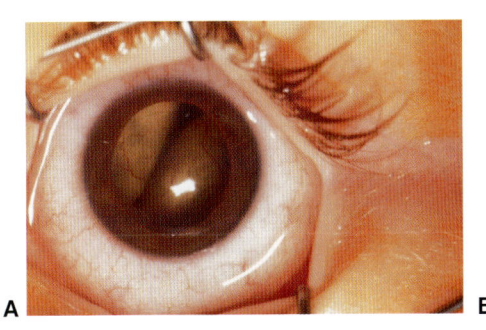

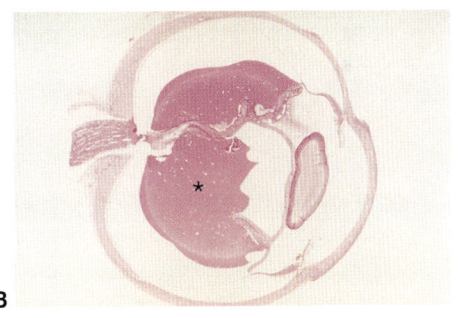

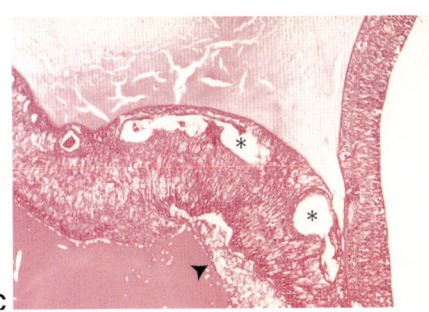

Figure 11-4 **A,** Leukocoria as a result of Coats disease. **B,** Total exudative retinal detachment in Coats disease. Note the dense subretinal proteinaceous fluid *(asterisk)*. **C,** Telangiectatic vessels *(asterisks)* and "foamy" macrophages *(arrowhead)* typical of Coats disease. *(Courtesy of Hans E. Grossniklaus, MD.)*

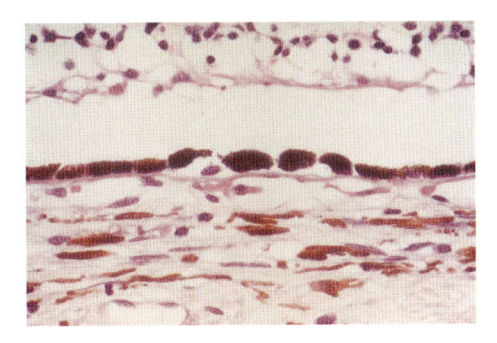

Figure 11-5 In CHRPE, the RPE cells are larger than normal and contain more densely packed melanin granules. For clinical images of CHRPE, see Figure 17-11 in Chapter 17. *(Courtesy of Hans E. Grossniklaus, MD.)*

consistent with the loss of regulatory control of cell growth that gives rise to the other soft-tissue changes in this syndrome.

> Kasner L, Traboulsi EI, Delacruz Z, Green WR. A histopathologic study of the pigmented fundus lesions in familial adenomatous polyposis. *Retina.* 1992;12:35–42.

Inflammations

Infectious

Viral

Multiple viruses may cause retinal infections, including rubella, measles, human immunodeficiency virus (HIV), herpes simplex, herpes zoster, and cytomegalovirus (CMV). Two of the clinically most important entities are discussed here: acute retinal necrosis (ARN) and CMV infection.

Acute retinal necrosis is a clinically descriptive term that has been applied to the findings in patients with acute retinal infection caused by herpes simplex virus types 1 and 2 and herpes zoster. In at least 1 case, CMV has also been reported as a causative agent. The histopathologic findings are diffuse uveitis, vitritis, retinal vasculitis, and necrotizing retinitis (Fig 11-6). Electron microscopy has demonstrated viral inclusions in retinal cells. The involvement of the viruses just named in ARN has been demonstrated by culture, polymerase chain reaction (PCR), and immunohistochemistry.

CMV infection of the retina occurs as an opportunistic infection in approximately 37% of patients with AIDS and less commonly in patients immunosuppressed for other reasons (Fig 11-7). This infection is histopathologically characterized by retinal necrosis, which leads to a thin fibroglial scar with healing. Acute lesions show large neurons (20–30 μm) that contain large eosinophilic intranuclear or intracytoplasmic inclusion bodies. At the cellular level, CMV may infect vascular endothelial cells, retinal neurons, and macrophages.

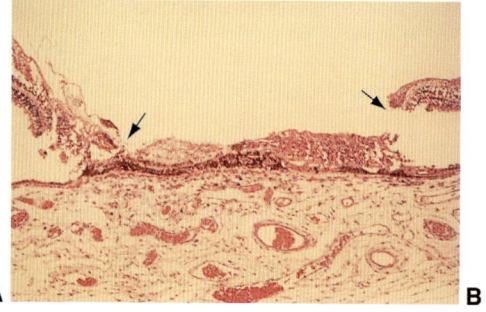

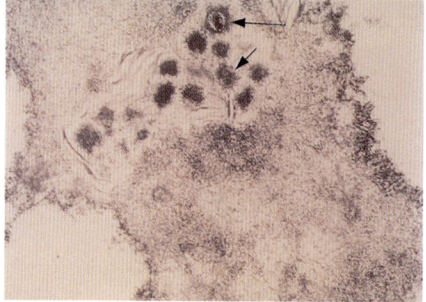

Figure 11-6 **A,** Acute retinal necrosis (ARN) is characterized by full-thickness necrosis of the retina *(between arrows).* **B,** Electron microscopy demonstrates viral particles *(arrows)* within retinal cells. *(Courtesy of Hans E. Grossniklaus, MD.)*

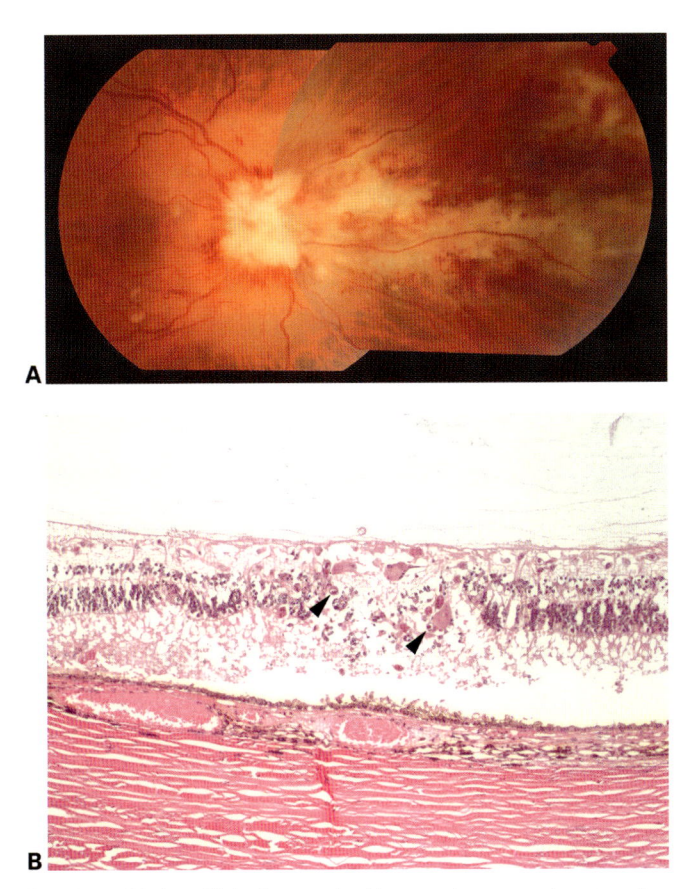

Figure 11-7 **A,** CMV retinitis/papillitis. Intraretinal hemorrhages and areas of opaque retina are present nasal to the optic disc. Note the marked optic disc and peripapillary retinal swelling and cotton-wool spots temporal to the optic disc. **B,** Histopathologically, full-thickness retinal necrosis, cytomegalo cells, and intranuclear *(arrowheads)* and/or intracytoplasmic inclusions are present. *(Part A courtesy of R. Doug Davis, MD; part B courtesy of Robert H. Rosa, Jr, MD.)*

Bacterial

See the discussion of endophthalmitis in Chapter 10. See also BCSC Section 9, *Intraocular Inflammation and Uveitis*.

Fungal

Fungal infections of the retina are uncommon, occurring almost exclusively in immunosuppressed patients as a result of fungemia. These infections usually begin as single or multiple foci of choroidal and retinal infection (Fig 11-8). The most common causative fungi are *Candida* species. Less common agents include *Aspergillus* species and *Cryptococcus neoformans*.

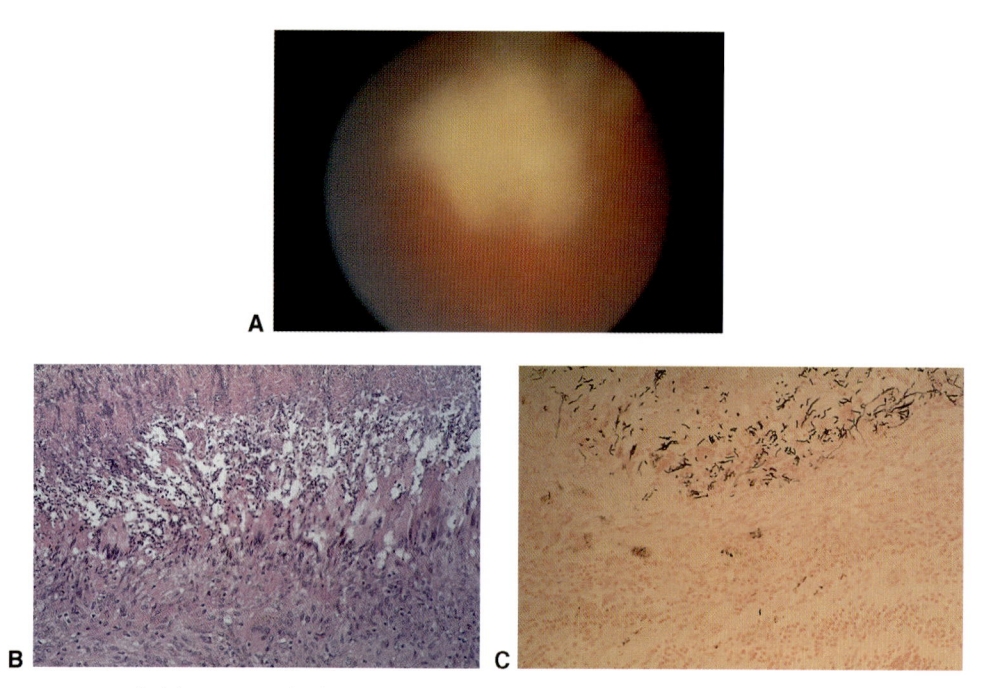

Figure 11-8 **A,** Vitreous, retinal, and choroidal infiltrate in a patient with fungal chorioretinitis. **B,** Granulomatous infiltration surrounding central area of necrosis. **C,** Gomori methenamine–silver nitrate stain of section parallel to **B** shows numerous fungal hyphae. *(Courtesy of David J. Wilson, MD.)*

Histopathologically, fungal infections are typified by necrotizing granulomatous inflammation. A central zone of necrosis is typically surrounded by granulomatous inflammation, and a surrounding infiltrate of lymphocytes is common. With treatment, the lesions heal with a fibrous scar. The causative agent can usually be identified by culture or by the specific features of the fungal hyphae in histopathologic material.

Toxoplasmosis

Most cases of toxoplasmosis represent reactivation of a transplacentally acquired retinal infection. Less commonly, toxoplasmic retinitis occurs as an acquired retinal infection in immunosuppressed patients. Microscopic examination of active toxoplasmic retinitis reveals necrosis of the retina, a prominent infiltrate of neutrophils and lymphocytes, and *Toxoplasma* organisms in the form of cysts and tachyzoites (Fig 11-9). There is generally a prominent lymphocytic infiltrate of the vitreous and the anterior segment. Healing brings resolution of the inflammatory cell infiltrate with encystment of the organisms in the retina adjacent to the chorioretinal scar.

Noninfectious

Noninfectious inflammatory retinal conditions include birdshot retinochoroidopathy, pars planitis, Eales disease, and cancer-associated retinopathy (CAR). See BCSC Section 9,

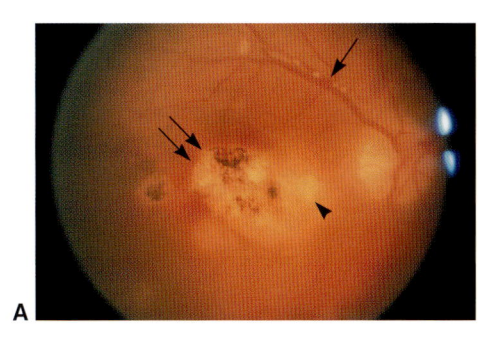

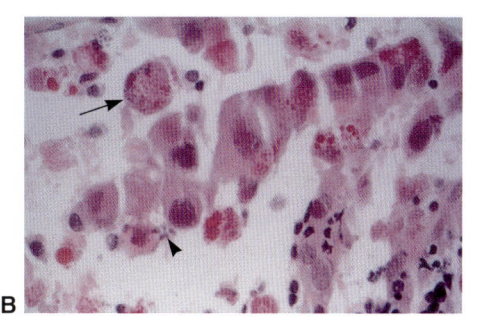

Figure 11-9 A, Chorioretinal scars with pigmentation *(double arrow)* typical of prior infection with toxoplasmosis. Active retinitis *(arrowhead)* and perivascular sheathing *(arrow)* are present. **B,** Cysts *(arrow)* and released organisms (bradyzoites, *arrowhead*) in active toxoplasmosis. *(Courtesy of Hans E. Grossniklaus, MD.)*

Intraocular Inflammation and Uveitis, and Section 12, *Retina and Vitreous,* for discussion of these conditions.

Sarcoidosis

Sarcoidosis, a systemic inflammatory process, is characterized by granulomatous inflammation without a demonstrable infectious cause (see Fig 12-8). Sarcoidosis can affect virtually any tissue within the eye, including the retina. Retinal involvement is characterized histopathologically by the presence of noncaseating granulomas. These are generally small, but when they are large, exudative retinal detachment may be present. Associated retinal findings include retinal periphlebitis, which corresponds to the clinical *taches de bougie,* or candlewax drippings; cystoid macular edema; retinal vascular occlusive disease; and retinal and optic nerve head neovascularization.

Degenerations

Typical and Reticular Peripheral Cystoid Degeneration

Typical peripheral cystoid degeneration (TPCD) is a universal finding in the eyes of people over the age of 20. In TPCD, cystic spaces develop in the outer plexiform layer. *Reticular peripheral cystoid degeneration (RPCD)* is less common. In RPCD, the cystic spaces are present in the NFL. When present, RPCD occurs posterior to areas of TPCD (Fig 11-10).

Typical and Reticular Degenerative Retinoschisis

Coalescence of the cystic spaces of TPCD forms typical degenerative retinoschisis. *Retinoschisis* is said to be present when the fluid-filled space in the outer plexiform layer is 1.5 mm or greater in diameter. *Typical degenerative retinoschisis* is present in approximately 1% of adults and is usually inferotemporal in location. *Reticular degenerative retinoschisis* is present in 1.6% of adults. In reticular degenerative retinoschisis, the splitting of retinal layers occurs in the NFL, so the inner layer of the schisis cavity is thinner than in typical

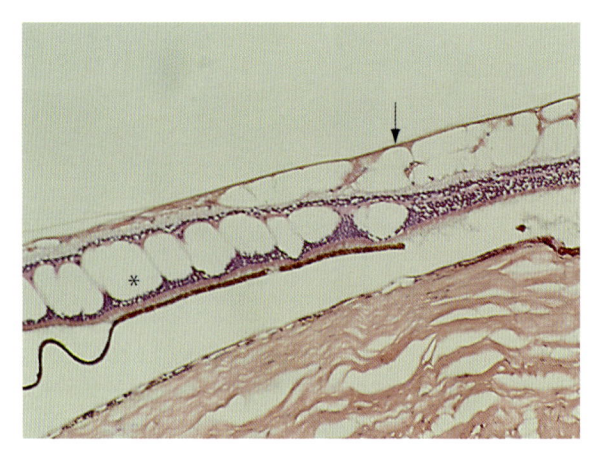

Figure 11-10 Retinal degeneration. Typical peripheral cystoid degeneration consists of cystoid spaces in the outer plexiform layer *(asterisk)* on the lower left (anterior retina). In the upper right (posterior retina), reticular peripheral cystoid degeneration *(arrow)* is present.

degenerative retinoschisis. Reticular degenerative retinoschisis tends to be more bullous than typical degenerative retinoschisis and is more likely to be associated with outer layer breaks and a more posterior location.

Lattice Degeneration

Lattice degeneration may be a familial condition (Fig 11-11). It is found in 8%–10% of the general population, but only a small number of affected persons develop retinal detachment. In contrast, lattice degeneration is seen in 20%–40% of all rhegmatogenous detachments. The most important histopathologic features of lattice degeneration include

- discontinuity of the internal limiting membrane of the retina
- an overlying pocket of liquefied vitreous
- sclerosis of the retinal vessels, which remain physiologically patent
- condensation and adherence of vitreous at the margins of the lesion
- variable degrees of atrophy of the inner layers of the retina

Although atrophic holes often develop in the center of the lattice lesion, they are rarely the cause of retinal detachment because the vitreous is liquefied over the surface of the lattice, and thus no vitreous traction occurs. Retinal detachment associated with lattice degeneration is generally the result of vitreous adhesion at the margin of lattice degeneration, leading to retinal tears in this location with vitreous detachment.

Radial perivascular lattice degeneration is a special type that has the same histopathologic features as typical lattice degeneration but occurs posteriorly along the course of retinal vessels. Radial perivascular lattice degeneration is more common in hereditary vitreoretinal degenerations such as Stickler syndrome and can be associated with severe forms of retinal detachment.

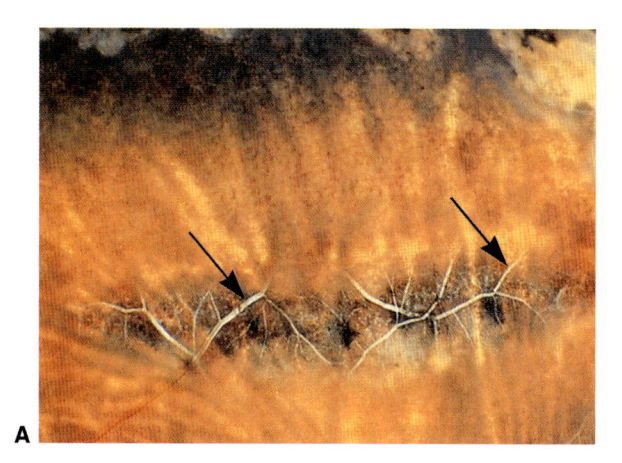

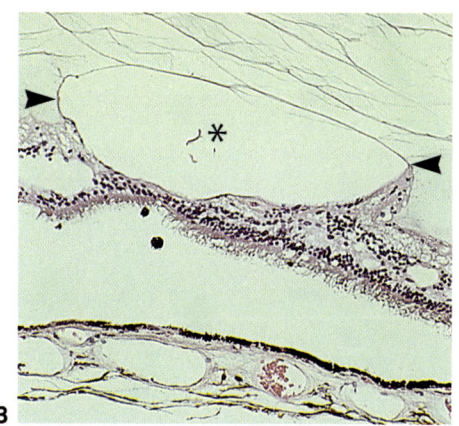

CHAPTER 11: Retina and Retinal Pigment Epithelium • 149

Figure 11-11 Retinal lattice degeneration. **A,** Lattice degeneration may present as prominent sclerotic vessels *(arrows)* in a wicker or lattice pattern. The clinical presentation has many variations. **B,** The vitreous directly over lattice degeneration is liquefied *(asterisk)*, but formed vitreous remains adherent at the margins *(arrowheads)* of the degenerated area. The internal limiting membrane is discontinuous, and the inner retinal layers are atrophic.

Paving-Stone Degeneration

In contrast to retinal vascular occlusion, which leads to inner retinal ischemia, occlusion of the choriocapillaris can lead to loss of the outer retinal layers and RPE. This type of atrophy, called *cobblestone,* or *paving-stone, degeneration,* is very common in the retinal periphery. The well-demarcated, flat, pale lesions seen clinically correspond to circumscribed areas of retinal and RPE atrophy in which the inner nuclear layer is adherent to Bruch's membrane (Fig 11-12).

Ischemia

There are many causes of retinal ischemia, including

- diabetes
- retinal artery and vein occlusion
- radiation retinopathy
- retinopathy of prematurity
- sickle cell retinopathy
- vasculitis
- carotid occlusive disease

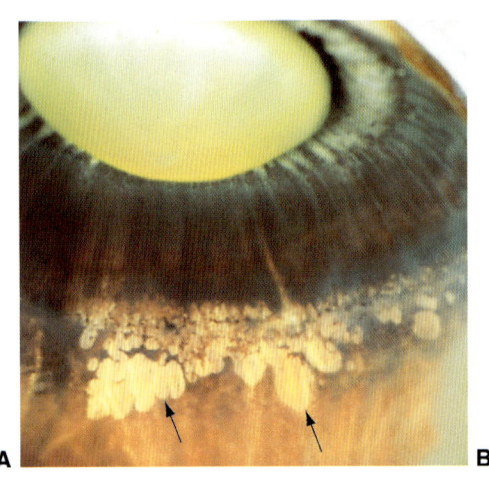

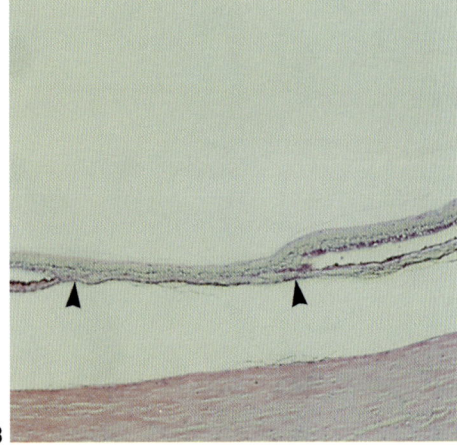

Figure 11-12 **A,** Paving-stone degeneration appears as areas of depigmentation *(arrows)* in the periphery of the retina near the ora serrata. **B,** Histopathologically, paving-stone degeneration consists of atrophy of the outer retinal elements and chorioretinal adhesion to the remaining inner retinal elements. A sharp boundary *(arrowheads)* exists between normal and atrophic retina, corresponding to the clinical appearance of paving-stone degeneration.

Figure 11-13 Inner retinal ischemia. The photoreceptor nuclei (outer nuclear layer, *ON*) and the outer portion of the inner nuclear layer *(IN)* are identifiable. The inner portion of the inner nuclear layer is absent. There are no ganglion cells, and the NFL is absent. This pattern of ischemia corresponds to the supply of the retinal arteriolar circulation and may be observed in arterial and venular occlusions.

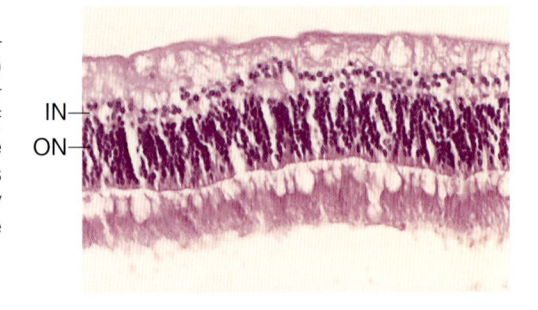

The specific aspects of some of these diseases are discussed later in the chapter. However, certain histopathologic findings are common to all the disorders that result in retinal ischemia. The retinal changes that occur with ischemia can be grouped into cellular responses and vascular responses.

Cellular responses

The neurons in the retina are highly active metabolically, requiring, on a per gram of tissue basis, large amounts of oxygen for production of adenosine triphosphate (ATP) (see also BCSC Section 2, *Fundamentals and Principles of Ophthalmology,* Part IV, Biochemistry and Metabolism). This makes them highly sensitive to interruption of their blood supply. With prolonged oxygen deprivation (greater than 90 minutes in experimental studies), the neuronal cells become pyknotic, and they are subsequently phagocytosed and disappear. The extent and location of the area of atrophic retina resulting from ischemia depends on the size of the occluded vessel and on whether it is a retinal or a choroidal blood vessel. As described earlier, the retinal circulation supplies the inner retina, and the choroidal circulation supplies the outer retina and RPE. Infarctions of the retinal circulation lead to *inner ischemic retinal atrophy* (Fig 11-13), and infarctions of the choroidal circulation lead to *outer ischemic retinal atrophy* (Fig 11-14).

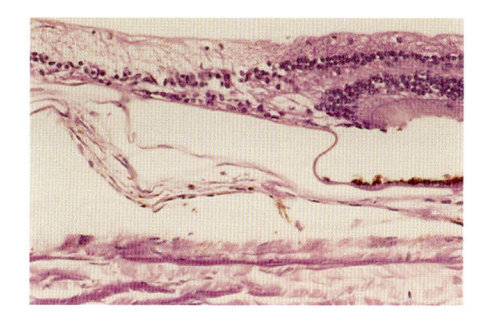

CHAPTER 11: Retina and Retinal Pigment Epithelium • 151

Figure 11-14 Begin at the right edge of the photograph and trace the ganglion cell and the inner nuclear layer toward the left. In this case, there is loss of the nuclei of the photoreceptor layer (outer nuclear layer), the photoreceptor inner and outer segments, and the RPE. This is the pattern of outer retinal atrophy, secondary to interruption in the choroidal vascular blood supply. Compare with Figure 11-13.

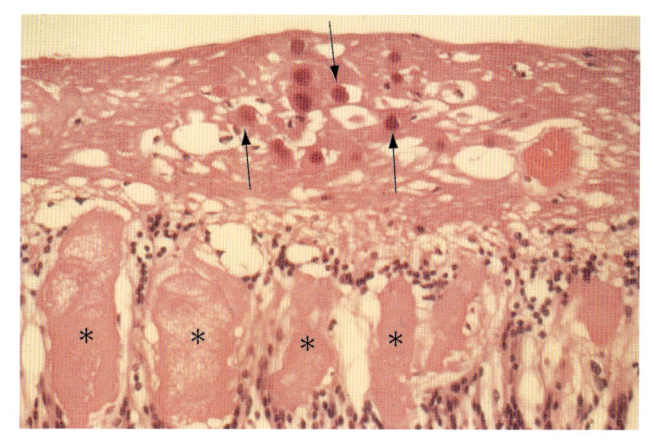

Figure 11-15 Cytoid bodies *(arrows)* within the NFL. Cystoid spaces *(asterisks)* are filled with proteinaceous fluid. *(Courtesy of W. Richard Green, MD.)*

The neuronal cells of the retina have no capacity for regeneration after ischemic damage. Following ischemic damage to the nerve fibers of the ganglion cells, *cytoid bodies* (swollen axons) become apparent histopathologically (Fig 11-15). These are localized accumulations of axoplasmic material that are present in ischemic infarcts of the NFL. *Cotton-wool spots* are the clinical correlate of ischemic infarcts of the NFL that resolve over 4–12 weeks, leaving an area of inner ischemic atrophy.

Glial cells, like axons, degenerate in areas of infarction. Proliferation of the glial cells may occur adjacent to local areas of infarction or in areas of ischemia without infarction, resulting in a glial scar.

Microglial cells are actually tissue macrophages rather than true glial cells. These cells are involved with the phagocytosis of necrotic cells as well as of extracellular material, such as lipid and blood, that accumulates in areas of ischemia. Microglial cells are fairly resistant to ischemia.

Vascular responses

Many of the vascular changes in retinal ischemia are mediated by vascular endothelial growth factor (VEGF). This growth factor is a potent mediator of vascular permeability and angiogenesis. It has been shown to play a role in numerous ocular conditions associated with vascularization.

152 • Ophthalmic Pathology and Intraocular Tumors

In addition to the vascular changes secondary to ischemia itself, vascular changes may also be caused by the specific disease process responsible for the ischemia. Edema and hemorrhages are common with acute retinal ischemia. Retinal capillary closure, microaneurysms, lipid exudates, and neovascularization may develop with chronic retinal ischemia.

Edema, one of the earliest manifestations of retinal ischemia, is a result of transudation across the inner blood–retina barrier (Fig 11-16). Fluid and serum components accumulate in the extracellular space, and the fluid pockets are delimited by the surrounding neurons and glial cells. Exudate accumulating in the outer plexiform layer of the macula (Henle's layer) produces a star figure because of the orientation of the nerve fibers in this layer (Fig 11-17). In cases of chronic edema, the extracellular deposits will become richer in protein and lipids, as the water component of the exudate is more efficiently removed, resulting in so-called *hard exudates.* Histologically, retinal exudates appear as eosinophilic, sharply circumscribed spaces within the retina (Fig 11-18). Chronic edema may result in intraretinal lipid deposits that are contained within the microglial cells.

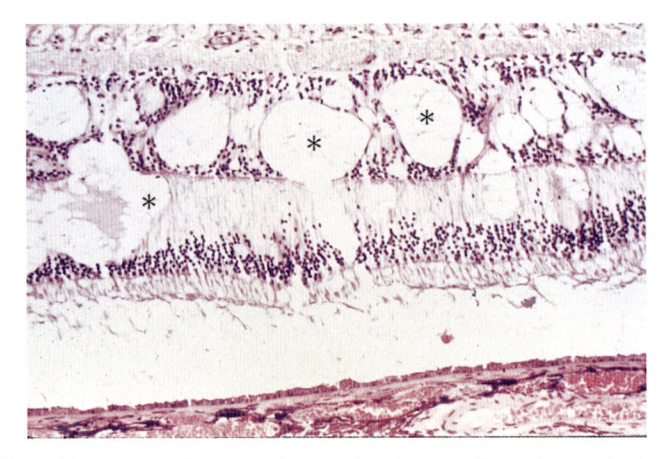

Figure 11-16 Cystoid spaces in inner nuclear and outer plexiform layers *(asterisks)*. *(Courtesy of W. Richard Green, MD.)*

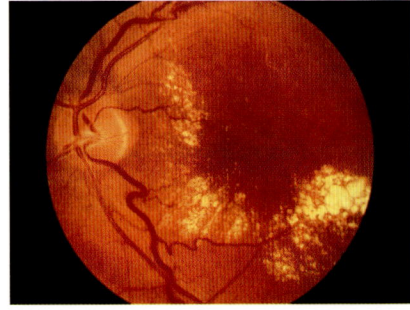

Figure 11-17 Intraretinal lipid deposits, or hard exudates. *(Courtesy of David J. Wilson, MD.)*

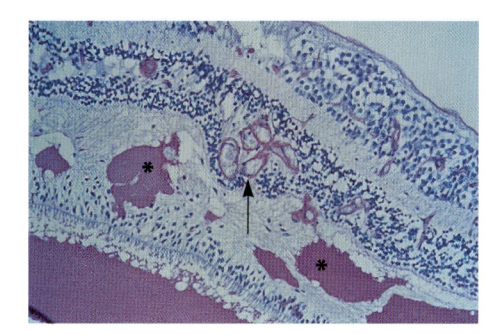

CHAPTER 11: Retina and Retinal Pigment Epithelium • 153

Figure 11-18 Intraretinal exudates *(asterisks)* surrounding intraretinal microvascular abnormalities *(arrow)*. *(Courtesy of W. Richard Green, MD.)*

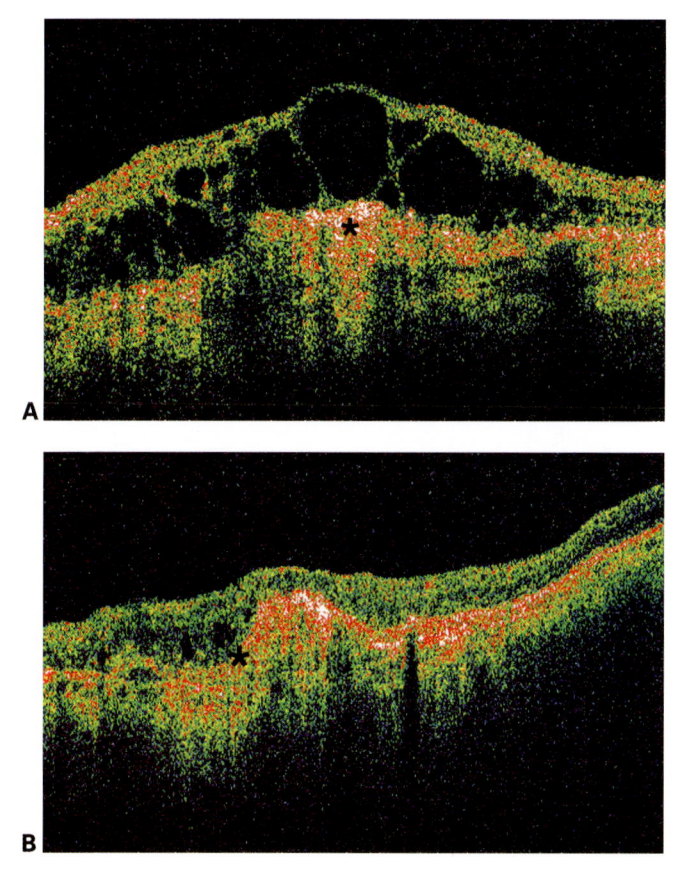

Figure 11-19 Cystoid macular edema and IVTA. OCT showing CME associated with choroidal neovascularization *(asterisk)* in exudative AMD before **(A)** and after **(B)** IVTA. *(Courtesy Robert H. Rosa, Jr, MD, and Terry Hanke, CRA.)*

Intravitreal triamcinolone acetonide (IVTA) has been employed in the treatment of various macular diseases associated with macular edema and choroidal neovascularization. Gain in visual acuity, which is mostly secondary to a decrease in macular edema, has been achieved with IVTA in such conditions as diffuse diabetic macular edema, central and branch retinal vein occlusions, pseudophakic cystoid macular edema, posterior uveitis, and choroidal neovascularization (Fig 11-19). Some studies have suggested that

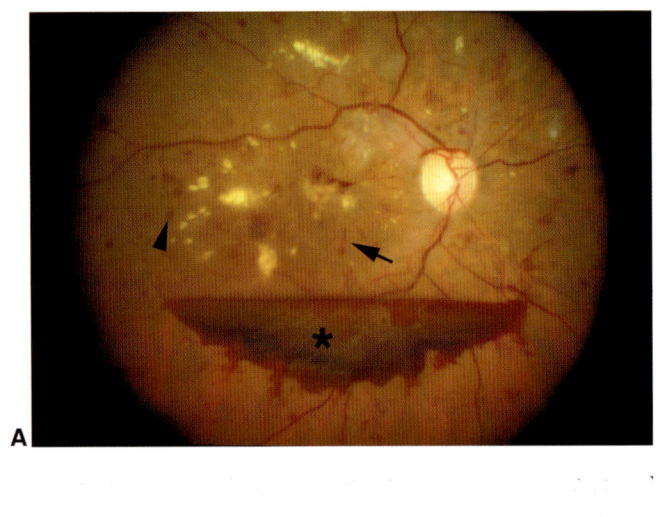

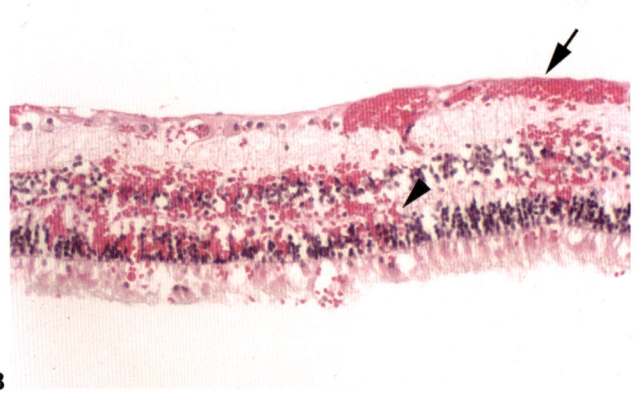

Figure 11-20 Intraretinal hemorrhage. **A,** Fundus photograph showing dot-and-blot *(arrowhead),* flame-shaped *(arrow),* and boat-shaped *(asterisk)* hemorrhages in diabetic retinopathy. **B,** Histopathologically, the dot-and-blot hemorrhage corresponds to blood in the middle layers (inner nuclear and outer plexiform layers) of the retina *(arrowhead).* The flame-shaped hemorrhage corresponds to blood in the NFL *(arrow),* and the boat-shaped hemorrhage corresponds to subhyaloid blood. *(Courtesy of Robert H. Rosa, Jr, MD.)*

IVTA may be useful as angiostatic therapy in eyes with iris neovascularization, proliferative ischemic retinopathies, and choroidal neovascularization. Hypotheses regarding the mechanism of action of IVTA include an anti-inflammatory effect, inhibition of VEGF, improvement in diffusion, and reestablishment of the blood–retina barrier through a reduction in permeability.

> Jonas JB. Intravitreal triamcinolone acetonide for treatment of intraocular oedematous and neovascular diseases. *Acta Ophthalmol Scand.* 2005;83:645–663.

Retinal hemorrhages also develop as a result of ischemic damage to the inner blood–retina barrier. As with edema and exudates, the shape of the hemorrhage conforms to the surrounding retinal tissue. Consequently, hemorrhages in the nerve fiber are

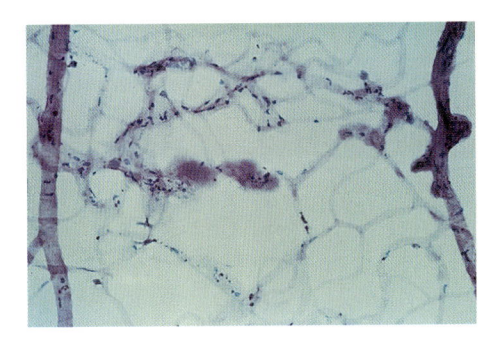

CHAPTER 11: Retina and Retinal Pigment Epithelium • 155

Figure 11-21 Trypsin digest preparation, illustrating acellular capillaries adjacent to dilated irregular vascular channels (IRMA). *(Courtesy of W. Richard Green, MD.)*

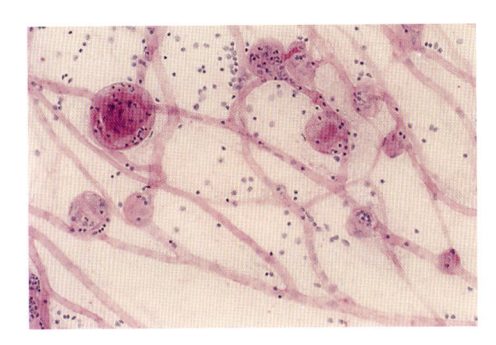

Figure 11-22 Retinal trypsin digest preparation, showing diabetic microaneurysms.

flame-shaped, whereas those in the nuclear or inner plexiform layer are circular, or "dot and blot" (Fig 11-20). Subhyaloid and sub-ILM hemorrhages have a boat-shaped configuration. White-centered hemorrhages *(Roth spots)* may be present in a number of conditions. The white centers of the hemorrhages can have a number of causes, including aggregates of white blood cells, platelets, and fibrin; or they may be due to retinal light reflexes. Hemorrhages clear over a period of time ranging from days to months.

Chronic retinal ischemia leads to architectural changes in the retinal vessels. The capillary bed becomes acellular in an area of vascular occlusion. Adjacent to acellular areas, dilated irregular vascular channels known as *intraretinal microvascular abnormalities (IRMA)* and microaneurysms often appear (Figs 11-21, 11-22). *Microaneurysms* are fusiform or saccular outpouchings of the retinal capillaries best seen clinically with fluorescein angiography and histologically with PAS-stained trypsin digest preparations. The density of the endothelial cells lining the microaneurysms and IRMA is frequently variable. Microaneurysms evolve from thin-walled hypercellular microaneurysms to hyalinized, hypocellular microaneurysms.

In some cases of retinal ischemia, neovascularization of the retina and the vitreous may occur, most commonly in diabetes and branch retinal vein occlusion. Retinal neovascularization generally consists of the growth of new vessels on the vitreous side of the ILM (Fig 11-23); only rarely does neovascularization occur within the retina itself. Hemorrhage may develop from retinal neovascularization as the associated vitreous exerts traction on the fragile new vessels. Retinal neovascularization should be distinguished from

Figure 11-23 Retinal neovascularization. The new blood vessels have broken through the internal limiting membrane.

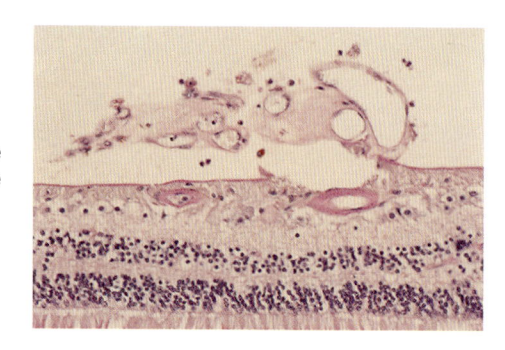

retinal collaterals and arteriovenous shunts, which represent dilation and increased flow in existing retinal vessels.

> Adamis AP, Miller JW, Bernal MT, et al. Increased vascular endothelial growth factor levels in the vitreous of eyes with proliferative diabetic retinopathy. *Am J Ophthalmol.* 1994;118:445–450.

Specific Ischemic Retinal Disorders

Central and branch retinal artery and vein occlusions

Central retinal artery occlusions (CRAO) result from

- localized arteriosclerotic changes
- an embolic event
- rarely, vasculitis (as in temporal arteritis)

As the retina becomes ischemic, it swells and loses its transparency. This swelling is best appreciated clinically and histopathologically in the posterior pole, where the NFL and the ganglion cell layer are the thickest (Fig 11-24). Because the ganglion cell layer and the NFL are thickest in the macula but absent in the fovea, the normal color of the choroid shows through in the fovea and produces a cherry-red spot, ophthalmoscopically suggesting CRAO. The retinal swelling eventually clears and leaves the classic histologic picture of inner ischemic atrophy (see Fig 11-13). Scarring and neovascularization are rare.

Branch retinal artery occlusion (BRAO) is usually the result of emboli that most frequently lodge at the bifurcation of a retinal arteriole. *Hollenhorst plaques,* which are cholesterol emboli within retinal arterioles, seldom occlude the vessel. Emboli may be the first or most important clue to a significant systemic disorder such as carotid vascular disease (Hollenhorst plaques), cardiac valvular disease (calcific emboli), or thromboembolism (platelet-fibrin emboli).

The histology of the acute phase of BRAO is characterized by swelling of the inner retinal layers with the death of all nuclei. As the edema resolves, a classic picture emerges of inner ischemic atrophy in the distribution of the retina supplied by the occluded arteriole. The NFL, the ganglion cell layer, the inner plexiform layer, and the inner nuclear layer are affected (see Fig 11-13). Arteriolar occlusions result in infarcts with complete postnecrotic atrophy of the affected layers.

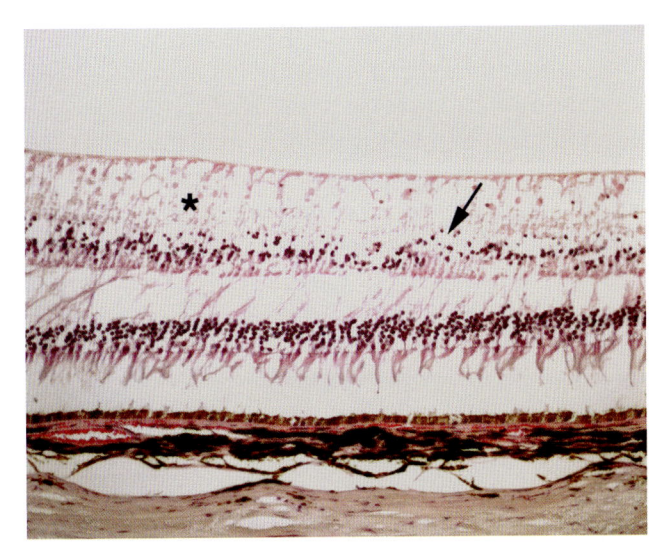

Figure 11-24 Acute central retinal artery occlusion. Histopathologically, necrosis occurs in the inner retina *(asterisk)* corresponding to the retinal whitening observed by ophthalmoscopic examination. Note the pyknotic nuclei *(arrow)* in the inner aspect of the inner nuclear layer. *(Courtesy of Robert H. Rosa, Jr, MD.)*

Central retinal vein occlusion (CRVO) occurs at the level of the lamina cribrosa. The pathophysiology of CRVO is the same as that of hemiretinal vein occlusion but different from that of branch retinal vein occlusion (see the following discussion). What has previously been called *papillophlebitis* represents a CRVO in a patient with good collateral circulation. Central retinal vein occlusions develop as a result of structural changes in the central retinal artery and the lamina cribrosa that lead to compression of the central retinal vein. This compression creates turbulent flow in the vein and predisposes to thrombosis. These structural changes occur in arteriosclerosis, hypertension, diabetes, and glaucoma.

CRVO is recognized clinically by the presence of retinal hemorrhages in all 4 quadrants. Usually, prominent edema of the optic nerve head occurs, along with dilation of the retinal veins and variable numbers of cotton-wool spots and amounts of macular edema. CRVO occurs in 2 forms: a milder perfused type and a more severe nonperfused type.

Nonperfused CRVO was defined in the CRVO study as a CRVO in which greater than 10 disc areas showed nonperfusion on fluorescein angiography. Nonperfused CRVOs typically have extensive retinal edema and hemorrhage. Marked venular dilation and a variable number of cotton-wool spots are found.

> Baseline and early natural history report. The Central Vein Occlusion Study. *Arch Ophthalmol.* 1993;111:1087–1095.

Acute ischemic CRVO is characterized histologically by the following:

- marked retinal edema
- focal retinal necrosis
- subretinal, intraretinal, and preretinal hemorrhage

Vein occlusions can produce ischemia, allowing glial cells to survive and respond to the insult by replication and intracellular deposition of filaments *(gliosis)*. The hemorrhage, hemosiderosis, disorganization of the retinal architecture, and gliosis seen in vein occlusions distinguish the final histologic picture from that seen in CRAO (Fig 11-25). Numerous microaneurysms are present in the retinal capillaries following CRVO, and acellular capillary beds are present to a variable degree. With time, dilated collateral vessels develop at the optic nerve head. Neovascularization of the iris is common following CRVO.

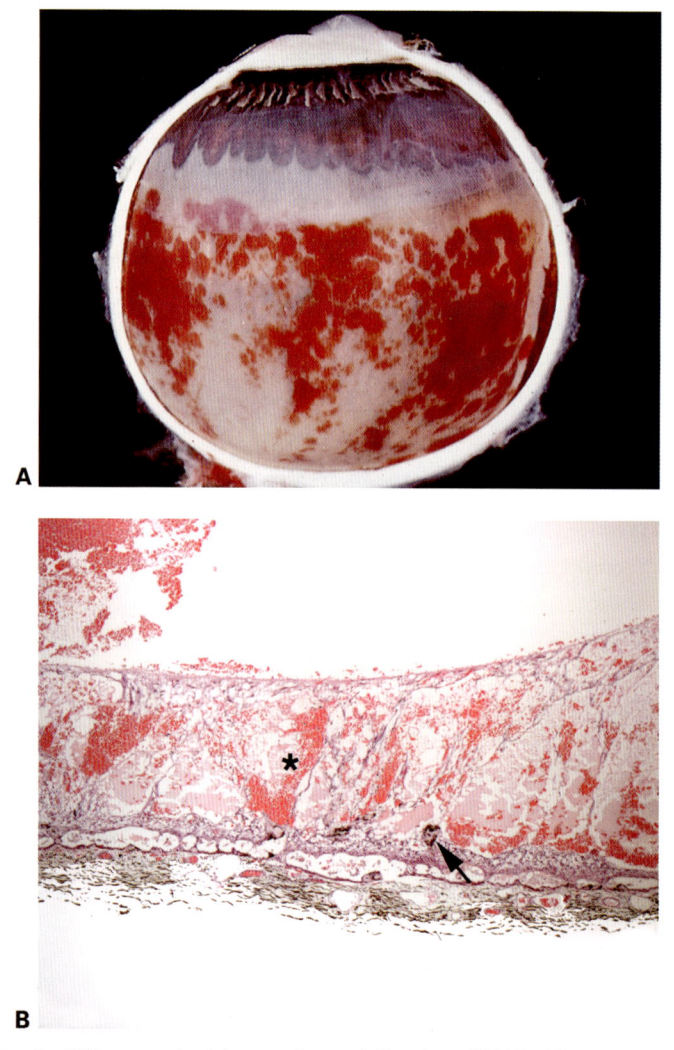

Figure 11-25 A, Diffuse retinal hemorrhage following CRVO. The damaged retina will be replaced by gliosis. **B,** Histopathology of longstanding CRVO shows loss of the normal lamellar architecture of the retina, marked edema with cystic spaces *(asterisk)* containing blood and proteinaceous exudate, vitreous hemorrhage, and nodular hyperplasia of the RPE *(arrow)*. *(Part B courtesy of Robert H. Rosa, Jr, MD.)*

Branch retinal vein occlusion (BRVO) is occlusion of a tributary retinal vein. These occlusions occur almost universally at the site of an arteriovenous crossing. At the crossing of a branch retinal artery and vein, the 2 vessels share a common adventitial sheath. With arteriosclerotic changes in the arteriole, the retinal venule may become compressed, leading to turbulent flow, which predisposes to thrombosis. This condition is more common in patients with arteriosclerosis and hypertension.

BRVO occurs most commonly in the superotemporal quadrant (63% of cases). The occlusion leads to retinal hemorrhages and cotton-wool spots. Because BRVO does not always result in total inner retinal ischemia and death of all tissue, neovascularization of the optic nerve and retina may develop. Overall, 50%–60% of patients with BRVO maintain a visual acuity of 20/40 or better after 1 year. Findings in eyes with permanent visual loss from BRVO include

- CME
- retinal nonperfusion
- pigmentary macular disturbance
- macular edema with hard lipid exudates
- subretinal fibrosis
- epiretinal membrane formation

Photocoagulation therapy is considered for chronic macular edema and neovascularization.

The histologic picture of BRVO resembles that seen in CRVO but is localized to the area of the retina in the distribution of the occluded vein. Inner ischemic retinal atrophy is a characteristic late histologic finding in both retinal arterial and venous occlusions (see Fig 11-13). Numerous microaneurysms and dilated collateral vessels may be present. Acellular retinal capillaries are present to a variable degree, correlating with retinal capillary nonperfusion on fluorescein angiography.

Diabetic Retinopathy

Diabetic retinopathy is 1 of the 4 most frequent causes of new blindness in the United States and the leading cause among 20- to 64-year-olds. Early in the course of diabetic retinopathy, certain physiologic abnormalities occur:

- impaired autoregulation of the retinal vasculature
- alterations in retinal blood flow
- breakdown of the blood–retina barrier

Histologically, the primary changes occur in the retinal microcirculation. These changes include

- thickening of the retinal capillary basement membrane
- selective loss of pericytes compared with retinal capillary endothelial cells
- microaneurysm formation (see Fig 11-22)
- retinal capillary closure (see Fig 11-21) (histologically recognized as acellular capillary beds)

Dilated intraretinal telangiectatic vessels, or intraretinal microvascular abnormalities (IRMA), may develop, as shown in Figure 11-21, and neovascularization may follow (see Fig 11-23). Intraretinal edema, hemorrhages, exudates, and microinfarcts of the inner retina may develop secondary to the primary retinal vascular changes. Acutely, microinfarcts of the inner retina are characterized clinically as cotton-wool spots (see Fig 11-15). Subsequently, focal inner ischemic atrophy appears (see Fig 11-13).

Other histologic changes in diabetes

In diabetes, the corneal epithelial basement membrane is thickened. This change is associated with inadequate adherence of the epithelium to the underlying Bowman's layer, predisposing diabetic patients to corneal abrasions and poor corneal epithelial healing. Lacy vacuolation of the iris pigment epithelium occurs in association with hyperglycemia; histologically, the intraepithelial vacuoles contain glycogen (PAS-positive and diastase-sensitive). Histopathologically, thickening of the ciliary epithelial basement membrane is almost universally present in diabetic eyes. The incidence of cataract formation is increased.

Laser photocoagulation is often used in eyes with diabetic retinopathy. Argon laser photocoagulation, the type most frequently employed, results in variable destruction of the outer retina, destruction of the RPE, and occlusion of the choriocapillaris (Fig 11-26). These lesions heal by proliferation of the adjacent RPE and glial scarring.

Retinopathy of Prematurity

Retinal ischemia also plays a role in retinopathy of prematurity (ROP). This ischemia develops not because of the occlusion of existing vessels but rather because of the absence of retinal vessels in the incompletely developed retinal periphery. A decrease in retinal blood flow from oxygen-induced vasoconstriction may also be a contributing factor.

The clinical and histologic features of ROP are somewhat different from those present in other retinal ischemic states. Retinal edema and exudates do not develop. Retinal hemorrhages and retinal vascular dilation develop only in the most severe cases *(plus* or

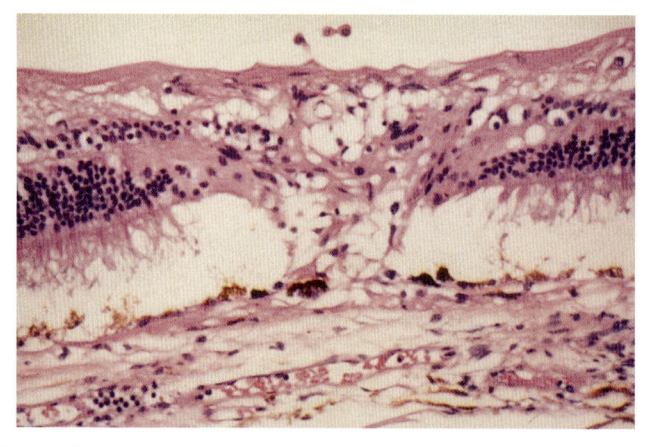

Figure 11-26 Laser photocoagulation scar characterized by absence of the RPE centrally with peripheral RPE hyperplasia and loss of the photoreceptors, the outer nuclear layer, and a portion of the inner nuclear layer. *(Courtesy of David J. Wilson, MD.)*

rush disease). Neovascularization of the retina and vitreous may develop as a result of proliferation of new vessels at the border between the vascularized and avascular peripheral retina. Fibrovascular proliferation into the vitreous at this site may lead to tractional retinal detachment, macular heterotopia, and high myopia.

Age-Related Macular Degeneration

Age-related macular degeneration (AMD) is the leading cause of new blindness in the United States. The precise pathogenesis of this disorder is not known, but genetic predisposition plays an important role. Environmental factors such as smoking and dietary intake of antioxidants may play a role in the pathogenesis of AMD. The retina seems particularly susceptible to oxidative stress because of its high concentration of oxygen, polyunsaturated fatty acids, and photosensitizers in combination with intense exposure to light. Randomized clinical trials have demonstrated a significant reduction in the risk of progression of AMD in elderly persons with a high dietary intake of antioxidants, including beta carotene, vitamins C and E, and zinc. In addition, laboratory studies have demonstrated the effects of different types of oxidative stress on the photoreceptors and RPE and suggested that the use of multiple antioxidants may be helpful in reducing oxidative damage to the photoreceptors/RPE. It is likely that AMD represents a general phenotype resulting from a variety of genetic mutations.

> Age-Related Eye Disease Study Research Group. A randomized, placebo-controlled, clinical trial of high-dose supplementation with vitamins C and E, beta carotene, and zinc for age-related macular degeneration and vision loss: AREDS report no. 8. *Arch Ophthalmol.* 2001;119:1417–1436.
>
> Lu L, Hackett SF, Mincey A, Lai H, Campochiaro PA. Effects of different types of oxidative stress in RPE cells. *J Cell Physiol.* 2006;206:119–125.
>
> van Leeuwen R, Boekhoorn S, Vingerling JR, et al. Dietary intake of antioxidants and risk of age-related macular degeneration. *JAMA.* 2005;294:3101–3107.

Several characteristic changes in the retina, RPE, Bruch's membrane, and choroid occur in AMD. Perhaps the first detectable pathologic change is the appearance of deposits between the basement membrane of the RPE and the elastic portion of Bruch's membrane (basal linear deposits) and similar deposits between the plasma membrane of the RPE and the basement membrane of the RPE (basal laminar deposits). These deposits are not clinically visible and may require electron microscopy to be distinguished. In advanced cases, these deposits may become confluent and can be seen at the light microscopic level (Fig 11-27). This appearance has been described as *diffuse drusen,* for which there is no exact clinical correlate.

The first clinically detectable feature of AMD is the appearance of drusen. The clinical term *drusen* has been correlated pathologically to large PAS-positive deposits between the RPE and Bruch's membrane. Many eyes with clinically apparent drusen (especially soft drusen) are found to have basal laminar and/or basal linear deposits and diffuse drusen on histopathologic analysis. Drusen, which may be transient, have been classified clinically as follows:

- *hard (hyaline) drusen:* the typical discrete, yellowish lesions that are PAS-positive nodules composed of hyaline material between the RPE and Bruch's membrane (Fig 11-28)

162 • Ophthalmic Pathology and Intraocular Tumors

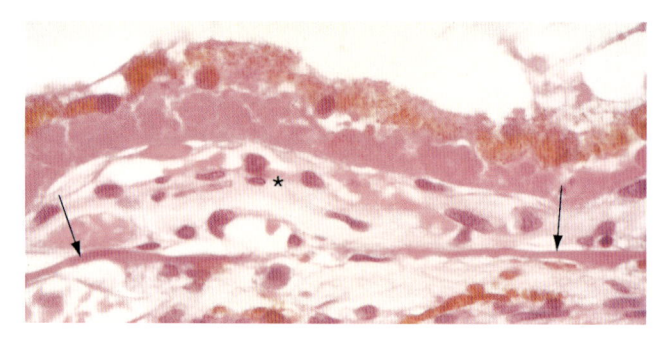

Figure 11-27 Diffuse drusen. There is diffuse deposition of eosinophilic material beneath the RPE. CNV *(asterisk)* is present between the diffuse drusen and the elastic portion of Bruch's membrane *(arrows)*. *(Courtesy of Hans E. Grossniklaus, MD.)*

Figure 11-28 Hard drusen *(arrow)*. Note the periodic acid–Schiff staining of the dome-shaped, nodular, hard druse. *(Reproduced with permission from Spraul CW, Grossniklaus HE. Characteristics of drusen and Bruch's membrane changes in postmortem eyes with age-related macular degeneration. Arch Ophthalmol. 1997;115:267–273. © 1997, American Medical Association.)*

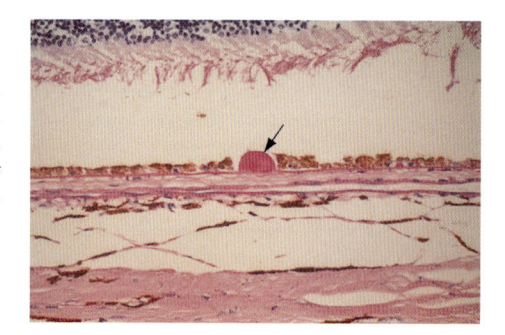

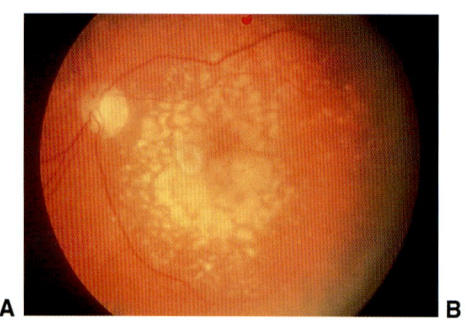

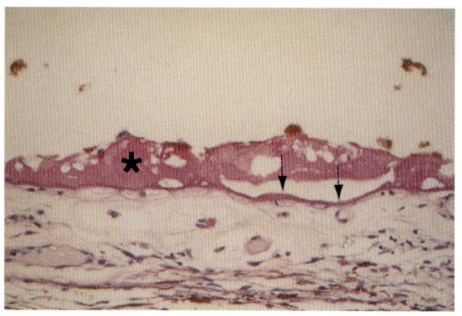

Figure 11-29 A, Clinical photograph of multiple confluent drusen. **B,** Thick eosinophilic deposits *(asterisk)* between the RPE and the elastic portion *(arrows)* of Bruch's membrane. *(Reproduced with permission from Spraul CW, Grossniklaus HE. Characteristics of drusen and Bruch's membrane changes in postmortem eyes with age-related macular degeneration. Arch Ophthalmol. 1997;115:267–273. © 1997, American Medical Association.)*

- *soft drusen*: drusen with amorphous, poorly demarcated boundaries, usually >63 µm in size; histologically, they represent cleavage of the RPE and basal laminar or linear deposits from Bruch's membrane (Fig 11-29)
- *small drusen*: <63 µm
- *intermediate drusen*: 63–125 µm
- *large drusen*: >125 µm

- *basal laminar or cuticular drusen:* diffuse, small, regular, and nodular deposits of drusenlike material in the macula
- *calcific drusen:* sharply demarcated, glistening, refractile lesions usually associated with RPE atrophy

Photoreceptor atrophy occurs to a variable degree in macular degeneration. It is not clear whether this atrophy is a primary abnormality of the photoreceptors or is secondary to the underlying changes in the RPE and Bruch's membrane. In addition to photoreceptor atrophy, large zones of atrophy may appear in the RPE (Fig 11-30). When this occurs centrally, it is termed *central areolar atrophy of the RPE*. Drusen, photoreceptor atrophy, and RPE atrophy may all be present to varying degrees in *dry,* or *nonexudative, AMD*.

Eyes with choroidal neovascularization *(wet,* or *exudative, AMD)* have fibrovascular tissue present between the inner and outer layers of Bruch's membrane, beneath the

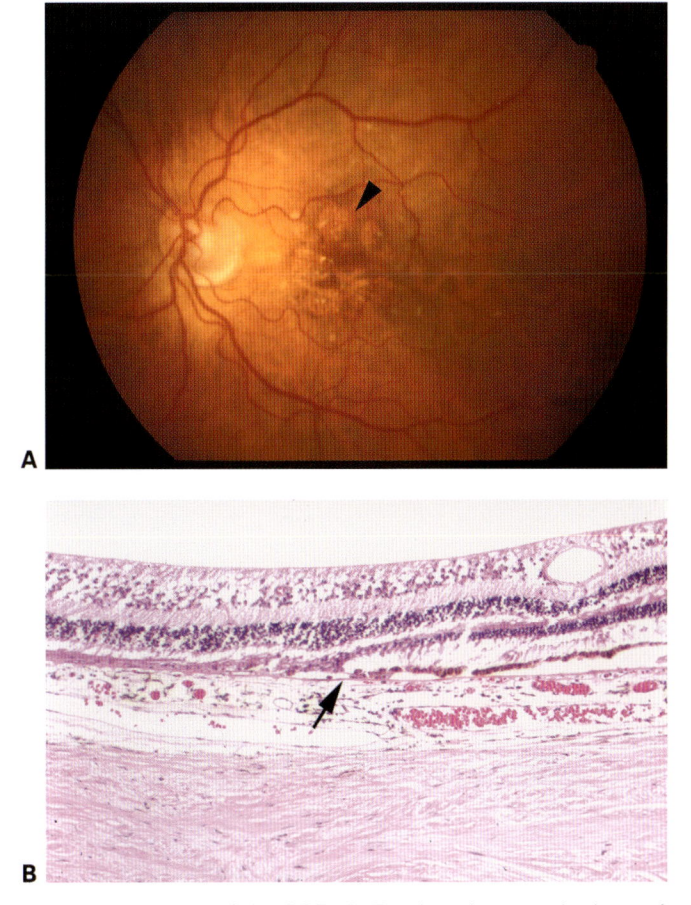

Figure 11-30 Geographic atrophy of the RPE. **A,** Fundus photograph shows focal geographic atrophy of the RPE *(arrowhead)* and drusen in nonexudative AMD. **B,** Histopathologically, there is loss of the photoreceptor cell layer, RPE, and choriocapillaris *(left of arrow)* with an abrupt transition zone *(arrow)* to a more normal-appearing retina/RPE *(right of arrow)*. Note the thickened ganglion cell layer identifying the macular region. *(Courtesy of Robert H. Rosa, Jr, MD.)*

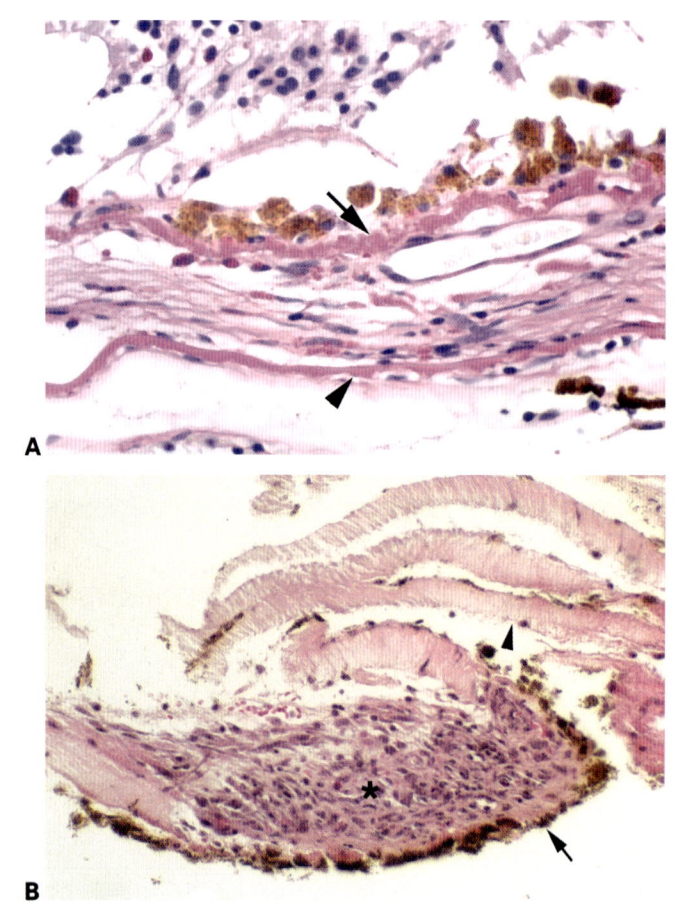

Figure 11-31 A, CNV located between the inner *(arrow)* and outer *(arrowhead)* layers of Bruch's membrane (sub-RPE, type 1 CNV). Note loss of the overlying photoreceptor inner and outer segments, RPE hyperplasia, and the PAS-positive basal laminar deposit *(arrow).* **B,** Surgically excised CNV (subretinal, type 2 CNV) composed of fibrovascular tissue *(asterisk)* lined externally by RPE *(arrow)* with adherent photoreceptor outer segments *(arrowhead). (Courtesy of Robert H. Rosa, Jr, MD.)*

RPE, or in the subretinal space (Fig 11-31), which leads to the exudative consequences of wet AMD. Choroidal neovascularization is associated with the presence of basal laminar deposits and diffuse drusen. The new blood vessels leak fluid, producing serous retinal detachments, and they rupture easily, leading to subretinal and intraretinal hemorrhages.

Subretinal neovascular membranes have been classified as type 1 or type 2, based on their pathologic and clinical features. *Type 1 neovascularization* (Fig 11-31A) is characterized by neovascularization within Bruch's membrane in the sub-RPE space. In this type of neovascularization, the RPE is often abnormally oriented or absent across a broad expanse of the inner portion of Bruch's membrane. *Type 2 neovascularization* (Fig 11-31B) occurs in the subretinal space and generally features only a small defect in which the RPE is abnormally oriented or absent. Type 1 neovascularization is more characteristic of AMD, whereas type 2 is more characteristic of ocular histoplasmosis. Type 2 membranes are more amenable to surgical removal than type 1 membranes because native RPE would be excised with a type 1 membrane, leaving an atrophic lesion (without RPE) in the area of membrane excision.

> Grossniklaus HE, Gass JD. Clinicopathologic correlations of surgically excised type 1 and type 2 submacular choroidal neovascular membranes. *Am J Ophthalmol.* 1998;126:59–69.

Surgically excised choroidal neovascular membranes (see Fig 11-31) are composed of vascular channels, RPE, and various other components of the RPE–Bruch's membrane complex. These latter may include photoreceptor outer segments, basal laminar and linear deposits, hyperplastic RPE, and inflammatory cells.

> Grossniklaus HE, Miskala PH, Green WR, et al. Histopathologic and ultrastructural features of surgically excised subfoveal choroidal neovascular lesions: submacular surgery trials report no. 7. *Arch Ophthalmol.* 2005;123:914–921.

Polypoidal Choroidal Vasculopathy

Polypoidal choroidal vasculopathy (PCV), previously described as *posterior uveal bleeding syndrome* and *multiple recurrent serosanguineous RPE detachments,* is a disorder in which dilated, thin-walled vascular channels (Fig 11-32), apparently arising from the short posterior ciliary arteries, penetrate into Bruch's membrane. Associated choroidal neovascularization is often present in these lesions, as observed in several histologic specimens. Ophthalmoscopically, the polypoidal lesions appear as elevated orange-red polyplike and

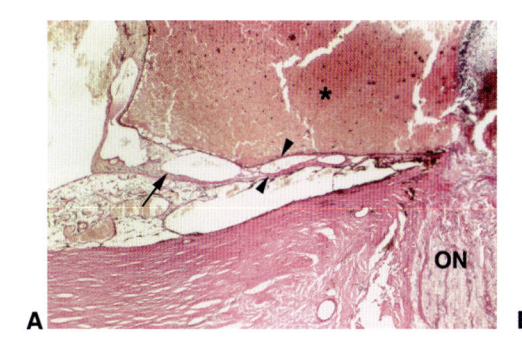

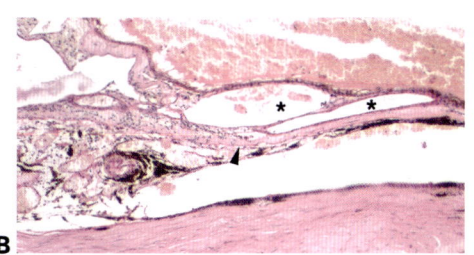

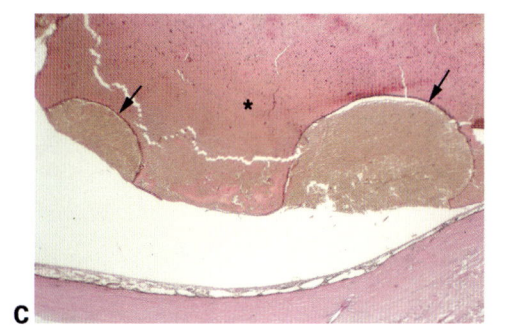

Figure 11-32 Polypoidal choroidal vasculopathy (PCV). **A,** Peripapillary dilated vascular channels *(arrow)* between the RPE and outer aspect of Bruch's membrane *(arrowheads).* Note the dense subretinal hemorrhage *(asterisk).* Optic nerve, *ON.* **B,** Higher-power view of thin-walled vascular channels *(asterisks)* interposed between the RPE and Bruch's membrane *(arrowhead).* **C,** Hemorrhagic RPE detachments *(arrows)* and serosanguineous subretinal fluid *(asterisk).* *(Courtesy of Robert H. Rosa, Jr, MD.)*

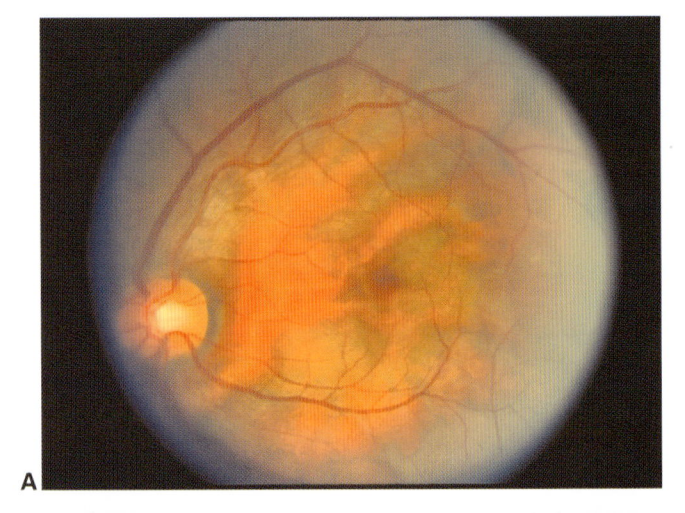

Figure 11-33 Polypoidal choroidal vasculopathy (PCV). **A,** Elevated, red-orange, nodular and tubular lesions in the peripapillary and macular regions. **B,** Late fluorescein angiogram (860 seconds) shows hyperfluorescent polypoidal lesions *(arrows)* without apparent leakage. **C,** Dense subretinal hemorrhage in same patient as in **A** and **B**. Note the persistent red-orange lesions nasal and superior to the optic disc. *(Courtesy of Robert H. Rosa, Jr, MD.)*

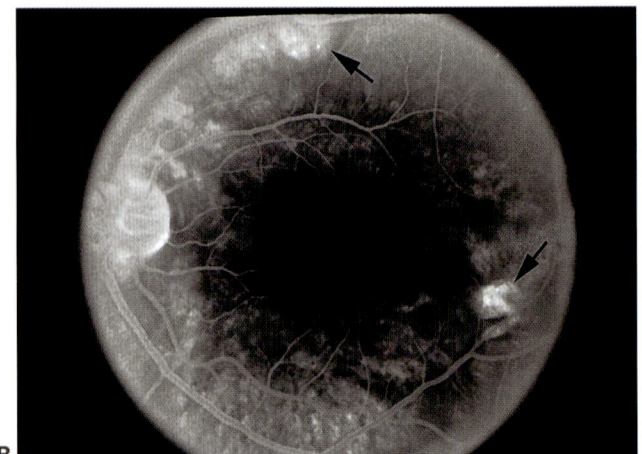

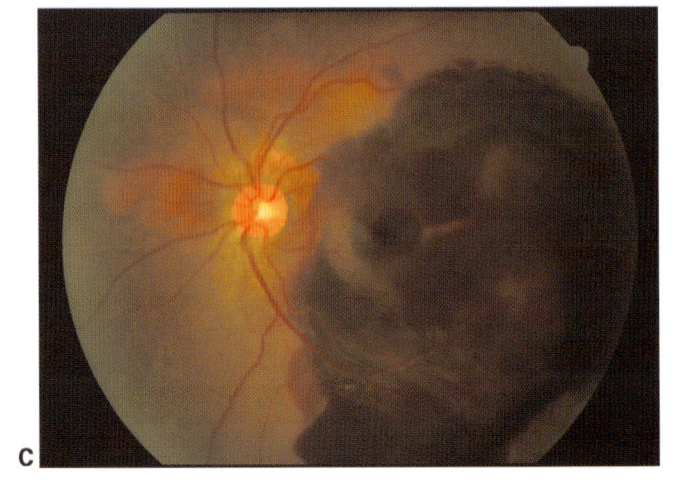

tubular subretinal lesions (Fig 11-33); they are often associated with serosanguineous detachments of the retina and RPE. The lesions may simulate hemorrhage from CNV associated with AMD. In Japanese and Chinese patients, the condition primarily affects men (~80%) and is generally unilateral (~85%); in Europe and the Americas, it preferentially affects darker pigmented patients (79%), with a female preponderance (96%), is more often bilateral (68%), and may be associated with hypertension (43%). More recently, polypoidal lesions have been identified in Caucasian patients, most of whom also have exudative AMD.

> Rosa RH Jr, Davis JL, Eifrig CW. Clinicopathologic reports, case reports, and small case series: clinicopathologic correlation of idiopathic polypoidal choroidal vasculopathy. *Arch Ophthalmol.* 2002;120:502–508.

Macular Dystrophies

Fundus flavimaculatus and Stargardt disease

Fundus flavimaculatus and Stargardt disease are thought to represent 2 ends of the spectrum of a disease process characterized by yellowish flecks at the level of the RPE (Fig 11-34A; see also Fig 9-7, BCSC Section 12, *Retina and Vitreous*), a generalized vermillion color to the fundus on clinical examination, a dark choroid on fluorescein angiography (Fig 11-34B; see also Fig 9-8, BCSC Section 12, *Retina and Vitreous*), and gradually decreasing visual acuity. The inheritance pattern is generally autosomal recessive, but autosomal dominant forms have been reported as well. Several genetic mutations have been observed in patients with a Stargardt-like phenotype, including the *ABCA4*, *STGD4*, *ELOV4*, and *RDS/peripherin* genes. ABCA4 gene mutations are responsible for the majority of cases of Stargardt disease. The *ABCA4* gene encodes a protein called RIM protein, which is a member of the adenosine triphosphate (ATP)-binding cassette transporter family. It is expressed in the rims of rod and cone photoreceptor disc membranes and is involved in the transport of vitamin A derivatives to the RPE. The most striking feature on light and electron microscopy is the marked engorgement of RPE cells (Fig 11-34C and D; see also Fig 9-9, BCSC Section 12, *Retina and Vitreous*) with lipofuscin-like, PAS-positive material, with apical displacement of the normal RPE melanin granules.

Best disease

Best disease, or Best vitelliform macular dystrophy, is a dominantly inherited, early-onset macular degenerative disease that exhibits some histopathologic similarities to AMD. The diagnosis of Best disease is based on the presence of a vitelliform lesion (see Fig 9-10, BCSC Section 12, *Retina and Vitreous*) or pigmentary changes in the central macula and a reduced ratio of the light peak to dark trough in the electro-oculogram. Recently, mutations in the *VMD2* gene on chromosome 11q13 encoding the bestrophin protein were identified in Best disease. The gene product, bestrophin, localizes to the basolateral plasma membrane of the RPE and represents a newly identified family of chloride ion channels. Investigators have reported that bestrophins are volume-sensitive and may play a role in cell volume regulation in the RPE cells.

> Fischmeister R, Hartzell HC. Volume sensitivity of the bestrophin family of chloride channels. *J Physiol.* 2005;562:477–491.

168 • Ophthalmic Pathology and Intraocular Tumors

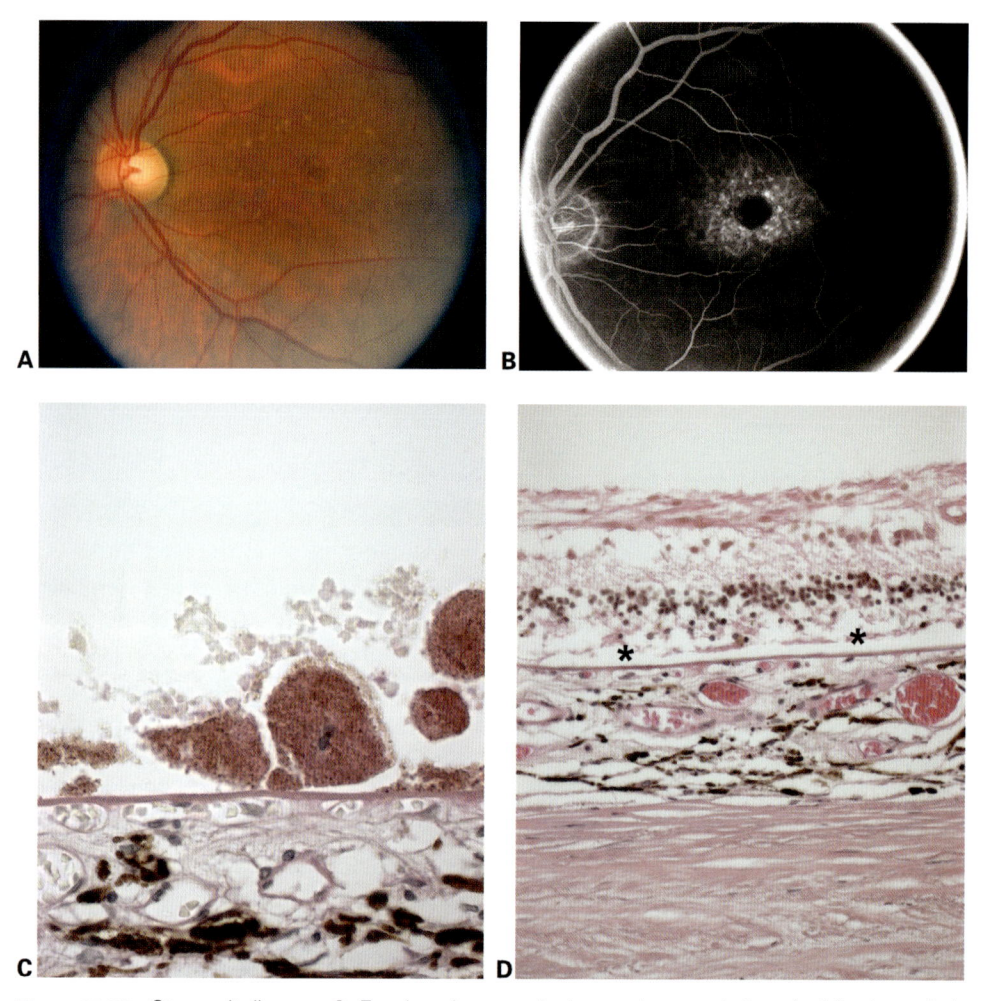

Figure 11-34 Stargardt disease. **A,** Fundus photograph shows characteristic retinal flecks and pigment mottling in the macular region. **B,** Fluorescein angiogram (midphase) shows late hyperfluorescence in a "bull's-eye" pattern in the central macula. Note the dark choroid (eg, absence of normal background choroidal blush), which is characteristic of Stargardt disease. **C,** Histopathology with periodic acid–Schiff (PAS) stain discloses hypertrophic RPE cells with numerous PAS-positive cytoplasmic granules containing lipofuscin. This histopathologic finding corresponds to the retinal flecks seen clinically. **D,** In advanced stages of Stargardt disease, geographic RPE atrophy with loss of the photoreceptor cell layer *(asterisks)* may be observed. *(Courtesy of Sander Dubovy, MD.)*

> Marmorstein AD, Marmorstein LY, Rayborn M, Wang X, Hollyfield JG, Petrukhin K. Bestrophin, the product of the Best vitelliform macular dystrophy gene (VMD2), localizes to the basolateral plasma membrane of the retinal pigment epithelium. *Proc Natl Acad Sci USA.* 2000;97:12758–12763.

Pattern dystrophy

Pattern dystrophy is a heterogeneous group of retinal dystrophies that includes butterfly-shaped pattern dystrophy (BPD) and adult-onset foveomacular vitelliform dystrophy (AFMVD). BPD is characterized by a butterfly-shaped, irregular, depigmented lesion at the level of the RPE. AFMVD is characterized by the presence of slightly elevated, symmetric, solitary, round to oval, yellow lesions at the level of the RPE (Fig 11-35; see also

CHAPTER 11: Retina and Retinal Pigment Epithelium • 169

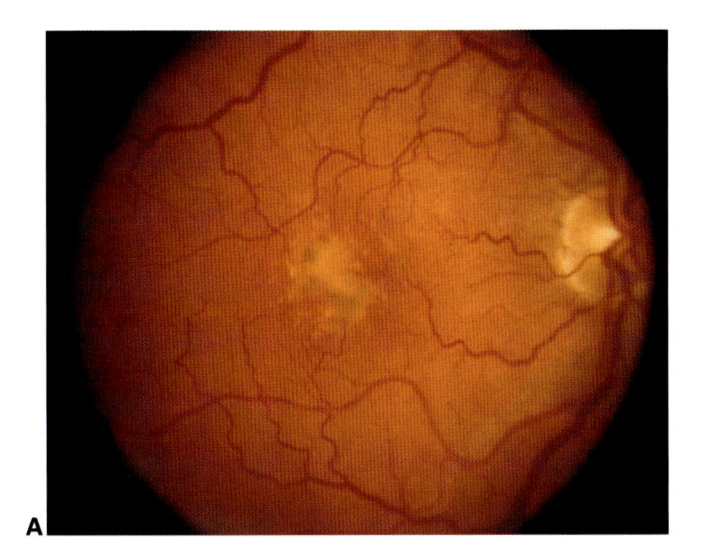

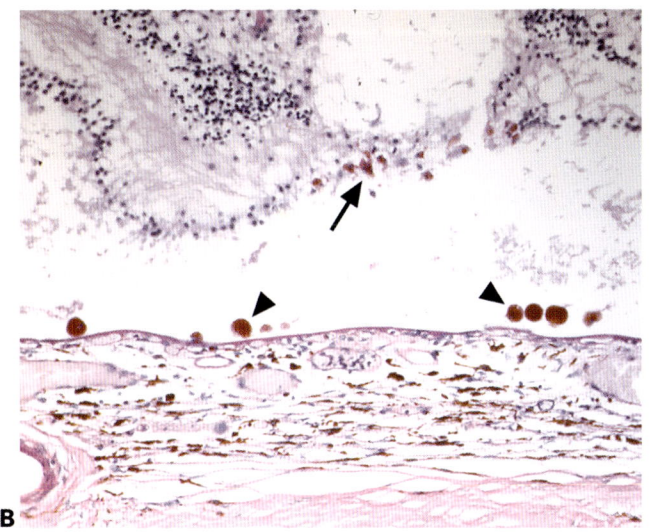

Figure 11-35 Adult-onset foveomacular vitelliform dystrophy. **A,** Yellowish, egg yoke–like lesion in the central macula. **B,** Histopathologic findings include pigment-containing cells in the subretinal space *(arrowheads)* and outer neurosensory retina *(arrow).* **C,** Electron microscopy shows pigment-containing cells filled with lipofuscin *(arrowheads). (Courtesy of Sander Dubovy, MD.)*

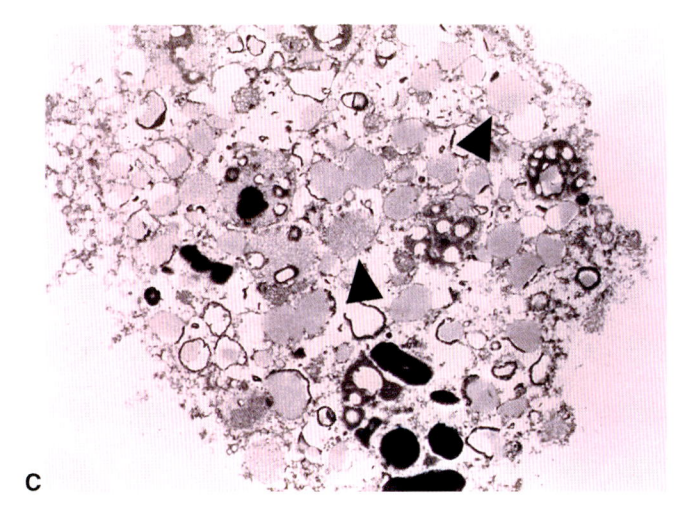

170 • Ophthalmic Pathology and Intraocular Tumors

Fig 9-11, BCSC Section 12, *Retina and Vitreous*). Optical coherence tomography (OCT) has demonstrated elevation of the photoreceptor layer, with localization of the dystrophic material between the photoreceptors and RPE. The most common genetic mutation associated with the pattern dystrophies is in the *RDS/peripherin* gene. Histopathologic studies reveal central loss of the RPE and photoreceptor cell layer, with a moderate number of pigment-containing macrophages in the subretinal space and outer retina (see Fig 11-35). To either side, the RPE is distended with lipofuscin. Basal laminar and linear deposits are present throughout the macular region. The pathologic finding of pigmented cells with lipofuscin in the subretinal space correlates clinically with the vitelliform appearance.

> Dubovy SR, Hairston RJ, Schatz H, et al. Adult-onset foveomacular pigment epithelial dystrophy: clinicopathologic correlation of three cases. *Retina*. 2000;20:638–649.

See BCSC Section 12, *Retina and Vitreous,* for further discussion and illustrations of macular dystrophies.

Figure 11-36 Retinitis pigmentosa. **A,** Fundus photograph shows mild optic atrophy, marked retinal arteriolar narrowing and bone spicule pigmentation in the fundus. **B,** Histopathologically, note the marked loss of photoreceptor cells and RPE pigment migration into the retina in a perivascular distribution, corresponding to the bone spicule–like pattern seen clinically. The retina is artifactitiously detached. *(Part A courtesy of Robert H. Rosa, Jr, MD.)*

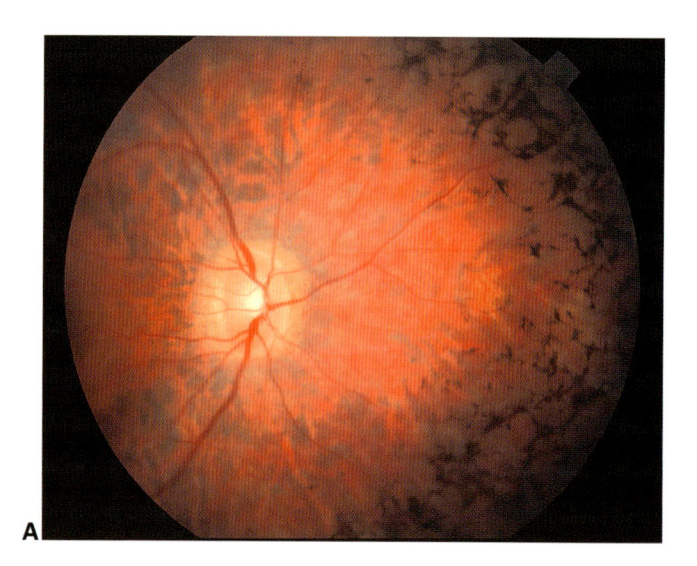

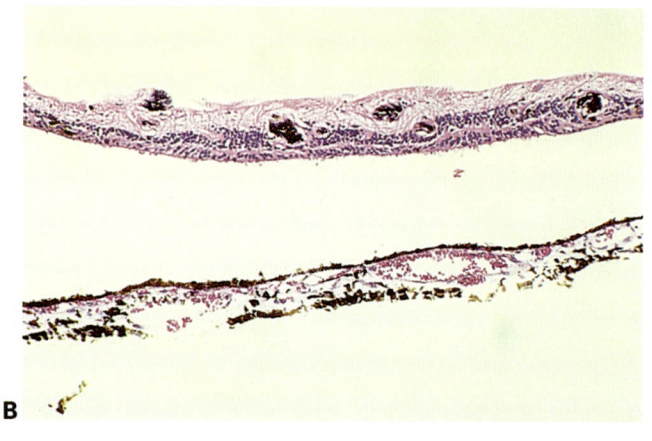

Generalized Chorioretinal Degeneration

The term *retinitis pigmentosa* is a misnomer, because clear evidence of inflammation is lacking. Retinitis pigmentosa (RP) is a group of inherited progressive retinal diseases affecting about 1 in 3500 people worldwide. The genetics of RP are complex. It can be sporadic, autosomal dominant, autosomal recessive, or X-linked. A large number of mutations can cause RP: deletions, insertions, or substitutions—all of which can cause missense, mutations, or truncations. The *RHO, RP1,* and *RPGR* genes contribute the greatest number of known mutations associated with RP. Mutations in the rhodopsin gene *(RHO)* are the most common cause of autosomal dominant RP. The disease is characterized primarily by the loss of rod photoreceptor cells by apoptosis. Cones are seldom directly affected by the identified mutations; however, they degenerate secondarily to rods.

Ophthalmoscopic findings include pigment arranged in a bone spicule–like configuration around the retinal arterioles, arteriolar narrowing, and optic disc atrophy (Fig 11-36). Microscopically, photoreceptor cell loss occurs, as well as RPE hyperplasia with migration into the retina around retinal vessels. The arterioles, although narrowed clinically, show no histologic abnormality initially. Later, thickening and hyalinization of the vessel walls appear. The optic nerve may show diffuse or sectoral atrophy, with gliosis as a late change.

Ben-Arie-Weintrob Y, Berson EL, Dryja TP. Histopathologic-genotypic correlations in retinitis pigmentosa and allied diseases. *Ophthalmic Genet.* 2005;26:91–100.

Neoplasia

Retinoblastoma

Retinoblastoma is the most common primary intraocular malignancy in childhood, occurring in 1 in 14,000–20,000 live births; the incidence varies slightly from country to country. Chapter 19 in this volume discusses retinoblastoma at length, from a more clinical point of view. Several other volumes of the BCSC cover various aspects of this topic as well; consult the *Master Index.* For American Joint Committee on Cancer (AJCC) definitions and staging of retinoblastoma, see Table A-3 in the appendix.

Pathogenesis

Although retinoblastoma was once considered to be of glial origin (lesions clinically simulating retinoblastoma were formerly called *pseudogliomas*), the neuroblastic origin of this tumor from the nucleated layers of the retina has now been established. Immunohistochemical studies have demonstrated that tumor cells stain positive for neuron-specific enolase, rod–outer segment photoreceptor–specific S antigen, and rhodopsin. Tumor cells also secrete an extracellular substance known as *interphotoreceptor retinoid-binding protein,* a product of normal photoreceptors. Recently, retinoblastoma tumor cells grown in culture have been shown to express a red and a green photopigment gene, as well as cone cell alpha subunits of transducin. These findings further support the concept that retinoblastoma may be a neoplasm of cone cell lineage. However, continuing immunohistochemical and molecular studies are adding data that complicate the hypothesis that a single cell type is the progenitor of retinoblastoma. The presence of small amounts of glial tissue within retinoblastoma suggests that tumor cells may possess the ability to differentiate into astroglia or that the resident glial cells proliferate in response to primary neoplastic cells.

The so-called *retinoblastoma gene,* localized to the long arm of chromosome 13, is deceptively named, as it does not actively cause retinoblastoma. The normal gene *suppresses* the development of retinoblastoma (and possibly other tumors, such as osteosarcoma). Retinoblastoma develops when both homologous loci of the suppressor gene become nonfunctional either by a deletion error or by mutation. Although 1 normal gene is sufficient to suppress the development of retinoblastoma, the presence of 1 normal gene and 1 abnormal gene is apparently an unstable situation that may lead to mutation in the normal gene and the loss of tumor suppression, thus allowing retinoblastoma to develop.

> Dryja TP, Cavenee W, White R, et al. Homozygosity of chromosome 13 in retinoblastoma. *N Engl J Med.* 1984;310:550–553.

Histologic features

Histologically, retinoblastoma consists of cells with round, oval, or spindle-shaped nuclei that are approximately twice the size of a lymphocyte (Fig 11-37). Nuclei are hyperchromatic and surrounded by an almost imperceptible amount of cytoplasm. Mitotic activity is usually high, although pyknotic nuclei may make this difficult to assess. As tumors expand into the vitreous or subretinal space, they frequently outgrow their blood supply, creating a characteristic pattern of necrosis; calcification is a common finding in areas of necrosis (Fig 11-38). Cuffs of viable cells course along blood vessels with regions of ischemic necrosis beginning 90–120 μm from nutrient vessels. DNA released from necrotic cells may be detected within tumor vessels and within blood vessels in tissues remote from the tumor, such as the iris. Neovascularization of the iris can complicate retinoblastoma (Fig 11-39).

Cells shed from retinoblastoma tumors remain viable in the vitreous and subretinal space, and they may eventually give rise to implants throughout the eye. It may be difficult to determine histologically whether multiple intraocular foci of the tumor represent multiple

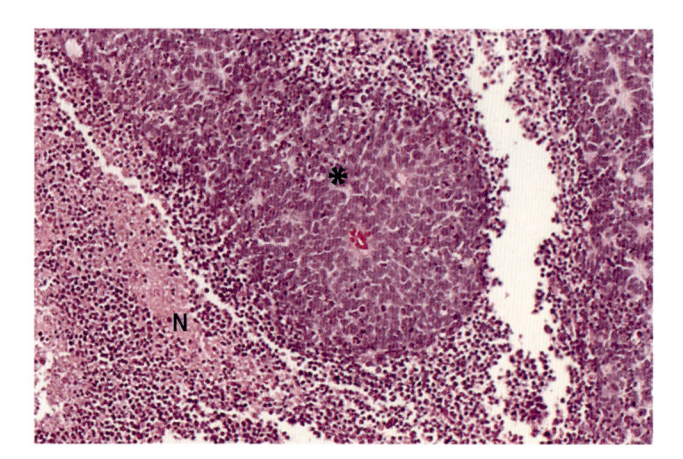

Figure 11-37 Retinoblastoma. Note the viable tumor *(asterisk)* aggregated around a blood vessel, and the alternating zones of necrosis *(N).*

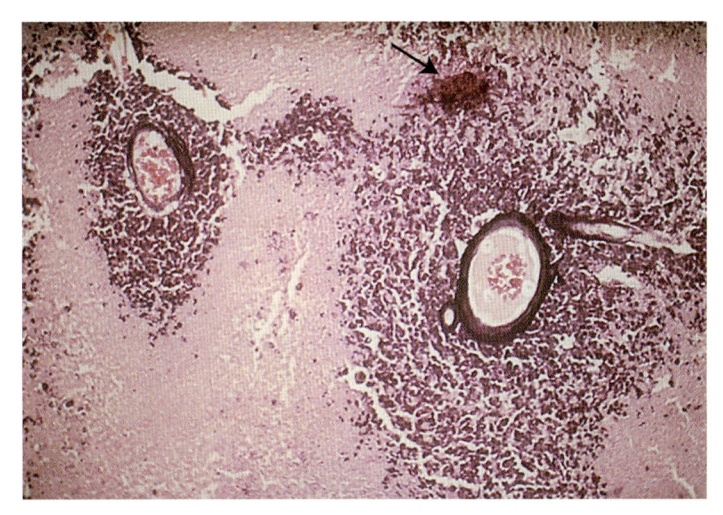

CHAPTER 11: Retina and Retinal Pigment Epithelium • 173

Figure 11-38 Retinoblastoma. Zones of viable tumor (usually surrounding blood vessels) alternate with zones of tumor necrosis. Calcium *(arrow)* is present in the necrotic area. The basophilic material surrounding the blood vessels is DNA, presumably liberated from the necrotic tumor.

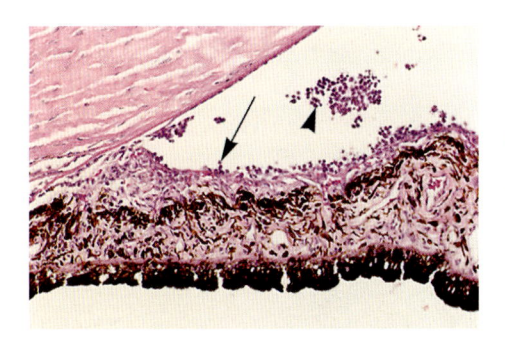

Figure 11-39 Retinoblastoma. Note the thick iris neovascular membrane *(arrow)* and the free-floating tumor cells *(arrowhead)* in the anterior chamber.

primary tumors, implying a systemic distribution of the abnormal gene, or tumor seeds (see Fig 19-6 in Chapter 19).

The formation of highly organized *Flexner-Wintersteiner rosettes* is a characteristic feature of retinoblastoma that does not occur in other neuroblastic tumors, with the rare exception of some pinealoblastomas and ectopic intracranial retinoblastomas. Flexner-Wintersteiner rosettes are expressions of retinal differentiation. The cells of these rosettes surround a central lumen lined by a refractile structure. The refractile lining corresponds to the external limiting membrane of the retina that represents sites of attachments between photoreceptors and Müller cells. The rosette is characterized by a single row of columnar cells with eosinophilic cytoplasm and peripherally situated nuclei (Fig 11-40A). The chromatin of cell nuclei in rosettes is usually looser than that of nuclei from undifferentiated cells in adjacent tumor.

A less commonly encountered rosette, without features of retinal differentiation, known as the *Homer Wright rosette,* can be found in other neuroblastic tumors, such as neuroblastoma and medulloblastoma of the cerebellum, as well as in retinoblastoma. The

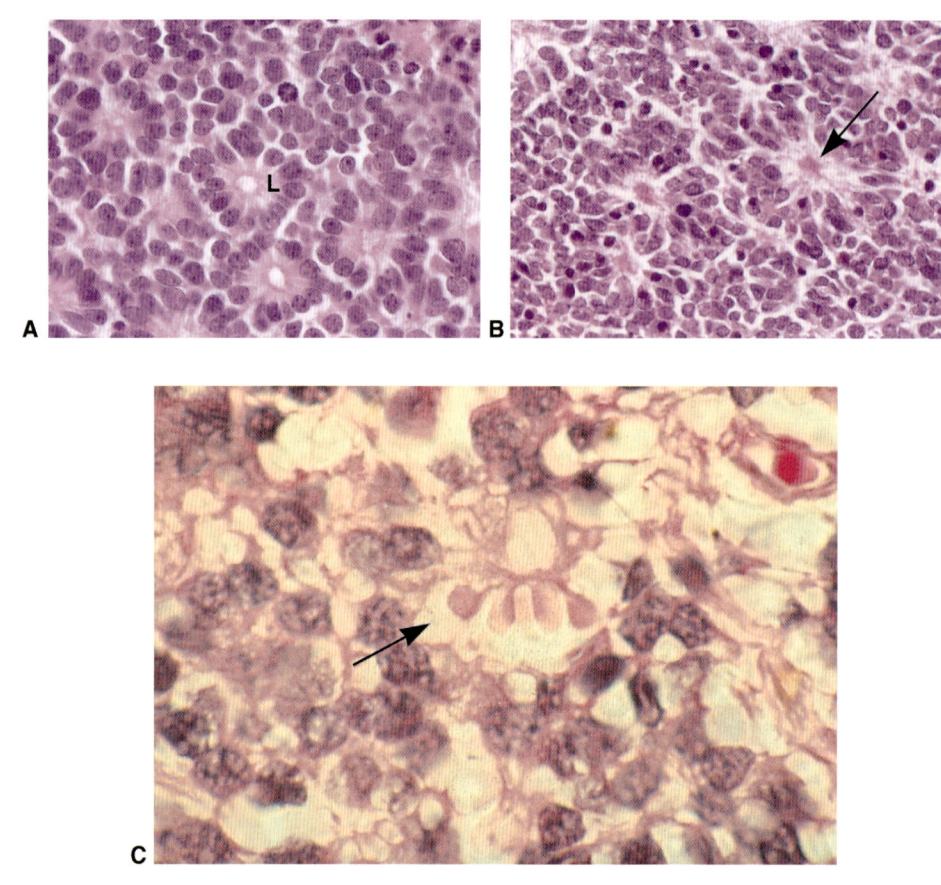

174 • Ophthalmic Pathology and Intraocular Tumors

Figure 11-40 Retinoblastoma rosettes. **A,** Flexner-Wintersteiner rosettes: note the central lumen *(L)*. **B,** Homer Wright rosettes: note the neurofibrillary tangle *(arrow)* in the center of these structures. **C,** The fleurette *(arrow)* demonstrates bulbous cellular extension of retinoblastoma cells that represent differentiation along the lines of photoreceptor inner segments.

lumen of a Homer Wright rosette is filled with a tangle of eosinophilic cytoplasmic processes (Fig 11-40B).

Evidence of photoreceptor differentiation has also been documented for another flowerlike structure known as a *fleurette*. Fleurettes are curvilinear clusters of cells composed of rod and cone inner segments that are often attached to abortive outer segments (Fig 11-40C). The fleurette expresses a greater degree of retinal differentiation than does the Flexner-Wintersteiner rosette. In a typical retinoblastoma, the undifferentiated tumor cells greatly outnumber the fleurettes and Flexner-Wintersteiner rosettes, and differentiation is not an important prognostic indicator.

Progression

The most common route for retinoblastoma tumor to escape from the eye is by way of the optic nerve. Direct infiltration of the optic nerve can lead to extension into the brain. Cells that spread into the leptomeninges can gain access to the subarachnoid space, with the

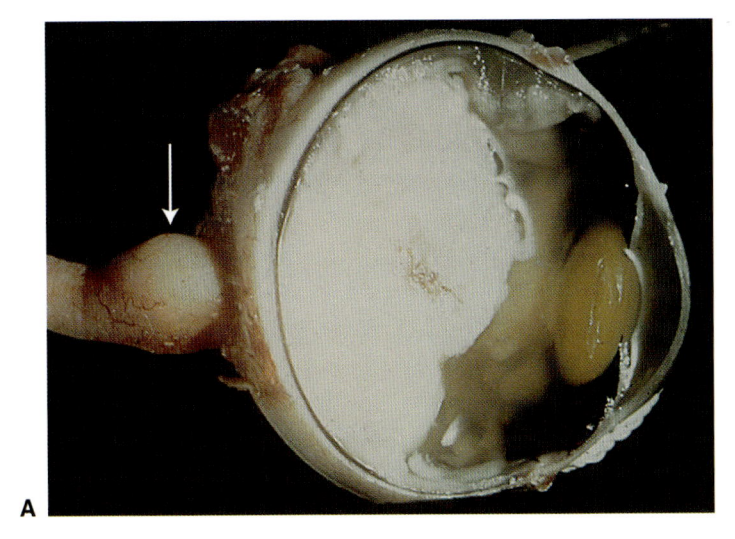

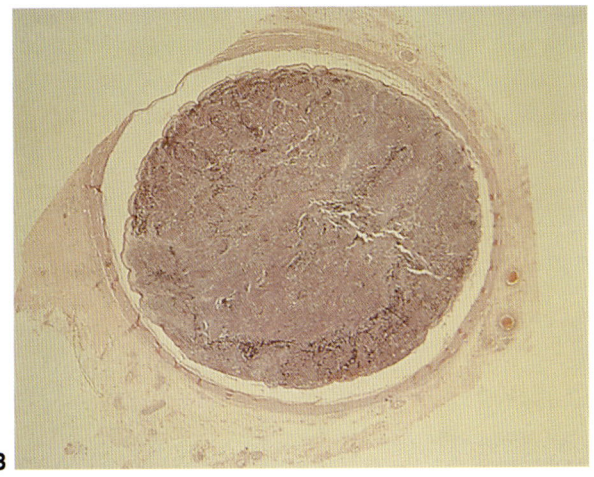

CHAPTER 11: Retina and Retinal Pigment Epithelium • 175

Figure 11-41 Retinoblastoma. **A,** Massive invasion of the globe posteriorly by retinoblastoma with bulbous enlargement of the optic nerve *(arrow)* caused by direct extension. **B,** A cross section of the optic nerve taken at the surgical margin of transection. Tumor is present in the nerve at this point, and the prognosis is poor.

potential for seeding throughout the central nervous system (Fig 11-41). Invasion of the optic nerve is a poor prognostic sign (Fig 11-42). See Chapter 19 for a discussion of prognosis.

Massive uveal invasion, in contrast, theoretically increases the risk of hematogenous dissemination. Spread to regional lymph nodes may be seen when a tumor involving the anterior segment grows into the conjunctival substantia propria, especially when the filtration angle is involved.

Spontaneous regression of retinoblastoma
Spontaneous regression of retinoblastoma is discussed in Chapter 19.

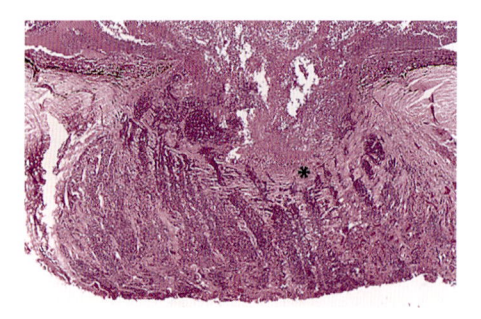

Figure 11-42 Retinoblastoma has invaded the optic nerve and extended to the margin of resection posterior to the lamina cribrosa *(asterisk)*. This is an extremely poor prognostic sign.

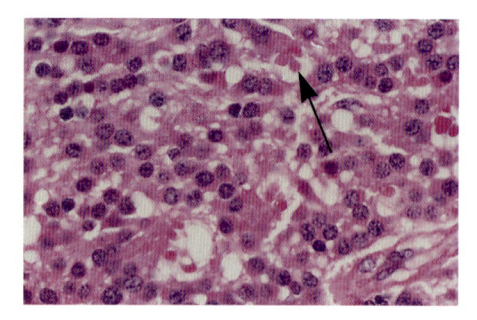

Figure 11-43 Retinocytoma. Note the exquisite degree of photoreceptor differentiation with apparent stubby inner segments *(arrow)*.

Retinocytoma

Retinocytoma is characterized histologically by numerous fleurettes admixed with individual cells that demonstrate varying degrees of photoreceptor differentiation (Fig 11-43). Retinocytoma should be distinguished from the spontaneous regression of retinoblastoma that is the end result of coagulative necrosis. See the discussion in Chapter 19.

Also referred to as *retinoma,* retinocytoma differs from retinoblastoma in the following ways:

- Retinocytoma cells have more cytoplasm and more evenly dispersed nuclear chromatin than do retinoblastoma cells. Mitoses are not observed in retinocytoma.
- Although calcification may be identified in retinocytoma, necrosis is usually absent.

Trilateral retinoblastoma

Trilateral retinoblastoma is discussed in Chapter 19.

Secondary malignancies

Patients with the genetic form of retinoblastoma have an increased risk for the development of secondary malignancies. The most common secondary malignancy is osteosarcoma. External-beam radiation therapy increases the risk of secondary malignancy. See Chapter 19 for more complete discussion of both genetic counseling for and management of retinoblastoma.

Medulloepithelioma

Also known as *diktyoma,* medulloepithelioma is a congenital neuroepithelial tumor arising from primitive medullary epithelium. This tumor usually occurs in the ciliary body but has also been documented in the retina and optic nerve. Clinically, medulloepithelioma may appear as a lightly pigmented or amelanotic, cystic mass in the ciliary body, with erosion into the anterior chamber and iris root (see Fig 23-1 in Part II, Intraocular Tumors). Although the tumor develops before the medullary epithelium shows substantial signs of differentiation, cells are organized into ribbonlike structures that have a distinct cellular

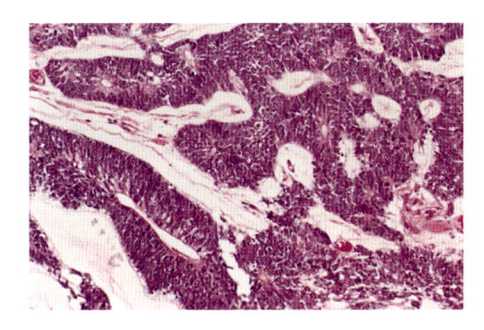

Figure 11-44 Medulloepithelioma. Histopathology shows ribbons and cords of tumor cells that seem to recapitulate the morphology of the ciliary epithelium.

polarity (Fig 11-44). These ribbonlike structures are composed of undifferentiated round to oval cells possessing little cytoplasm. Cell nuclei are stratified in 3 to 5 layers, and the entire structure is lined on one side by a thin basement membrane. One surface secretes a mucinous substance, rich in hyaluronic acid, that resembles primitive vitreous. Stratified sheets of cells are capable of forming mucinous cysts that are clinically characteristic. Homer Wright rosettes can also be seen.

Medulloepitheliomas that contain solid masses of neuroblastic cells indistinguishable from retinoblastoma are more difficult to classify. Medulloepitheliomas that have substantial numbers of undifferentiated cells with high mitotic rates and that demonstrate tissue invasion are considered malignant, although patients treated with enucleation have high survival rates, and "malignant" medulloepithelioma typically follows a relatively benign course if the tumor remains confined to the eye.

Heteroplastic tissue, such as cartilage or smooth muscle, may be found in medulloepitheliomas. Tumors composed of cells from 2 different embryonic germ layers are referred to as *teratoid medulloepitheliomas*. Malignant teratoid medulloepitheliomas demonstrate either solid areas of undifferentiated neuroblastic cells or sarcomatous transformation of heteroplastic elements.

Fuchs Adenoma

Fuchs adenoma, an acquired tumor of the nonpigmented epithelium of the ciliary body, may be associated with sectoral cataract and may simulate other iris or ciliary body neoplasms. Fuchs adenomas consist of hyperplastic, nonpigmented ciliary epithelium arranged in sheets and tubules with alternating areas of PAS-positive basement membrane material.

Combined Hamartoma of the Retina and RPE

A combined hamartoma of the retina and RPE is characterized clinically by the presence of a slightly elevated, variably pigmented mass involving the RPE, peripapillary retina, optic nerve, and overlying vitreous (see Fig 17-15). Frequently, a preretinal membrane is present that distorts the tumor's inner retinal surface. The lesion is often diagnosed in childhood, supporting a probable hamartomatous origin, but it is possible that the vascular changes are primary, with secondary changes in the adjacent RPE.

The tumor is characterized by thickening of the optic nerve head and peripapillary retina, with an increased number of vessels. The RPE is hyperplastic and frequently migrates into a perivascular location. Vitreous condensation and fibroglial proliferation may be present on the surface of the tumor.

Other Retinal Tumors

Other tumors of the retina are very rare. Massive gliosis of the retina may occur secondary to chronic retinal detachment or chronic inflammation. Various retinal tumors occur in association with some phakomatoses, including astrocytic hamartomas in tuberous sclerosis and hemangioblastomas in von Hippel–Lindau disease. The phakomatoses are discussed in BCSC Section 5, *Neuro-Ophthalmology,* and Section 6, *Pediatric Ophthalmology and Strabismus.*

Adenomas and Adenocarcinomas of the RPE

Neoplasia of the RPE is uncommon and is distinguished from hyperplasia of the RPE principally by the absence of a history or pathologic features suggesting prior trauma or eye disease. *Adenomas* of the RPE typically retain characteristics of RPE cells, including basement membranes, cell junctions, and microvilli. *Adenocarcinomas* are distinguished from adenomas by greater anaplasia, mitotic activity, and invasion of the choroid or retina. No metastases have ever been documented to occur in patients with RPE adenocarcinomas.

Spencer WH, ed. *Ophthalmic Pathology: An Atlas and Textbook.* 4th ed. Philadelphia: Saunders; 1997:1291–1313.

CHAPTER 12

Uveal Tract

Topography

The *iris, ciliary body,* and *choroid* constitute the uveal tract (Fig 12-1). The uveal tract is embryologically derived from mesoderm and neural crest. Firm attachments between the uveal tract and the sclera exist at only 3 sites:

1. scleral spur
2. exit points of the vortex veins
3. optic nerve

Iris

The iris is located in front of the crystalline lens. It separates the anterior segment of the eye into 2 compartments, the anterior chamber and the posterior chamber, and forms a circular aperture (pupil) that controls the amount of light transmitted into the eye. The iris is composed of 5 layers:

1. anterior border layer
2. stroma
3. muscular layer
4. anterior pigment epithelium
5. posterior pigment epithelium

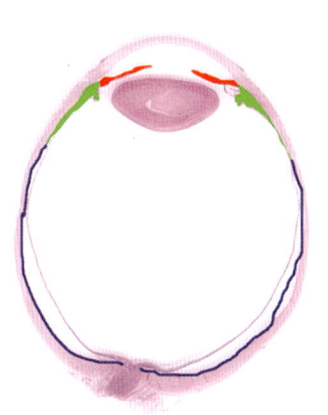

Figure 12-1 Uveal topography. The uveal tract consists of the iris *(red)*, the ciliary body *(green)*, and the choroid *(blue)*. *(Courtesy of Nasreen A. Syed, MD.)*

The anterior border layer represents a condensation of iris stroma and melanocytes and is coarsely ribbed with numerous crypts (Fig 12-2). The stroma contains blood vessels, nerves, melanocytes, fibrocytes, and clump cells. The clump cells are both macrophages containing phagocytosed pigment (type I, or clump cells of Koganei) and variants of smooth muscle cells (type II clump cells). The vessels within the stroma appear thick-walled because of a thick collar of collagen fibrils. The dilator and sphincter muscle make up the muscular layer. The posterior portion of the iris is lined by the anterior and posterior pigment epithelium, which is composed of a double layer of pigment epithelium arranged in an apex-to-apex configuration. The cell body of the anterior pigment epithelium gives rise to the dilator muscle. The color of the iris is determined by the number and size of the melanin pigment granules in the stromal melanocytes.

Ciliary Body

The ciliary body, which is approximately 6.0–6.5 mm wide, extends from the base of the iris and becomes continuous with the choroid at the ora serrata. The ciliary body is composed of 2 areas:

1. the *pars plicata*, which contains the ciliary processes
2. the *pars plana*

The inner portion of the ciliary body is lined by a double layer of epithelial cells, the inner nonpigmented layer and the outer pigmented layer (Fig 12-3). The zonular fibers of the lens attach to the ciliary body processes. The ciliary muscle has 3 types of fibers:

1. longitudinal fibers (Brücke's muscle)
2. radial fibers
3. the innermost circular fibers (Müller's muscle)

These fiber groups function as a group during accommodation.

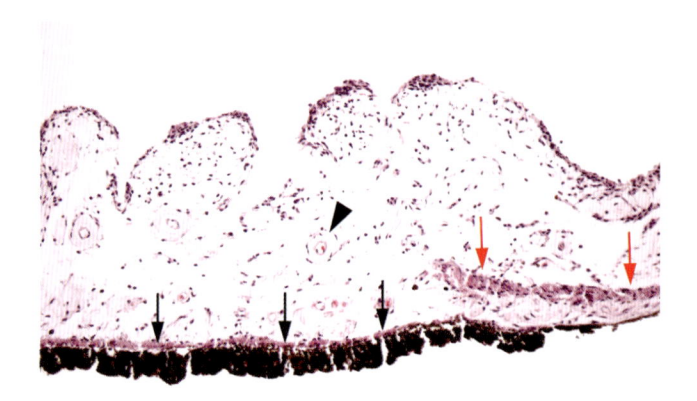

Figure 12-2 Histologic appearance of the iris: the anterior border layer is thrown into numerous crypts and folds. The sphincter muscle *(red arrows)* is present at the papillary border, whereas the dilator muscle *(black arrows)* lies just anterior to the posterior pigment epithelium. Normal iris vessels demonstrate a thick collagen cuff *(arrowhead)*. *(Courtesy of Nasreen A. Syed, MD.)*

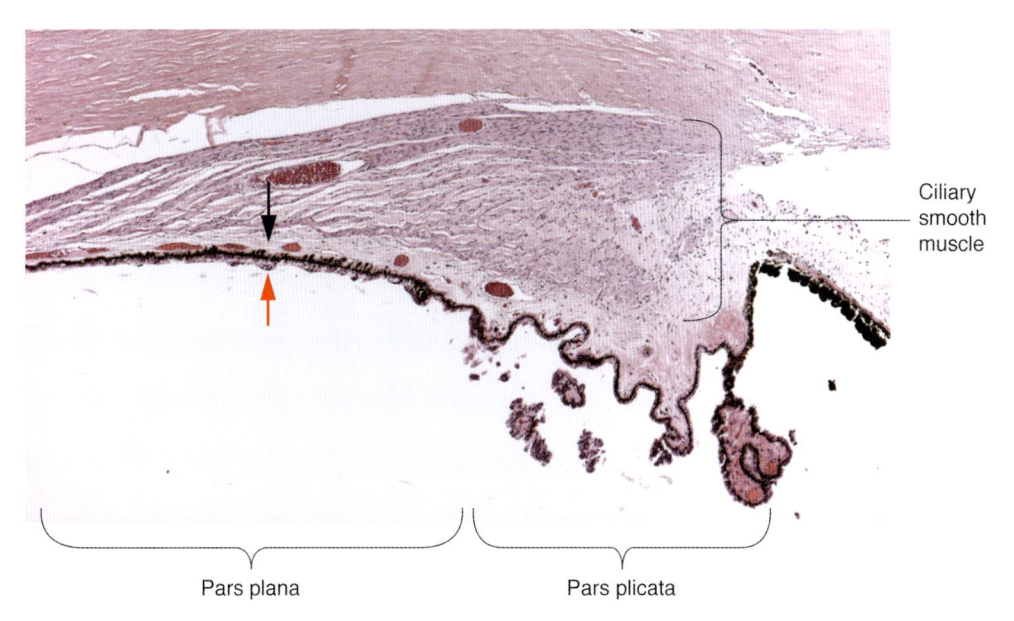

Figure 12-3 Normal ciliary body. The ciliary body is lined with a double layer of epithelium. The inner layer is nonpigmented *(red arrow)* and the outer layer is pigmented *(black arrow)*. *(Courtesy of Nasreen A. Syed, MD.)*

Choroid

The choroid is the pigmented vascular tissue that forms the middle coat of the posterior part of the eye. It extends from the ora serrata anteriorly to the optic nerve posteriorly and consists of 3 principal layers:

1. lamina fusca (suprachoroid layer)
2. stroma
3. choriocapillaris

The choriocapillaris provides nutrients for the retinal pigment epithelium (RPE) and the outer retinal layers (Fig 12-4).

Congenital Anomalies

The entities described in the following sections are discussed in detail in BCSC Section 2, *Fundamentals and Principles of Ophthalmology,* and Section 6, *Pediatric Ophthalmology and Strabismus.*

Aniridia

True aniridia, or complete absence of the iris, is rare. Most cases of aniridia are incomplete, and a narrow rim of rudimentary iris tissue is present peripherally. Aniridia is usually bilateral, although it may be asymmetric. Histologically, the rudimentary iris consists

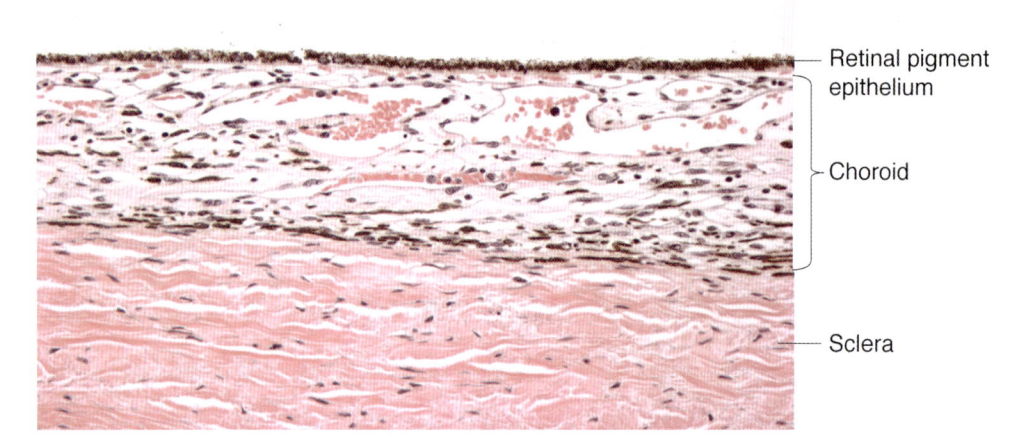

Figure 12-4 The choroid is a vascular, pigmented structure present between the retina and the sclera. The layer closest to the pigment epithelium is composed of capillaries and is known as the *choriocapillaris.* *(Courtesy of Nasreen A. Syed, MD.)*

of underdeveloped ectodermal–mesodermal neural crest elements. The anterior chamber angle is often incompletely developed, and peripheral anterior synechiae with an overgrowth of corneal endothelium are often present. These changes are most likely responsible for the high incidence of glaucoma associated with aniridia. Other ocular findings in aniridia include cataract, corneal pannus, and foveal hypoplasia.

Both autosomal dominant and recessive inheritance patterns for aniridia have been described. An association between sporadic aniridia and an increased incidence of Wilms tumor has been linked to 11p13 deletions and to mutations in the *PAX6* gene located in the same region. Microcephaly, mental retardation, and genitourinary abnormalities have also been described in association with aniridia.

> Hanson IM, Seawright A, Hardman K, et al. PAX6 mutations in aniridia. *Hum Mol Genet.* 1993;2:915–920.

Coloboma

A coloboma—the absence of part or all of an ocular tissue—may affect the iris, ciliary body, choroid, or all 3 structures. Colobomas may occur as isolated defects or as portions of more complex malformations. Typical colobomas occur as a result of faulty closure of the fetal fissure (optic groove) anywhere from the optic disc to the pupil in the inferonasal meridian. Atypical colobomas occur in locations outside the region of the fetal fissure. More than half of typical colobomas are bilateral, although they may be asymmetric.

Inflammations

BCSC Section 9, *Intraocular Inflammation and Uveitis,* discusses the conditions described in the following sections and also explains in depth the immunologic processes involved.

Infectious

The uveal tract may be involved in infectious processes that either seem restricted to a single intraocular structure or that may be part of a generalized inflammation affecting several or all coats of the eye. If the source of the infectious agent is introduced from outside the body, as with posttraumatic bacterial infection, the infection is termed *exogenous*. If, however, the infection originates elsewhere in the body, such as with a ruptured diverticulum, and subsequently spreads hematogenously to involve the uveal tract, the infection is referred to as *endogenous*. A wide variety of organisms have been shown to cause infections of the uveal tract, including bacteria, fungi, viruses, and protozoa. Obtaining a careful clinical history usually helps guide the physician in the consideration of causative agents.

Histopathology often shows a mixed acute and chronic inflammatory infiltrate within the choroid, ciliary body, or iris stroma. In cases of viral, fungal, or protozoal (eg, toxoplasmosis) agents, a granulomatous pattern of inflammation may be observed. Special tissue stains for microorganisms (tissue Gram, Gomori methenamine silver nitrate, PAS, Ziehl-Neelsen) are often helpful in identifying organisms admixed within the inflammatory reaction.

Noninfectious

Sympathetic ophthalmia

Sympathetic ophthalmia is a rare bilateral granulomatous panuveitis that occurs after accidental or surgical injury to 1 eye (the *exciting*, or *inciting*, *eye*) followed by a latent period and development of uveitis in the uninjured globe (the *sympathizing eye*). The inflammation in the sympathizing eye may occur as early as 10 days or as late as 50 years following the suspected triggering incident, but 4–8 weeks is the typical period of latency.

Histologically, a diffuse granulomatous inflammatory reaction appears within the uveal tract composed of lymphocytes and epithelioid histiocytes containing phagocytosed melanin pigment (Figs 12-5, 12-6). Typically, the choriocapillaris is spared. Varying degrees of

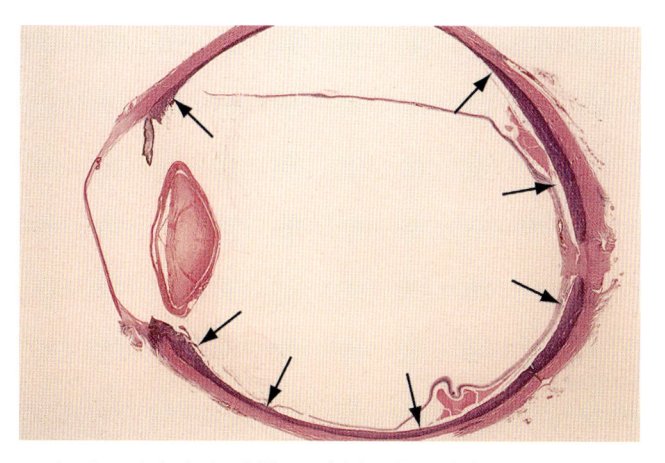

Figure 12-5 Sympathetic ophthalmia. Diffuse thickening of the uveal tract *(arrows)*. *(Courtesy of Hans E. Grossniklaus, MD.)*

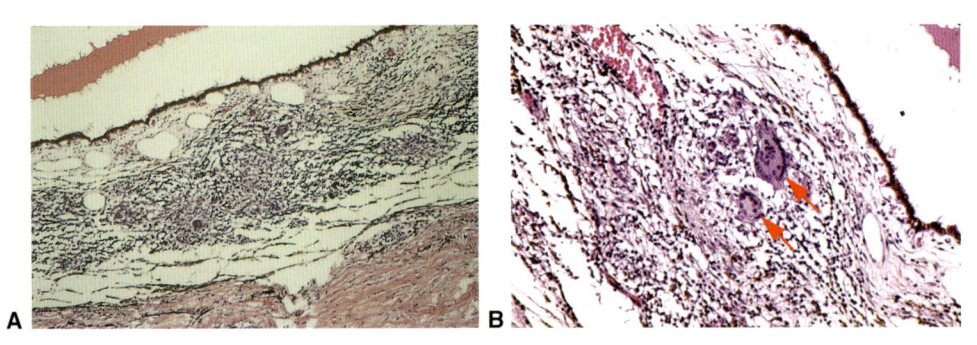

Figure 12-6 Sympathetic ophthalmia. **A,** Diffuse granulomatous inflammation within the choroid. **B,** Higher magnification shows the presence of multinucleated giant cells *(red arrows)*. *(Courtesy of Hans E. Grossniklaus, MD.)*

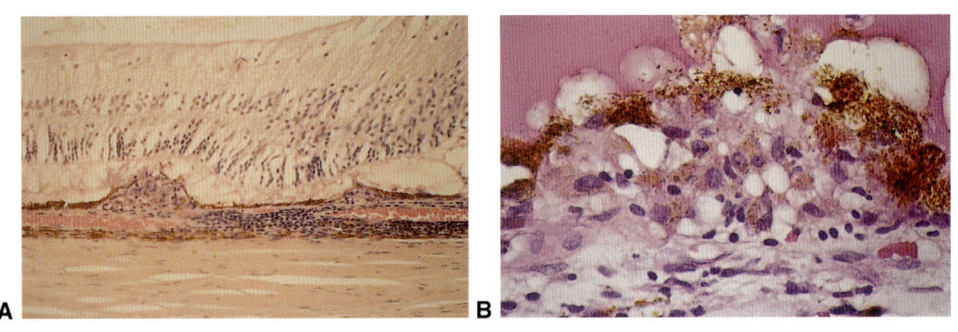

Figure 12-7 Dalen-Fuchs nodules in sympathetic ophthalmia. **A,** Focal collections of inflammatory cells are located between the RPE and Bruch's membrane. **B,** Higher magnification demonstrates the presence of epithelioid histiocytes within the nodules. *(Courtesy of Hans E. Grossniklaus, MD.)*

inflammation may be present in the anterior chamber, as evidenced by collections of histiocytes deposited on the corneal endothelium *(mutton-fat keratic precipitates)*. *Dalen-Fuchs nodules,* which are collections of epithelioid histiocytes and lymphocytes between the RPE and Bruch's membrane, may be seen in some cases (Fig 12-7). However, Dalen-Fuchs nodules may be present in other diseases, such as Vogt-Koyanagi-Harada syndrome, and thus are not pathognomonic of sympathetic ophthalmia.

Although the etiology of sympathetic ophthalmia is not known, the pathogenesis may involve a hypersensitivity to melanin pigment, retinal S-antigen, or other retinal or uveal proteins. Experimental animal studies suggest that the penetrating ocular injury allows antigens to gain access to the lymphatic system, where they are processed and subsequently incite an immune response.

Vogt-Koyanagi-Harada syndrome

Vogt-Koyanagi-Harada (VKH) syndrome is a rare cause of posterior or diffuse uveitis that may have both ocular and systemic manifestations. The syndrome occurs more commonly in patients with Asian or Native American ancestry and usually affects individuals between 30 and 50 years of age. Ocular symptoms include bilateral decreased visual acuity, pain, redness, and photophobia. Systemic manifestations include alopecia, poliosis (loss of pigmentation of eyebrows and eyelashes), vitiligo, dysacusis, headaches, and seizures.

A chronic, diffuse granulomatous uveitis resembles that seen in sympathetic ophthalmia. In classic cases, the entire choroid is involved by the inflammatory reaction, however, without sparing of the choriocapillaris. The granulomatous inflammation may extend to involve the retina. Because the disease is one of exacerbation and remission, chorioretinal scarring and RPE hyperplasia may also be observed. Choroidal neovascularization has been described in some cases, and exudative retinal detachments may occur. The etiology of VKH syndrome is unknown. A proposed mechanism involves an immune reaction to uveal melanin-associated protein, melanocytes, or pigment epithelium. There is a strong association between HLA-DR4 and VKH syndrome.

Sarcoidosis

Sarcoidosis is a multisystem granulomatous disease characterized by inflammatory nodules, which can occur in various organs and tissues. These nodules are composed of collections of noncaseating epithelioid histiocytes admixed with lymphocytes (Fig 12-8). The uveal tract is the most common site of ocular involvement by sarcoidosis. Anteriorly, inflammatory nodules of the iris may be seen, either at the pupillary margin *(Koeppe nodules)* or elsewhere on the iris *(Busacca nodules)*. In the posterior segment, chorioretinitis, periphlebitis, and chorioretinal nodules may be seen. Periphlebitis may appear clinically as inflammatory lesions described as *candlewax drippings*. The optic nerve may be edematous due to inflammatory infiltration. Histologically, the involved tissues show infiltration by noncaseating granulomatous inflammation. Multinucleated giant cells are often present, and *asteroid bodies* (star-shaped, acidophilic bodies) and *Schaumann bodies* (spherical, basophilic, often calcified bodies) may be seen within the giant cells. Neither asteroid nor Schaumann bodies are pathognomonic for sarcoidosis, however.

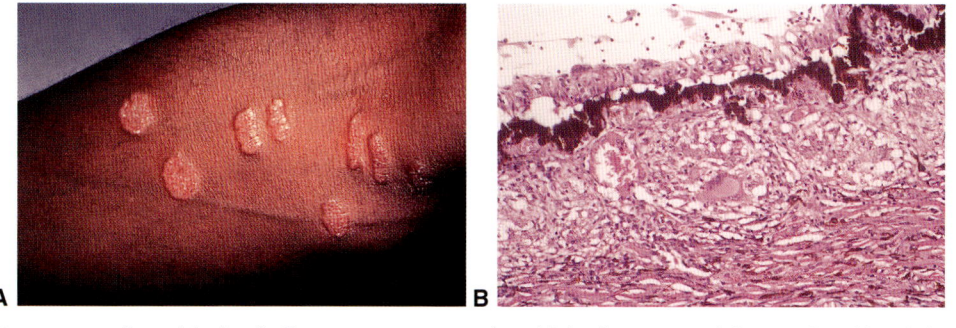

Figure 12-8 Sarcoidosis. **A,** Gross appearance of multiple discrete nodules on the skin of the upper extremity. **B,** Histopathology of sarcoid nodule showing epithelioid histiocytes and multinucleated giant cells. *(Part A courtesy of Curtis E. Margo, MD; part B courtesy of Hans E. Grossniklaus, MD.)*

Degenerations

Rubeosis Iridis

Rubeosis iridis, or neovascularization of the iris, is a common finding in surgically enucleated blind eyes. It may be associated with a wide variety of conditions (Table 12-1). Histopathologically, new vessels grow on the anterior surface of the iris and may extend to involve the angle, causing *neovascular glaucoma,* a secondary type of glaucoma. Initially, the vessels lack supporting tissue and do not possess the encircling thick fibrous cuff seen in normal iris vessels. The anterior surface of the iris leaflets often becomes flattened.

Less commonly, vessels may arise from the posterior surface of the iris. Fibrous tissue develops around the new vessels, creating fibrovascular membranes that line the anterior surface of the iris and cover the chamber angle. Myofibroblasts in the fibrovascular tissue may contract and lead to *ectropion uveae,* a displacement or dragging of the posterior iris pigment epithelium anterior to the level of the sphincter muscle. In the chamber angle, these fibrovascular membranes contribute to the formation of peripheral anterior synechiae. In advanced cases, atrophy of the dilator muscle, attenuation of the pigment epithelium, and stromal fibrosis occur.

A nonprogressive form of rubeosis iridis, consisting of small iris neovascular tufts at the pupillary margin, has also been described. The neovascular tissue may be isolated to 1 sector of the pupillary margin, or it may involve the entire margin. This condition has been described in patients with adult-onset diabetes mellitus and with myotonic dystrophy.

Table 12-1 Conditions Associated With Rubeosis Iridis

Vascular Disorders
Central retinal vein occlusion
Central retinal artery occlusion
Branch retinal vein occlusion
Carotid occlusive disease

Ocular Diseases
Intraocular inflammation
　Infectious (eg, severe corneal ulcer)
　Noninfectious (eg, uveitis)
Retinal detachment
Coats disease
Secondary glaucoma

Surgery and Radiation Therapy
Retinal detachment surgery
Radiation

Systemic Diseases
Diabetes mellitus
Sickle cell disease

Neoplastic Disease
Retinoblastoma
Melanoma of the choroid/iris
Metastatic carcinoma

Trauma

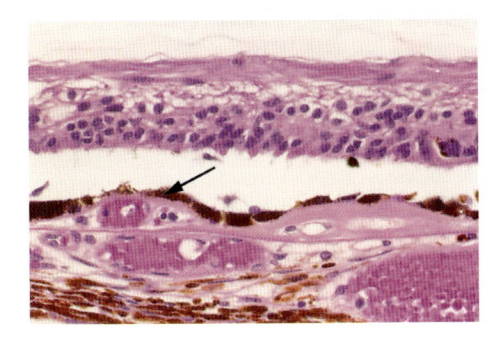

Figure 12-9 Sub-RPE neovascularization. A new blood vessel *(arrow)* lies between the RPE and Bruch's membrane.

Hyalinization of the Ciliary Body

Over time, the ciliary body processes become hyalinized and fibrosed. The thin, delicate processes become blunted and attenuated, and the stroma becomes more eosinophilic. This process is a normal aging change of the ciliary body and is not considered pathologic, although it does contribute functionally to the development of presbyopia.

Choroidal Neovascularization

New blood vessels may grow between the RPE and Bruch's membrane, a condition called *choroidal neovascularization*. Any condition that produces a disruption or break in Bruch's membrane, including age-related macular degeneration (AMD), angioid streaks, ocular histoplasmosis, and trauma, may predispose the eye to choroidal neovascularization. Complications of choroidal neovascularization include serous or hemorrhagic detachment of the RPE or retina, leading to fibrous tissue proliferation and disciform scarring (Fig 12-9). Choroidal neovascularization is discussed at length in BCSC Section 12, *Retina and Vitreous*.

Neoplasia

Iris

Nevus

An *iris nevus* represents a localized proliferation of melanocytic cells that generally appears as a darkly pigmented lesion of the iris stroma with minimal distortion of the iris architecture (see Fig 17-1). In some cases, the nevus may cause a distortion of the pupil or, less commonly, a sectoral cataract. Patients with neurofibromatosis have an increased incidence of iris nevi. There are conflicting data as to whether iris nevi occur more commonly in eyes containing posterior choroidal melanomas.

Iris nevi appear histologically as accumulations of branching dendritic cells or collections of bland-appearing spindle cells. A variety of growth patterns and cytologic appearances is possible, but cellular atypia and significant mitotic activity are not present. If the nevus is located near the pupillary margin, it may cause anterior displacement of the associated posterior pigment epithelium (ectropion uveae).

No treatment is indicated for iris nevi. They should be observed carefully over time, either through the use of photographs or with detailed drawings, to ascertain growth. See Chapter 17 for further discussion.

188 • Ophthalmic Pathology and Intraocular Tumors

Melanoma

Melanomas arising in the iris tend to follow a nonaggressive clinical course compared to posterior melanomas arising in the ciliary body and choroid. The majority of iris melanomas occur in the inferior sectors of the iris (see Fig 17-3). The lesions can be quite vascularized and may occasionally cause spontaneous hyphema. Iris melanomas are uncommon, accounting for between 3.3% and 16.6% of all uveal melanomas. The average age of presentation of patients with iris melanomas is 10–20 years younger than that of patients with posterior melanomas, which ranges between 40 and 50 years. Iris melanomas may occur in the pediatric age group, however.

The modified Callender classification for posterior melanomas (see the discussion later in the chapter) may not be applicable to iris melanomas in terms of prognostic significance, because even iris melanomas containing epithelioid melanoma cell types have a relatively benign course compared with their posterior melanoma counterparts.

Although iris melanomas may grow in a localized aggressive fashion, they rarely metastasize. One exception occurs when melanomas grow to diffusely involve the entire iris stroma (Fig 12-10). In such cases, the melanoma may extend posteriorly into the chamber angle and involve the ciliary body, giving rise to the so-called *ring melanoma*. Cataract and secondary glaucoma may develop as complications of the tumor growth.

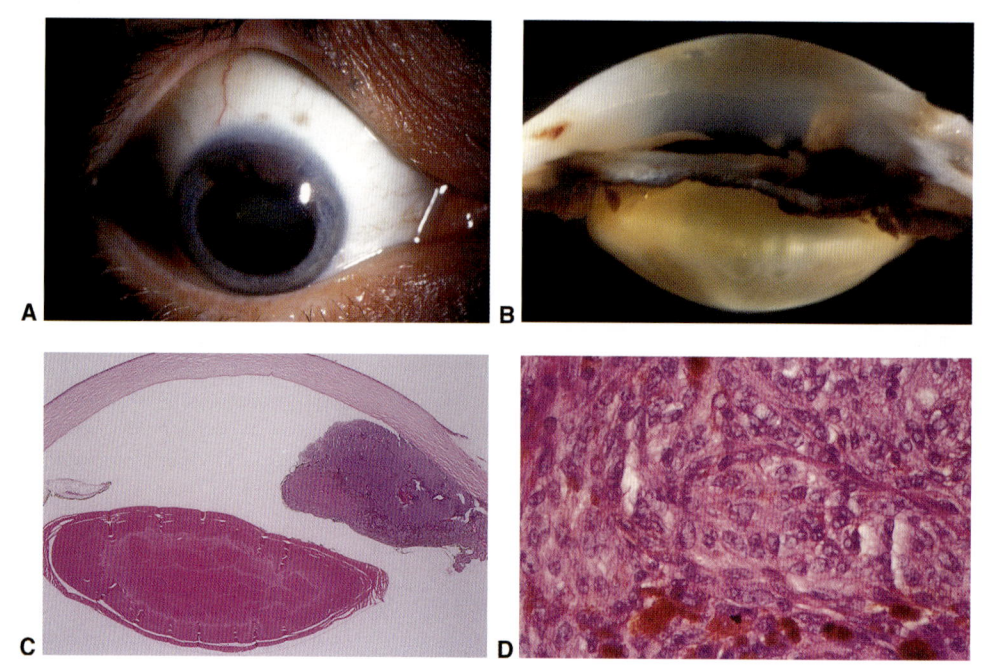

Figure 12-10 **A,** Clinical appearance of iris melanoma. The pigmented tumor is seen occupying the iris superiorly. **B,** Gross appearance of pigmented iris mass. **C,** Low magnification shows the iris melanoma completely replacing the normal iris stroma, extending into the anterior chamber, and touching the posterior cornea. **D,** Histopathology of iris melanoma shows numerous plump epithelioid melanoma cells containing prominent nucleoli. *(Courtesy of Hans E. Grossniklaus, MD.)*

Choroid and Ciliary Body

Nevus

Most nevi of the uveal tract occur in the choroid (see Fig 17-2). One review of 100 nevi showed that fewer than 6% involved the ciliary body; the remainder were present in the choroid. Four types of nevus cells have been described:

1. plump polyhedral
2. slender spindle (Fig 12-11)
3. plump fusiform dendritic
4. balloon cells

Depending on the size and location of the nevus, it may exert nonspecific effects on adjacent ocular tissues. The associated choriocapillaris may become compressed or obliterated, and drusen may be seen overlying the nevus. Less commonly, localized serous detachments of the overlying RPE or neurosensory retina develop.

The majority of choroidal nevi remain stationary over long periods of observation. However, the presence of nevus cells associated with some melanomas supplies evidence that melanomas may arise from previous choroidal nevi.

Melanocytoma

The melanocytoma is a specific type of uveal tract nevus (magnocellular nevus) that warrants separate consideration. These jet black lesions may occur anywhere in the uveal tract, but they most commonly appear in the peripapillary region (see Fig 17-12).

Histologically, a melanocytoma is composed of plump polyhedral cells with small nuclei and abundant cytoplasm. Because the nevus cells are so heavily pigmented, it is usually necessary to obtain bleached sections to accurately study the cytologic features. Areas of cystic degeneration or necrosis may be observed.

Melanoma

Choroidal melanoma is the most common primary intraocular malignancy in adults. The incidence in the United States is approximately 6 cases per million. The tumor is rare in children and primarily affects patients between 50 and 70 years old. Melanomas occur most commonly in whites or other lightly pigmented individuals. Ocular melanocytic conditions

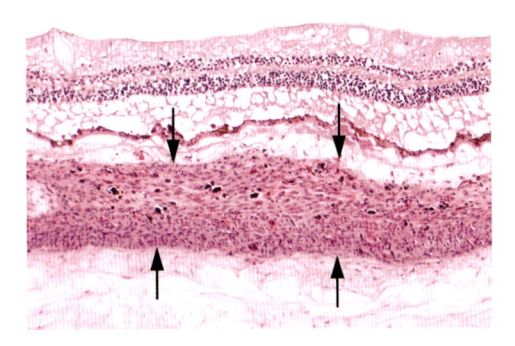

Figure 12-11 Spindle cell nevi *(between arrows)* are composed of slender, spindle-shaped cells with thin, homogeneous nuclei. *(Courtesy of Nasreen A. Syed, MD.)*

such as ocular and oculodermal melanocytosis (nevus of Ota) have been shown to be risk factors for the development of choroidal melanoma.

Ciliary body melanomas may be asymptomatic in their early stages, as they can remain hidden behind the iris. As they enlarge, they may cause displacement of the lens and sectoral cataracts. Ciliary body tumors may erode through the iris root and present as a peripheral iris mass. Other ciliary body melanomas can extend directly through the sclera, creating an epibulbar mass. Dilated episcleral vessels, *sentinel vessels*, may be visible directly over the tumor (see Fig 17-6). In rare cases, the tumor may grow circumferentially to involve the entire ciliary body. This growth pattern is referred to as a *ring melanoma*.

The location and size of posterior choroidal melanomas determine the patient's presenting symptoms. A peripheral lesion may go undetected for a protracted period, whereas a posterior pole tumor affecting the macula and, therefore, vision, may present quite early.

Choroidal melanomas are typically brown, elevated, dome-shaped subretinal masses. The degree of pigmentation is variable, ranging from dark brown to completely amelanotic. Over time, the tumor may break through the overlying Bruch's membrane, producing a collar-button or mushroom-shaped configuration. Prominent clumps of orange pigment (lipofuscin) at the level of the RPE may be present overlying the melanomas, and localized serous detachment of the sensory retina is frequently present.

Several factors have been significantly correlated with survival in patients with choroidal and ciliary body melanomas. The 2 most important variables associated with survival are

1. the size of the largest tumor dimension in contact with the sclera
2. the cell type making up the tumor

The modified Callender classification is used for the cytologic classification of uveal melanomas:

- spindle cell nevus
- spindle cell melanoma
- epithelioid melanoma
- mixed-cell type (mixture of spindle and epithelioid cells)

Occasionally, a melanoma undergoes extensive necrosis, which precludes classification.

Spindle cell melanoma has the best prognosis and epithelioid melanoma the worst. Melanomas of mixed-cell type have an intermediate prognosis. Some authors have suggested that survival following enucleation decreases with increasing proportions of epithelioid cells in mixed-cell melanomas. Totally necrotic melanomas assume the same prognosis as mixed-cell melanomas.

The modified Callender classification has some disadvantages. First, there is continuing controversy about the minimum number of epithelioid cells needed for a melanoma to be classified as mixed-cell type. Second, the scheme is difficult to reproduce, even among experienced ophthalmic pathologists. This difficulty arises because the cytologic features of the melanoma cells reflect a continuous spectrum (Figs 12-12 through 12-14).

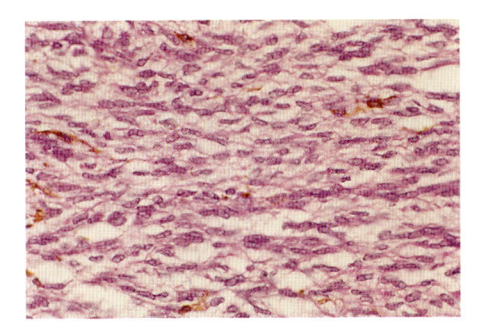

Figure 12-12 Spindle-A cells are characterized by low nuclear-to-cytoplasmic ratios. Neither nucleoli nor mitoses are observed, and a central stripe may be noted down the long axis of the nucleus. Tumors composed exclusively of spindle-A cells are considered to be nevi.

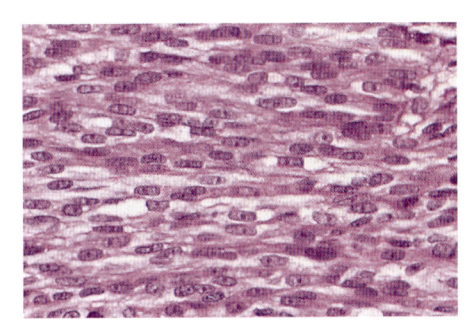

Figure 12-13 Spindle-B cells demonstrate a higher nuclear-to-cytoplasmic ratio; more coarsely granular chromatin; and plumper, large nuclei. Mitotic figures and nucleoli are present, although not in large numbers. Tumors composed of mixtures of spindle-A and spindle-B cells are designated spindle cell melanomas.

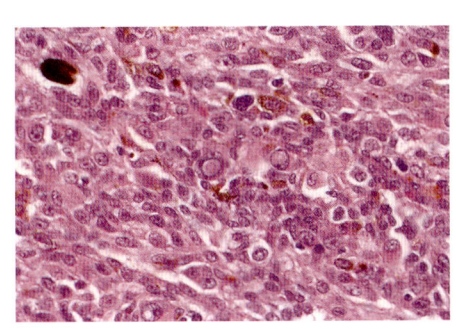

Figure 12-14 Epithelioid melanoma cells. Patients with this type of melanoma have the poorest prognosis. Cells resemble epithelium because of abundant eosinophilic cytoplasm and enlarged oval to polygonal nuclei. Epithelioid melanoma cells often lack cohesiveness and demonstrate marked pleomorphism, including the formation of multinucleated tumor giant cells. Nuclei have a conspicuous nuclear membrane, very coarse chromatin, and large nucleoli.

Cytomorphometric measurements of melanoma cells have been studied. One such measurement is the *mean of the 10 largest melanoma cell nuclei (MLN)*. This parameter has been shown to correlate well with mortality after enucleation. The correlation of morphometry is enhanced further when combined with the largest dimension of scleral contact by tumor.

Intrinsic tumor microvascular patterns have also been studied and shown to have prognostic significance. Tumors containing more complex microvascular patterns such as vascular closed loops or vascular networks (3 vascular loops located back-to-back) are associated with an increased incidence of the development of subsequent metastases (Fig 12-15).

As mentioned earlier, melanomas may break through the overlying Bruch's membrane and assume a mushroom-shaped configuration (Fig 12-16). Tumors may also contribute to serous detachments of the overlying and adjacent retina, with subsequent degenerative

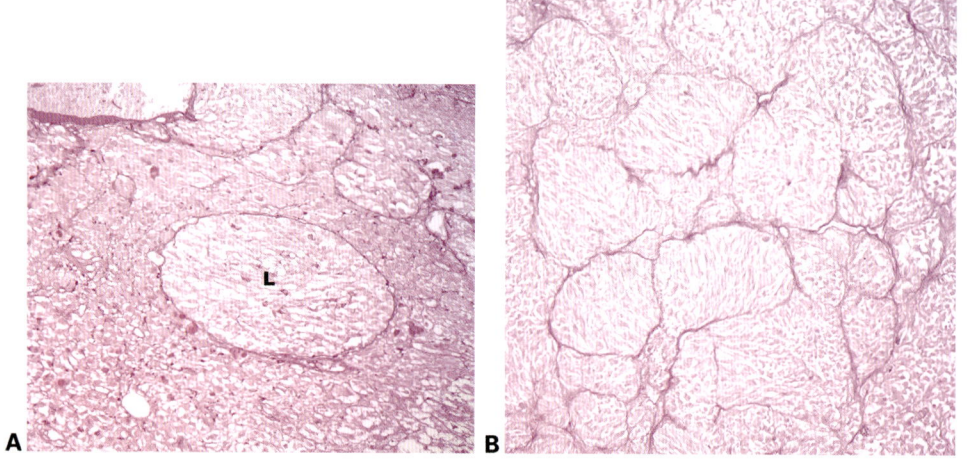

192 • Ophthalmic Pathology and Intraocular Tumors

Figure 12-15 Microvascular patterns in uveal melanoma. **A,** Microvascular closed loop *(L)*. **B,** Microvascular network: 3 or more back-to-back loops. *(Courtesy of Nasreen A. Syed, MD.)*

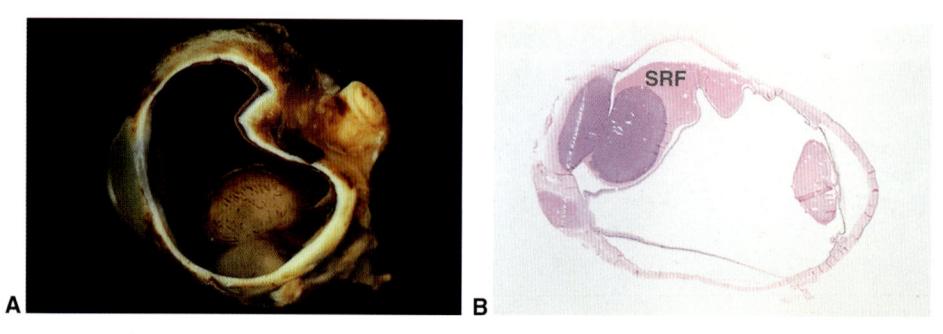

Figure 12-16 Choroidal melanoma with rupture through Bruch's membrane. **A,** Gross appearance. **B,** Microscopic appearance. Note the subretinal fluid *(SRF)* adjacent to the tumor.

changes in the outer segments of the photoreceptors. Melanomas may extend through scleral emissary channels to gain access to the episcleral surface and the orbit (Fig 12-17). Less commonly, aggressive melanomas may directly invade the underlying sclera or overlying retina (Fig 12-18).

Tumor necrosis can incite variable degrees of intraocular inflammation. Direct invasion of the anterior chamber may lead to secondary glaucoma. In addition, tumor necrosis may lead to the liberation of melanin pigment, which can then gain access to the anterior chamber and angle, causing a type of secondary glaucoma called *melanomalytic glaucoma*.

Lymphatic spread of ciliary body and choroidal melanomas is rare. Metastases almost invariably result from the hematogenous spread of melanoma to the liver. The reason for the propensity of melanomas to spread to the liver is unknown, although more than 95% of tumor-related deaths have liver involvement. In as many as one third of tumor-related deaths, the liver is the sole site of metastasis.

CHAPTER 12: Uveal Tract • 193

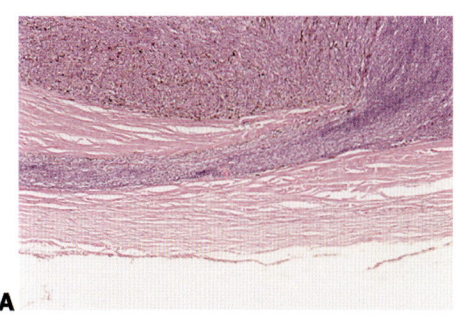

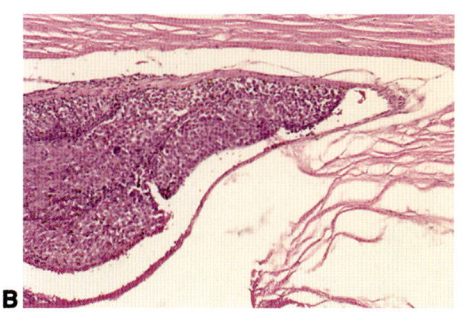

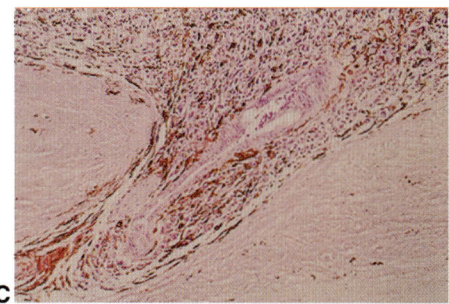

Figure 12-17 A, Note the melanoma cells tracking along scleral emissary canals. **B,** Melanoma is found within the vortex vein. **C,** Some melanomas track along the outer sheaths of vortex veins and nerves.

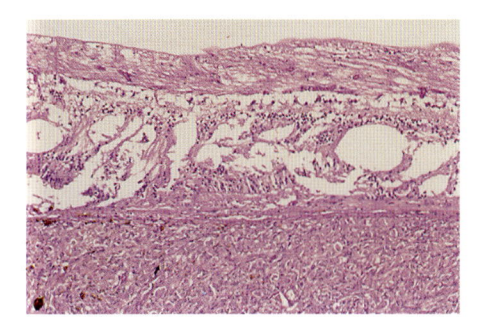

Figure 12-18 Note the retinal degeneration overlying this choroidal melanoma and the retinal invasion by tumor.

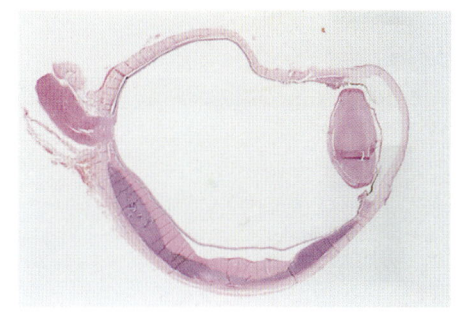

Figure 12-19 Some melanomas form diffuse, placoid growths.

Some types of uveal melanomas show biologic behavior that cannot be predicted according to the criteria just discussed. Survival rates of patients with diffuse ciliary body melanomas (ring melanoma) are particularly poor. These relatively flat tumors are almost always of mixed-cell type, and they may grow circumferentially without becoming significantly elevated. Diffuse choroidal melanomas similarly have a poor prognosis (Figs 12-19, 12-20).

For further discussion, see Chapter 17. For American Joint Committee on Cancer (AJCC) definitions and staging of uveal melanomas, see Table A-4 in the appendix.

Figure 12-20 By definition, a ring melanoma follows the major arterial circle of the iris circumferentially around the eye.

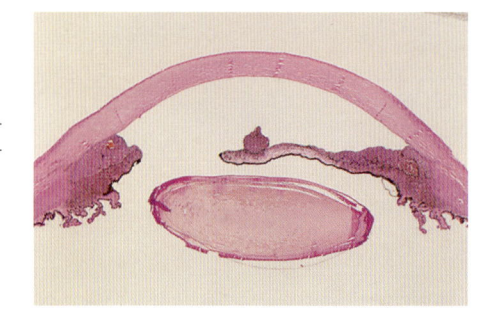

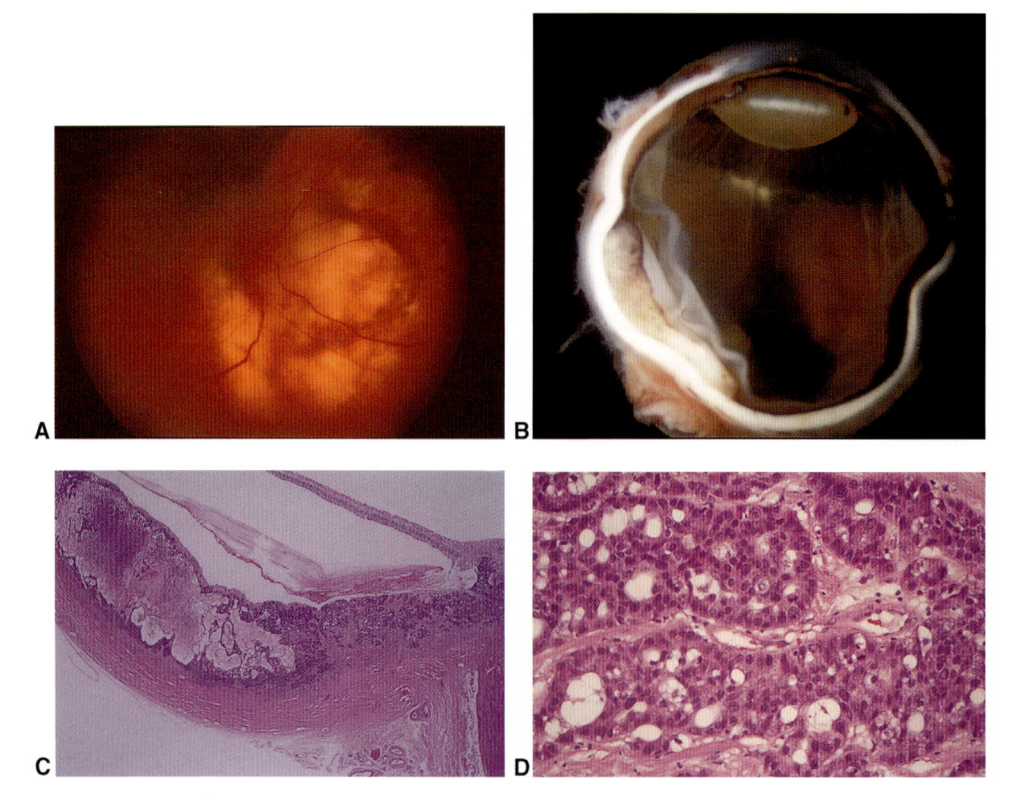

Figure 12-21 **A,** Clinical appearance of a metastatic lesion from a primary lung tumor. **B,** Gross appearance of lesion. **C,** Choroidal metastasis from lung adenocarcinoma; histopathology shows adenocarcinoma with mucin production. **D,** Higher magnification depicts a well-differentiated adenocarcinoma with distinct glandular appearance. *(Courtesy of Hans E. Grossniklaus, MD.)*

Metastatic Tumors

Metastatic lesions are the most common intraocular tumors in adults. These lesions most often involve the choroid, but any ocular structure can be affected. Unlike primary uveal melanoma, metastatic lesions are often multiple and may be bilateral. Although these lesions typically assume a flattened growth pattern, rare cases of collar-button or mushroom-shaped lesions have been reported. The most common primary tumors metastasizing to the eye are breast carcinoma in women and lung carcinoma in men (Fig 12-21).

Other primary tumors with reported metastases to the uveal tract include cutaneous melanoma, prostate adenocarcinoma, renal cell carcinoma, and carcinoid tumors. Histologically, metastatic tumors may recapitulate the appearance of the primary lesion, or they may appear less differentiated. Special histochemical and immunohistochemical stains can be helpful in diagnosing the metastatic lesion and determining its origin. The importance of a careful clinical history cannot be overemphasized. See Chapter 20 for further discussion and multiple photographs.

Other Uveal Tumors

Hemangioma

Hemangiomas of the choroid occur in 2 specific forms. The *localized* choroidal hemangioma typically occurs in patients without systemic disorders. It generally appears as a red or orange tumor located in the postequatorial zone of the fundus. Such tumors commonly produce a secondary retinal detachment. If the detachment extends into the foveal region, blurred vision, metamorphopsia, and micropsia may occur. These benign vascular tumors characteristically affect the overlying RPE and cause cystoid degeneration of the outer retinal layers.

The *diffuse* choroidal hemangioma is generally seen in patients with Sturge-Weber syndrome (encephalofacial angiomatosis). This choroidal tumor produces diffuse reddish orange thickening of the entire fundus, resulting in an ophthalmoscopic pattern commonly referred to as the *tomato catsup fundus*. Retinal detachment and glaucoma often occur in eyes with this lesion. (See also BCSC Section 5, *Neuro-Ophthalmology*; Section 6, *Pediatric Ophthalmology and Strabismus*; and Section 12, *Retina and Vitreous*.)

Histopathologically, both the diffuse and localized hemangiomas show collections of variably sized vessels within the choroid (Fig 12-22). The lesions may appear

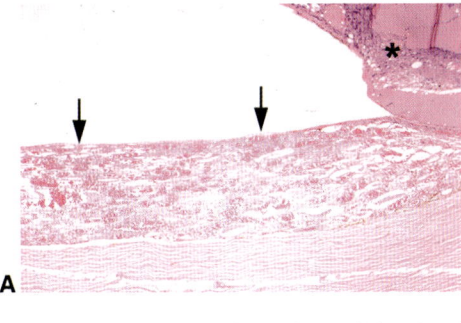

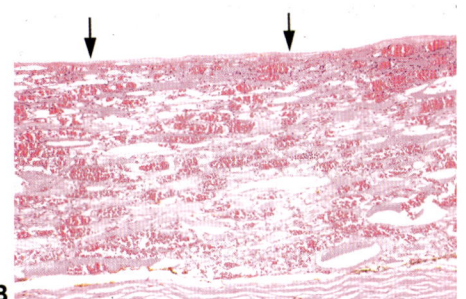

Figure 12-22 Choroidal hemangioma with a large number of thin-walled, variably sized vessels within the choroid. **A,** Low-magnification view illustrating exudative retinal detachment overlying the lesion *(asterisk)*. *Arrows* designate Bruch's membrane. **B,** Higher magnification; *arrows* designate Bruch's membrane. *(Courtesy of Nasreen A. Syed, MD.)*

as predominantly capillary hemangiomas, cavernous hemangiomas, or a mixed pattern of both. The adjacent and overlying choroid may show compressed melanocytes, hyperplastic RPE, and fibrous tissue proliferation.

When choroidal hemangiomas are asymptomatic, generally no treatment is indicated. The most common complication is serous detachment of the retina involving the fovea, with resultant visual loss. If this complication occurs, the surface of the tumor can be treated lightly with argon laser photocoagulation. The treatment goal is not to destroy the tumor but rather to create a chorioretinal adhesion that prevents further accumulation of fluid. If the retinal detachment is extensive, photocoagulation is usually unsuccessful. Recurrent detachments are common, and the long-term visual prognosis in patients with macular detachment or edema is guarded. See also Chapter 18 and Figures 18-1 and 18-2.

Choroidal osteoma

Choroidal osteomas are benign bony tumors that typically arise from the juxtapapillary choroid and are seen in adolescent to young adult patients, more commonly women than men. The characteristic lesion appears yellow to orange and has well-defined margins (see Fig 17-14). Histopathologically, the tumor is composed of unremarkable-appearing compact bone located in the peripapillary choroid. The intratrabecular spaces are filled with a loose connective tissue containing large and small blood vessels, vacuolated mesenchymal cells, and scattered mast cells. The bony trabeculae contain osteocytes, cement lines, and occasional osteoclasts.

Choroidal osteomas typically enlarge slowly over many years. If the tumor involves the macula, vision is generally impaired. Subretinal neovascularization is a common complication of macular choroidal osteoma. Both choroidal osteoma and hemangioma may mimic a choroidal melanoma clinically and should, therefore, be included in the differential diagnosis of choroidal melanoma.

Neural sheath tumors

Schwannomas (neurilemomas) and neurofibromas are rare tumors of the uveal tract. Multiple neurofibromas may occur in the ciliary body, iris, and choroid in patients with neurofibromatosis. The histopathologic features of neurofibromas are discussed in Chapter 14, Orbit.

Leiomyoma

Neoplasms arising from the smooth muscle of the ciliary body have been reported only rarely. By light and transmission electron microscopy, these tumors may exhibit both myogenic and neurogenic features. In such cases, the term *mesectodermal leiomyoma* is employed.

Lymphoid proliferation

The choroid may be the site of lymphoid proliferation, either as a primary ocular process or in association with systemic lymphoproliferative disease.

Uveal lymphoid infiltration (formerly *reactive lymphoid hyperplasia*) of the uveal tract is similar to the spectrum of low-grade lymphoid lesions that occur in the orbit (see Chapter 14, Orbit) and conjunctiva. There may be diffuse involvement of the uveal

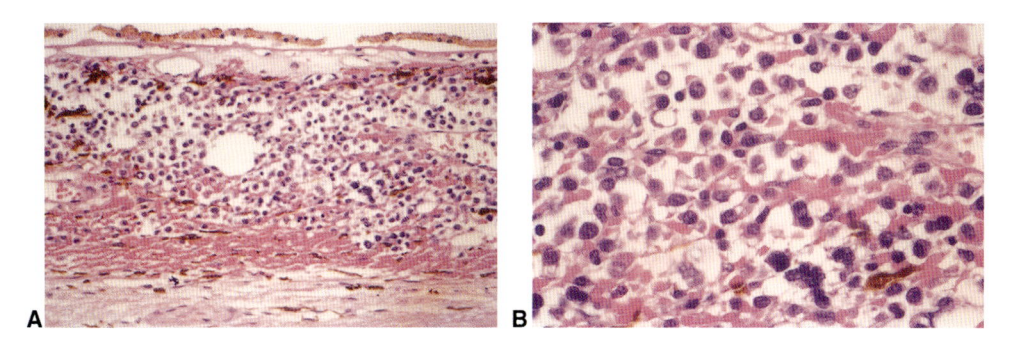

Figure 12-23 **A,** Diffuse expansion of choroid by lymphoma. **B,** Higher magnification depicts atypical lymphocytes. *(Courtesy of Hans E. Grossniklaus, MD.)*

tract by a mixture of lymphocytes and plasma cells, and lymphoid follicles may be present. Lymphocyte typing reveals a polymorphic population without clonal restriction; this finding distinguishes inflammatory pseudotumor from lymphoma.

> Grossniklaus HE, Martin DF, Avery R, et al. Uveal lymphoid infiltration: report of four cases and clinicopathologic review. *Ophthalmology.* 1998;105:1265–1273.

Lymphoma of the uveal tract occurs almost exclusively in association with systemic lymphoma (Fig 12-23). The classification of lymphomas is discussed in Chapter 14.

Trauma

The uveal tract is frequently involved in cases of ocular trauma. *Prolapse* of uveal tissue through a perforating ocular injury is a common association. *Rupture* of the choroid may occur as the result of a blunt or penetrating injury. The pattern of the rupture most frequently appears as semicircular lines circumscribing the peripapillary region. If the macula is involved, the prognosis for vision recovery is guarded. Subretinal neovascularization can occur as a late complication. More severe injury may cause rupture of both the choroid and retina, a condition termed *chorioretinitis sclopetaria.*

Choroidal detachment, either localized or diffuse, may occur after accidental or surgical trauma. Serous or hemorrhagic fluid accumulates in the suprachoroidal space between the choroid and the sclera. Depending on the etiology, the fluid may spontaneously resorb, allowing for reattachment of the choroid. In other cases, surgical drainage of the fluid may be required.

CHAPTER 13

Eyelids

Topography

The eyelids extend from the eyebrow superiorly to the cheek inferiorly and can be subdivided into orbital and tarsal components. At the level of the tarsus, the eyelid consists of 4 main histologic layers, from anterior to posterior:

- skin
- orbicularis oculi muscle
- tarsus
- palpebral conjunctiva

A surgical plane of dissection through an incision along the gray line of the eyelid margin is possible between the orbicularis and the tarsus, functionally dividing the eyelid into anterior and posterior lamellae (Fig 13-1). BCSC Section 7, *Orbit, Eyelids, and Lacrimal System,* covers the anatomy of the eyelids as well as the conditions discussed later in this chapter in detail.

The skin of the eyelids is thinner than that of most other body sites. It consists of an epidermis of keratinizing stratified squamous epithelium, which also contains melanocytes and antigen-presenting Langerhans cells; and a dermis of loose collagenous connective tissue, which contains the following:

- cilia and associated sebaceous glands (of Zeis)
- apocrine sweat glands (of Moll)
- eccrine sweat glands
- pilosebaceous units

Lid retraction is effected by the *levator palpebrae superioris,* which in the eyelid is an aponeurosis, and the *Müller muscle* (smooth muscle connecting the upper border of the tarsus with the levator). Forceful eyelid closure is accomplished by the *orbicularis oculi* (striated skeletal muscle). The *tarsal plate,* a thick plaque of dense, fibrous connective tissue, contains the sebaceous meibomian glands. Also present near the upper border of the superior tarsal plate (and less so along the lower border of the inferior tarsal plate) are the accessory lacrimal glands of Wolfring; the accessory lacrimal glands of Krause are located in the conjunctival fornices. The *palpebral conjunctiva* is tightly adherent to the posterior

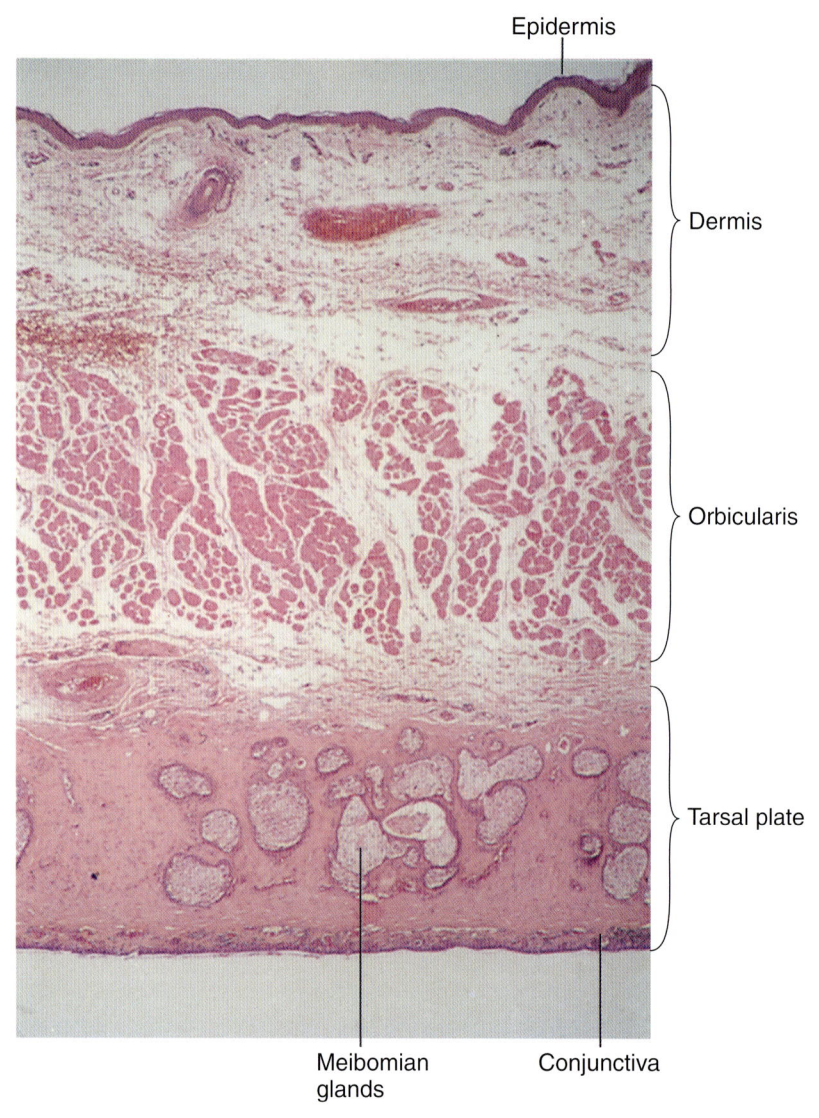

Figure 13-1 Cross section of a normal eyelid. Proceeding from top to bottom, note the epidermis, the dermis resting on the orbicularis, the tarsus surrounding the meibomian glands, and the palpebral (tarsal) conjunctiva.

Table 13-1 Glands of the Eyelid: Function and Pathology

Secretory Element	Normal Function	Pathology
Conjunctival goblet cells	Mucin secretion to enhance corneal wetting	Numbers diminished in some dry-eye states Present in mucoepidermoid carcinoma
Accessory lacrimal glands of Krause and Wolfring	Basal tear secretion of the aqueous layer	Sjögren syndrome Graft-vs-host disease Rare tumors (benign mixed tumor)
Meibomian glands	Secretion of lipid layer of tears to retard evaporation	Chalazion Sebaceous carcinoma
Sebaceous glands of Zeis	Lubrication of the cilia	External hordeolum Sebaceous carcinoma
Glands of Moll	Lubrication of the cilia	Ductal cyst (sudoriferous cyst, apocrine hidrocystoma) Apocrine carcinoma
Eccrine glands	Secretions for temperature control, electrolyte balance	Ductal cyst (sudoriferous cyst, eccrine hidrocystoma) Syringoma Sweat gland carcinoma

surface of the tarsus. Table 13-1 lists the normal functions of the eyelid glands and some of the pathologic conditions related to them.

Following are several terms used commonly in dermatopathology:

- *acanthosis:* increased thickness (hyperplasia) of the stratum malpighii (consisting of the strata basale, spinosum, and granulosum) of the epidermis
- *hyperkeratosis:* increased thickness of the stratum corneum of the epidermis
- *parakeratosis:* retention of nuclei within the stratum corneum with corresponding absence of the stratum granulosum
- *papillomatosis:* formation of fingerlike upward projections of epidermis lining fibrovascular cores
- *dyskeratosis:* premature individual cell keratinization within the stratum malpighii
- *acantholysis:* loss of cohesion (dissolution of intercellular bridges) between adjacent epithelial cells
- *spongiosis:* widening of intercellular spaces between cells in the stratum malpighii due to edema

Congenital Anomalies

BCSC Section 7, *Orbit, Eyelids, and Lacrimal System,* also discusses congenital anomalies, including those not mentioned here (eg, congenital ptosis).

Distichiasis

Distichiasis is the aberrant formation within the tarsus of cilia that exit the eyelid margin through the orifices of the meibomian glands. Although these lashes may rub against the eye, they are relatively well tolerated initially and may not cause symptoms of irritation until early childhood. Distichiasis is inherited in an autosomal dominant fashion and is usually the only congenital anomaly present. It may, however, be associated with other anomalies such as mandibulofacial dysostosis and trisomy 18. The pathogenesis of distichiasis is thought to be an anomalous formation within the tarsus of a complete pilosebaceous unit rather than the normal sebaceous (meibomian) gland.

Phakomatous Choristoma

A rare congenital tumor, phakomatous choristoma (Zimmerman tumor) is formed from the aberrant location of lens epithelium within the inferonasal portion of the lower eyelid. These cells may undergo cytoplasmic enlargement, identical to the "bladder" cell in a cataractous lens. PAS-positive basement membrane material is produced, recapitulating the lens capsule. The nodule formed is usually present at birth and enlarges slowly. Complete excision is the usual treatment.

Dermoid Cyst

Dermoid cysts may occur in the eyelid, but they are more common in the orbit and are discussed in Chapter 14.

Inflammations

Infectious

Depending on the causative agent, infections of the eyelids may produce disease that is localized (eg, hordeolum), multicentric (eg, papillomas), or diffuse (cellulitis). Routes of infection may be primary inoculation through a bite or wound, direct spread from a contiguous site such as a paranasal sinus infection, or hematogenous dissemination from a remote site. Infectious agents may be

- bacterial, such as *Staphylococcus aureus* in hordeolum and infectious blepharitis
- viral, as in papillomas caused by human papillomavirus (HPV)
- fungal, such as blastomycosis, coccidioidomycosis, or aspergillosis

Hordeolum

Also known as a *stye,* hordeolum is a primary, acute, self-limited inflammatory process typically involving the glands of Zeis and, less often, the meibomian glands of the upper eyelid. A small abscess, or focal collection of polymorphonuclear leukocytes and necrotic debris, forms at the site of infection. Healing occurs without visible scarring in most cases.

Cellulitis

The diffuse spread of acute inflammatory cells through tissue planes is known as *cellulitis.* The pathologic change is often accompanied by vascular congestion and edema (Fig 13-2).

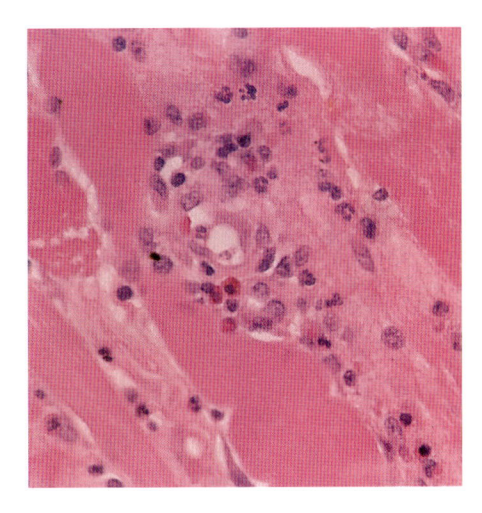

Figure 13-2 Polymorphonuclear leukocytes dissect between the skeletal muscle fibers of the orbicularis in this biopsy of a preseptal cellulitis of the eyelid.

Preseptal cellulitis involves the tissues of the eyelid anterior to the orbital septum, the fibrous membrane connecting the borders of the tarsal plates to the bony orbital rim. The condition most commonly affects the pediatric population and is most often secondary to upper respiratory tract infections caused by bacteria such as *Streptococcus pneumoniae*.

Viral infections

Examples of 2 types of viral infections involving the eyelids are viral papillomas and molluscum contagiosum. Virally induced *papillomas* of the eyelid are seen in young patients and are caused by HPV subtypes 6 and 11, those also associated with verruca. The papillomas are pedunculated growths along the eyelid margin composed of acanthotic and hyperkeratotic epidermis lining papillary fibrovascular cores. Koilocytotic cytoplasmic clearing of infected epithelial cells may be present. The growths may spontaneously regress over months to years if not surgically excised or ablated by cryotherapy. Lesions with a papillomatous appearance seen in middle-aged or elderly persons include seborrheic keratosis, actinic keratosis, intradermal nevus, and acrochordon (fibroepithelial polyp).

Molluscum contagiosum is caused by a member of the poxvirus family and also typically affects young or immunocompromised persons. Dome-shaped, waxy epidermal nodules with central umbilication form and, if present on the eyelid margin, may cause a secondary follicular conjunctivitis (Fig 13-3). Histopathologically, the lesions are distinctive, with a nodular proliferation of infected epithelium producing a central focus of necrotic cells that are extruded to the skin surface (Fig 13-4). As the replicating virus fills the cytoplasm, the nucleus is displaced peripherally and finally disappears as the cells are shed. Incision and curettage are usually curative.

Noninfectious

Chalazion

A chalazion is a chronic, often painless nodule of the eyelid that occurs when the lipid secretions of the meibomian glands or, less often, the glands of Zeis are discharged into the surrounding tissues, inciting a lipogranulomatous reaction (Fig 13-5). Because the lipid is dissolved by solvents during routine tissue processing, histologic sections show

204 • Ophthalmic Pathology and Intraocular Tumors

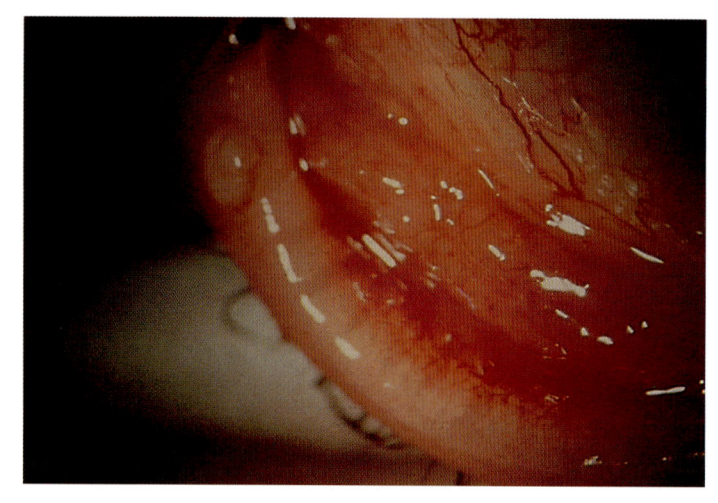

Figure 13-3 Molluscum contagiosum involving the eyelid margin. Note the associated follicular conjunctivitis.

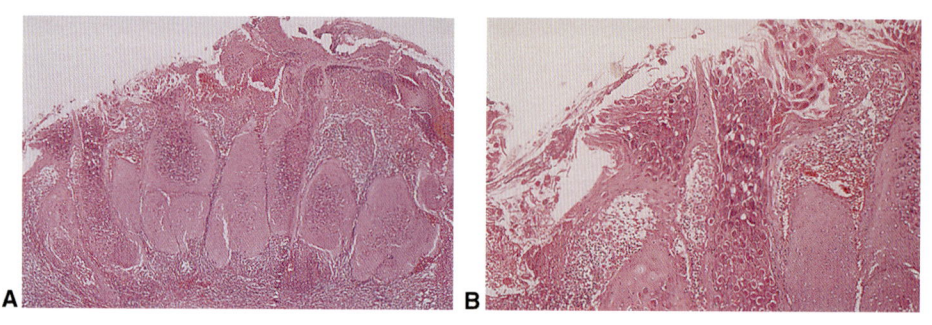

Figure 13-4 Molluscum contagiosum. **A,** Note the cup-shaped, thickened epidermis with a central crater. **B,** Note the eosinophilic inclusion bodies becoming basophilic as they migrate to the surface.

Figure 13-5 Chalazion. Granulomatous inflammation surrounds clear spaces formerly occupied by lipid (lipogranuloma).

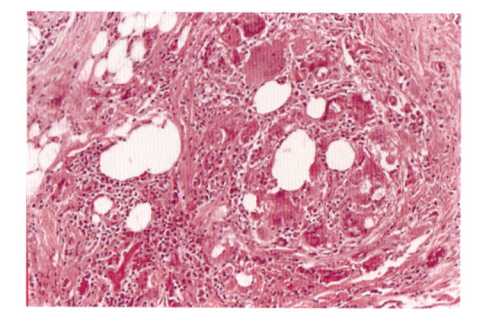

histiocytes and multinucleated giant cells enveloping optically clear spaces. Lymphocytes, plasma cells, and neutrophils may also be present.

Degenerations

Xanthelasma

Xanthelasmas are single or multiple soft yellow plaques occurring in the nasal aspect of the upper and lower eyelids in middle-aged to elderly individuals, predominantly females. Associated hyperlipoproteinemic states, particularly hyperlipoproteinemia types II and III, are present in 30%–40% of patients with xanthelasma. These eyelid xanthomas consist of collections of histiocytes with microvesicular foamy cytoplasm clustered around vessels and adnexal structures within the dermis (Fig 13-6). Associated inflammation is minimal to nonexistent. Treatment is either by surgical excision or by carbon dioxide laser ablation.

Amyloid

The term *amyloid* refers to a heterogeneous group of extracellular proteins that exhibit birefringence and dichroism under polarized light when stained with Congo red (see Fig 10-8). These features result from the 3-dimensional configuration of the proteins into a β-pleated sheet. Examples of proteins that may form amyloid deposits include

- immunoglobulin light chain fragments (AL amyloid) in plasma cell dyscrasias
- transthyretin mutations in familial amyloid polyneuropathy (FAP) types I and II (see Chapter 10, Vitreous)
- gelsolin mutations in FAP type IV (Meretoja syndrome [lattice corneal dystrophy type II])

Amyloid within the skin of the eyelid is highly indicative of a systemic disease process, either primary or secondary, whereas deposits elsewhere in the ocular adnexa but not in the eyelid are more likely a localized disease process. Other systemic diseases with eyelid manifestations are listed in Table 13-2.

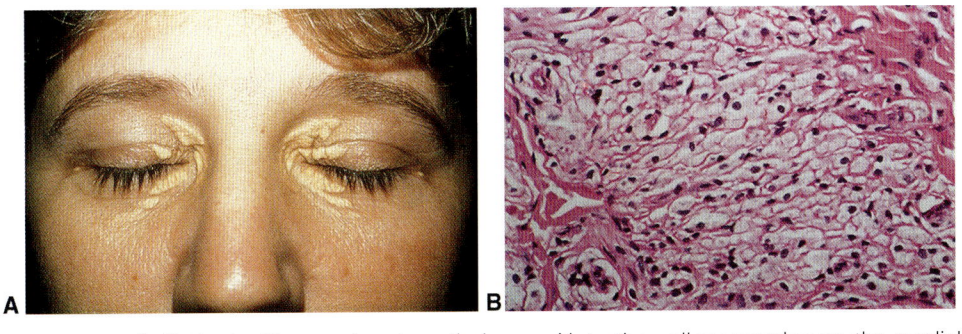

Figure 13-6 **A,** Patient with prominent xanthelasma. Note the yellow papules on the medial aspect of the upper and lower eyelids. **B,** Note the foam cells (filled with lipid) surrounding a venule at the left margin of this photograph. *(Part A from* External Disease and Cornea: A Multimedia Collection. *San Francisco: American Academy of Ophthalmology; 1994:slide 10.)*

206 • Ophthalmic Pathology and Intraocular Tumors

Table 13-2 Eyelid Manifestations of Systemic Diseases

Systemic Condition	Eyelid Manifestation
Erdheim-Chester disease	Xanthelasma, xanthogranuloma
Hyperlipoproteinemia	Xanthelasma
Amyloidosis	Waxy papules, ptosis, pupura
Sarcoidosis	Papules
Wegener granulomatosis	Edema, ptosis, lower eyelid retraction
Scleroderma	Reduced mobility, taut skin
Polyarteritis nodosa	Focal infarct
Systemic lupus erythematosus	Telangiectasias, edema
Dermatomyositis	Edema, erythema
Relapsing polychondritis	Papules
Carney complex	Myxoma
Fraser syndrome	Cryptophthalmos
Treacher Collins syndrome	Lower eyelid coloboma

Modified from Wiggs JL, Jakobiec FA. Eyelid manifestations of systemic disease. In: Albert DM, Jakobiec FA, eds. *Principles and Practice of Ophthalmology*. Philadelphia: Saunders; 1994:1859.

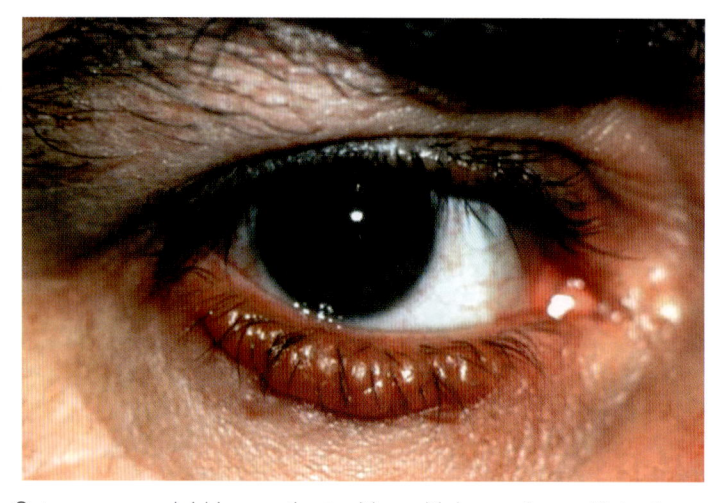

Figure 13-7 Cutaneous amyloid in a patient with multiple myeloma. Note the waxy elevation and the associated purpura. *(Courtesy of John B. Holds, MD.)*

Amyloid deposits in the skin are usually multiple, bilateral, symmetric, waxy yellow-white nodules. The deposition of amyloid within blood vessel walls in the skin causes increased vascular fragility and often results in intradermal hemorrhages, accounting for the purpura seen clinically (Fig 13-7). On routine histologic sections, amyloid appears as an amorphous to fibrillogranular, eosinophilic extracellular deposit, usually within vessel walls but also in connective tissue and around peripheral nerves and sweat glands. Other stains useful in demonstrating amyloid deposits include crystal violet and thioflavin T. Electron microscopy reveals the deposits to be composed of randomly oriented extracellular fibrils measuring 7.5–10.0 nm in diameter.

> Albert DM, Jakobiec FA, eds. *Principles and Practice of Ophthalmology.* 2nd ed. Philadelphia: Saunders; 2000.
> Garner A, Klintworth GK, eds. *Pathobiology of Ocular Disease: A Dynamic Approach.* 2nd ed. New York: Dekker; 1994:993–1007.

Neoplasia

Epidermal Neoplasms

Seborrheic keratosis

Seborrheic keratosis, a common benign epithelial proliferation, occurs in middle age. Clinically, 1 or more well-circumscribed, oval, dome-shaped to verrucoid "stuck-on" papules appear, principally on the trunk and face, varying from millimeters to centimeters in greatest dimension and from pink to brown in color. Histopathologically, several architectural patterns are possible, although all demonstrate hyperkeratosis, acanthosis, and some degree of papillomatosis. The acanthosis is a result of the proliferation of either polygonal or basaloid squamous cells without dysplasia.

A characteristic finding in most types of seborrheic keratoses is the formation of pseudohorn cysts, which are concentrically laminated collections of surface keratin within the acanthotic epithelium (Fig 13-8). Irritated seborrheic keratosis, also termed *inverted follicular keratosis* by some authors, shows nonkeratinizing squamous epithelial whorling, or squamous "eddies," instead of pseudohorn cysts (Fig 13-9). Heavy melanin phagocytosis by keratinocytes may impart a dark brown color to an otherwise typical seborrheic keratosis, which may then be confused clinically with malignant melanoma.

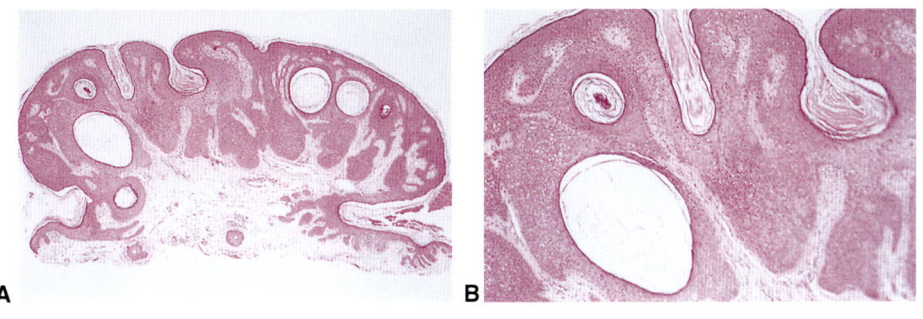

Figure 13-8 Seborrheic keratosis. **A,** The epidermis is acanthotic, and an excessive amount of keratin appears on the surface and within invaginations (hyperkeratosis). **B,** When serial histologic sections are studied, pseudohorn cysts within the epidermis are seen to represent crevices or infoldings of epidermis. *(Courtesy of Hans E. Grossniklaus, MD.)*

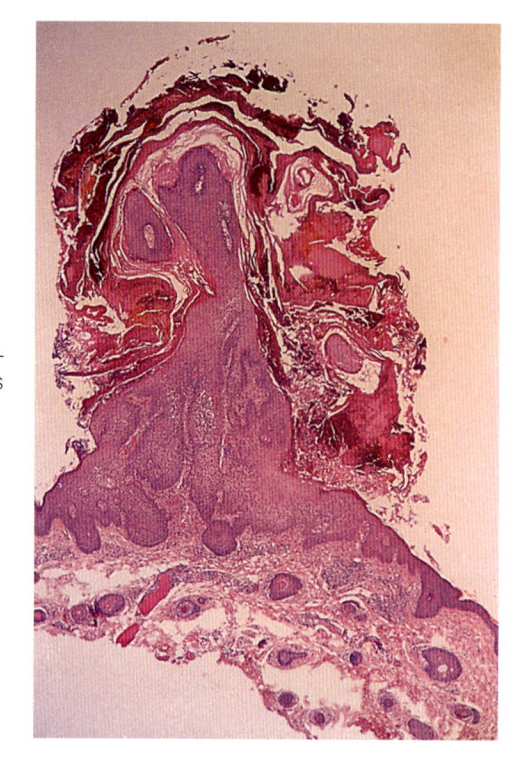

Figure 13-9 Inverted follicular keratosis. Clinically, this lesion appeared to be a cutaneous horn.

Table 13-3 Eyelid Neoplasms in Association With Systemic Malignancies

Syndrome	Eyelid Manifestation
Muir-Torre syndrome (visceral carcinoma, usually colon)	Keratoacanthoma, sebaceous neoplasm (adenoma, carcinoma)
Cowden disease (breast carcinoma; fibrous hamartomas of breast, thyroid, GI tract)	Multiple trichilemmomas
Basal cell nevus syndrome (medulloblastoma, fibrosarcoma)	Multiple basal cell carcinomas

Modified from Wiggs JL, Jakobiec FA. Eyelid manifestations of systemic disease. In: Albert DM, Jakobiec FA, eds. *Principles and Practice of Ophthalmology*. Philadelphia: Saunders; 1994:1859.

Sudden onset of multiple seborrheic keratoses is known as the *Leser-Trélat sign* and is associated with a malignancy, usually a gastrointestinal adenocarcinoma; these keratoses may in fact represent evolving acanthosis nigricans. Table 13-3 lists other systemic malignancies with cutaneous manifestations.

Keratoacanthoma

Keratoacanthoma is a rapidly growing epithelial proliferation with a potential for spontaneous involution that may be difficult to distinguish from squamous cell carcinoma both clinically and histopathologically. Recent evidence suggests that keratoacanthomas are a variant of a well-differentiated squamous cell carcinoma that has a tendency to regress. These studies are based on expression of proliferation markers (cyclins and cyclin-dependent kinases) and oncoproteins (mutated p53) that are expressed similarly by both entities. Dome-shaped nodules with a keratin-filled central crater may attain a considerable size, up to 2.5 cm in diameter, within a matter of 1–2 months (Fig 13-10). The natural history is typically spontaneous involution over several months, resulting in a slightly depressed scar. Histopathologically, keratoacanthomas show a cup-shaped invagination of well-differentiated squamous cells forming irregularly configured nests and strands and inciting a lymphoplasmacytic host response. The proliferating epithelial cells undermine the adjacent normal epidermis so that the edges of the lesion resemble the flying buttresses of a Gothic cathedral. At the deep aspect of the proliferating nodules, mitotic activity and nuclear atypia may occur, making the distinction between keratoacanthoma and invasive squamous cell carcinoma problematic. If unequivocal invasion is present, the lesion should be considered a well-differentiated squamous cell carcinoma. Many dermatopathologists and ophthalmic pathologists have ceased to use the term *keratoacanthoma* altogether and prefer to call it *well-differentiated keratinizing squamous cell carcinoma* because of the possible negative outcome of perineural invasion and metastasis. When the clinical differential diagnosis is keratoacanthoma versus squamous cell carcinoma, the lesion should be completely excised to permit optimal histopathologic examination of the lateral and deep margins of the tumor–host interface.

> Hurt MA. Keratoacanthoma vs. squamous cell carcinoma in contrast with keratoacanthoma is squamous cell carcinoma. *J Cutan Pathol.* 2004;31:291–292.
>
> Kerschmann RL, McCalmont TH, LeBoit PE. p53 oncoprotein expression and proliferation index in keratoacanthoma and squamous cell carcinoma. *Arch Dermatol.* 1994;130:181–186.
>
> Tran TA, Ross JS, Boehm JR, Carlson JA. Comparison of mitotic cyclins and cyclin-dependent kinase expression in keratoacanthoma and squamous cell carcinoma. *J Cutan Pathol.* 1999;26:391–397.

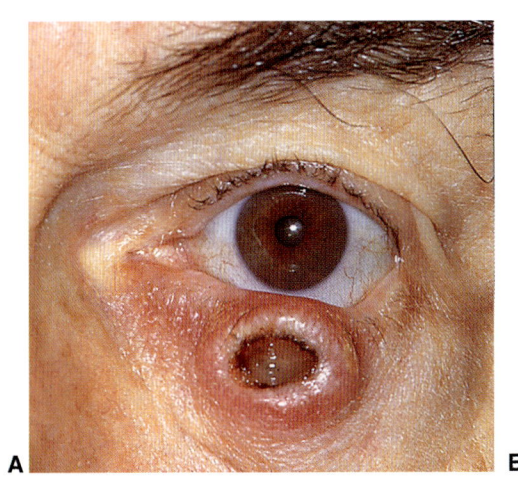

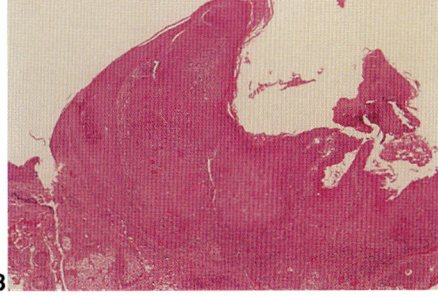

Figure 13-10 **A,** Patient with keratoacanthoma. Note the cuplike configuration. In this case, the central crater was originally filled with keratin. **B,** Histologic photograph.

Actinic keratosis

More specifically known as *solar keratosis,* actinic keratosis appears as erythematous, scaly macules or papules developing in middle age on sun-exposed skin, particularly the face and the dorsal surfaces of the hands. Actinic keratoses range from millimeters up to 1 cm in greatest dimension. Hyperkeratotic types may form a cutaneous horn, and hyperpigmented types may clinically simulate lentigo maligna. Squamous cell carcinoma may develop from preexisting actinic keratosis; thus, biopsy of suspicious lesions and long-term follow-up are necessary in patients with this condition. However, when squamous cell carcinoma arises in actinic keratosis, the risk of subsequent metastatic dissemination is very low (0.5%–3.0%).

Histopathologically, there are 5 subtypes, ranging from hypertrophic to atrophic; the sine qua non for diagnosis in all types is the presence of

- nuclear dysplasia
- nuclear enlargement
- nuclear hyperchromasia
- nuclear membrane irregularity
- increased nuclear-to-cytoplasmic ratio

Nuclear changes in actinic keratosis range from mild (involving only the basal epithelial layers) to frank carcinoma in situ, or full-thickness involvement of the epidermis.

Dyskeratosis (premature individual cell keratinization) and mitotic figures above the basal epithelial layer are often present (Fig 13-11). The underlying dermis shows solar elastosis (fragmentation, clumping, and loss of eosinophils; Fig 13-12) of dermal collagen and a lichenoid chronic inflammatory infiltrate of varying intensity. The base of the lesion must be examined histopathologically to determine whether invasive squamous cell carcinoma has supervened; as with keratoacanthoma, superficial shave biopsies not including the base of the lesion are contraindicated.

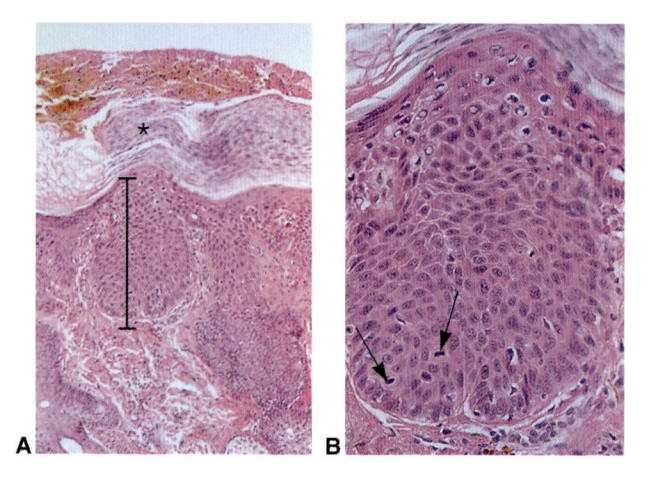

Figure 13-11 Actinic keratosis. **A,** Note the epidermal thickening (acanthosis *[I],* disorganization within the epidermis (dysplasia), parakeratosis *(asterisk),* and inflammation within the dermis. Solar elastosis is also noted in the dermis. **B,** Note the epidermal disorganization and mitotic figures *(arrows).*

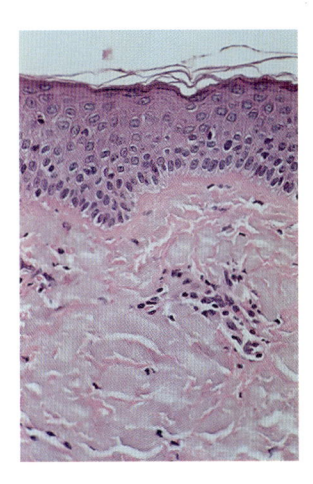

Figure 13-12 Solar elastosis. The collagen of the dermis appears blue in this H&E stain, instead of pink. This is a histopathologic marker of ultraviolet light–induced damage.

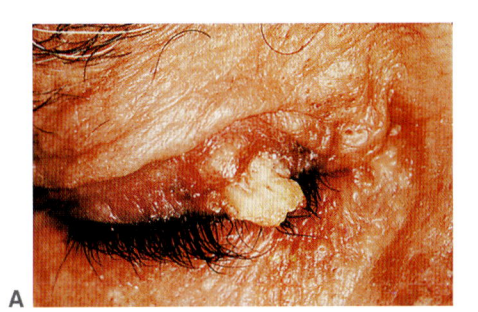

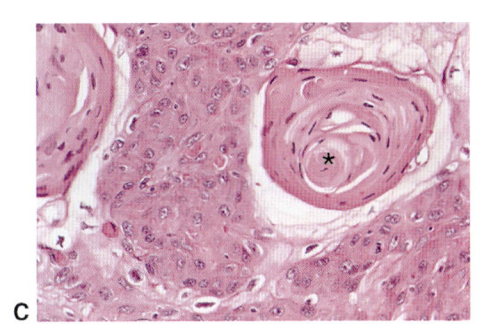

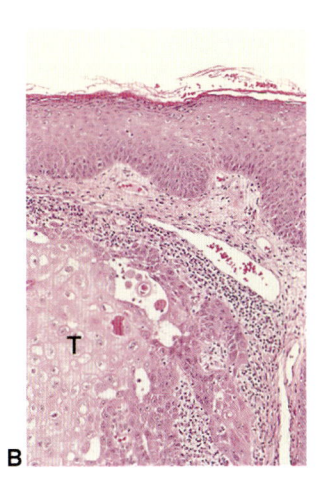

Figure 13-13 Squamous cell carcinoma. **A,** Clinical appearance. **B,** Note the tumor cells *(T)* invading the dermis. **C,** Keratin *(asterisk)* is produced in this well-differentiated squamous cell carcinoma.

Carcinoma

Although *squamous cell carcinoma* may occur in the eyelids, it is at least 10 and perhaps up to 40 times less common than basal cell carcinoma. Because the majority of squamous cell carcinomas arise in solar-damaged skin (actinic keratoses), the lower eyelid is more frequently involved than the upper. The clinical appearance is diverse, ranging from ulcers to plaques to fungating or nodular growths. Accordingly, the clinical differential diagnosis is a long list, and pathologic examination of excised tissue is necessary for accurate diagnosis. Histopathologic examination shows atypical squamous cells forming nests and strands, extending beyond the epidermal basement membrane, infiltrating the dermis, and inciting a desmoplastic fibrous tissue reaction (Fig 13-13).

Tumor cells may be

- well differentiated, forming keratin and easily recognizable as squamous
- moderately differentiated
- poorly differentiated, requiring ancillary studies to confirm the nature of the neoplasm

The presence of intercellular bridges between tumor cells should be sought when the diagnosis is in question. Perineural and lymphatic space invasion may be present and should be reported when identified microscopically. The use of frozen section (conventional or Mohs microsurgery) or permanent section margin control is indicated to treat this tumor adequately. Regional lymph node metastasis is reported to occur in 1%–21% of patients with squamous cell carcinoma of the eyelid.

Basal cell carcinoma is by far the most common malignant neoplasm of the eyelids, accounting for more than 90% of all eyelid malignancies. As with squamous cell carcinoma, exposure to sunlight is a risk factor. Lesions typically occur on the face, and the lower eyelid is more commonly involved than the upper. Tumors in the medial canthal area are more likely to be deeply invasive and to involve the orbit. The classic description is that of a "rodent" ulcer (*ulcus rodens,* or ulcer reminiscent of an object that has been chewed up by a rodent)— that is, a slowly enlarging ulcer with pearly, raised, rolled edges (Fig 13-14). The morpheaform, or fibrosing, basal cell carcinoma, however, is a flat or slightly depressed pale yellow indurated plaque; this type is often infiltrative, and its extent is difficult to determine clinically (Fig 13-15). Other growth patterns include nodular (most common) and multicentric.

As the name implies, basal cell carcinomas originate from the stratum basale, or stratum germinativum, of the epidermis. Tumor cells are characterized by relatively bland, monomorphous nuclei and a high nuclear-to-cytoplasmic ratio; anaplastic features and abnormal mitotic figures are uncommon. Basal cell carcinoma forms cohesive nests with nuclear palisading of the peripheral cell layer. A helpful diagnostic feature, albeit a presumed artifact of tissue processing, is the characteristic cleftlike separation of the tumor from its surround-

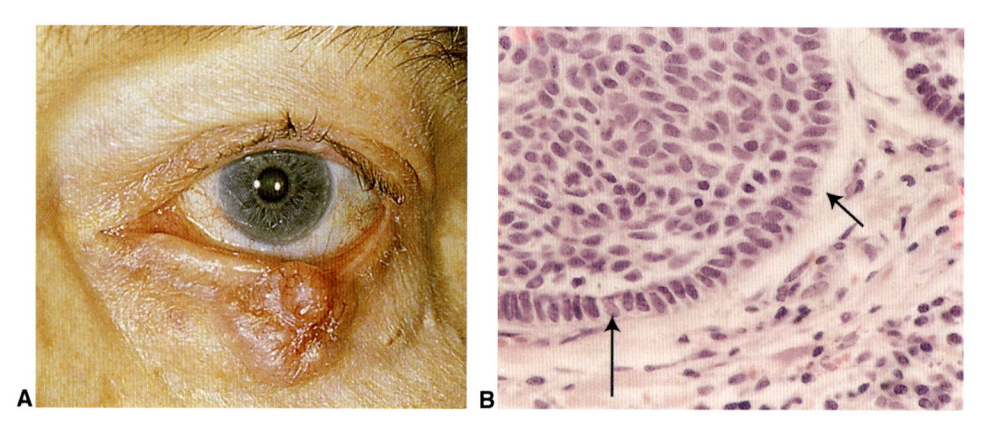

Figure 13-14 Basal cell carcinoma. **A,** Clinical appearance of a nodular "rodent" ulcer. **B,** Note the characteristic palisading of the cells around the outer edge of the tumor *(long arrow)* and the artifactitious separation between the nest of tumor cells and the dermis (cracking artifact, *short arrow*).

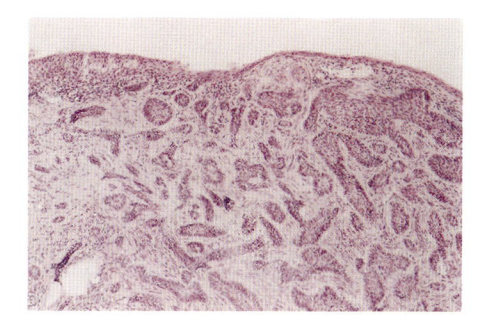

Figure 13-15 Basal cell carcinoma, morpheaform (sclerosing) type. Thin strands and cords of tumor cells are seen in a fibrotic (desmoplastic) dermis.

ing stroma (see Fig 13-14). Basal cell carcinomas may exhibit a variety of cytologic and architectural patterns, including squamous (metatypical), sebaceous, adenoid, and cystic differentiation. Fibrosing basal cell carcinomas are almost always undifferentiated.

Complete excision is the treatment of choice and margin control is required. Multicentric and infiltrating fibrosing basal cell carcinomas require frozen section examination of surgical margins or Mohs micrographic surgical technique for adequate excision. Morbidity in basal cell carcinomas is almost always the result of local spread; metastatic spread is extremely unusual.

Chévez-Barrios P. Frozen section diagnosis and indications in ophthalmic pathology. *Arch Pathol Lab Med.* 2005;129:1626–1634.

Dermal Neoplasms

Capillary hemangiomas are common in the eyelids of children. They usually appear at or shortly after birth as a red-purple nodule that may exhibit slow but worrisome growth over weeks to months. Spontaneous involution, however, is the rule, and lesions usually disappear by school age. Intervention is reserved for those lesions that diminish vision because of proptosis or astigmatism, promoting amblyopia. The histopathologic appearance depends on the stage of evolution of the hemangioma. Early lesions may be very cellular, with solid nests of plump endothelial cells and correspondingly little vascular luminal formation. Established lesions typically show well-developed, flattened, endothelium-lined capillary channels in a lobular configuration. Involuting lesions demonstrate increased fibrosis and hyalinization of capillary walls with luminal occlusion.

Appendage Neoplasms

A *sebaceous carcinoma* most commonly involves the upper eyelid of elderly persons. It may originate in the meibomian glands of the tarsus, the glands of Zeis in the skin of the eyelid, or the sebaceous glands of the caruncle. Clinical diagnosis is often missed or delayed because of this lesion's propensity to mimic a chalazion or chronic blepharoconjunctivitis (Fig 13-16). Histopathologically, well-differentiated sebaceous carcinomas are readily identified through the microvesicular foamy nature of the tumor cell cytoplasm (Fig 13-17). Moderately differentiated tumors may exhibit some degree of sebaceous differentiation. Poorly differentiated

214 • Ophthalmic Pathology and Intraocular Tumors

tumors, however, may be difficult to distinguish from the other, more common epithelial malignancies. The demonstration of lipid within the cytoplasm of tumor cells by special stains, such as oil red O or Sudan black, is diagnostic, but it must be performed on tissue prior to processing and paraffin embedding. Alternatively, osmium staining of tissue processed for electron microscopy will highlight intracytoplasmic lipid.

When sebaceous carcinoma is suspected clinically, the pathologist should be alerted so that frozen section slides can be generated for lipid stains. Another feature, characteristic of but not pathognomonic for sebaceous cell carcinoma, is the dissemination of individual tumor cells and clusters of tumor cells within the epidermis or conjunctival epithelium, known as *pagetoid spread* (see Fig 13-16). Another pattern in the conjunctiva is that of complete replacement of conjunctival epithelium by tumor cells. A rare variant of sebaceous carcinoma involves only the epidermis and conjunctiva without demonstrable invasive tumor.

Treatment recommendations include wide local excision of nodular lesions. Large or deeply invasive tumors may require exenteration. Suboptimal cytologic preservation and difficulty in distinguishing goblet cells from pagetoid spread of tumor cells may reduce

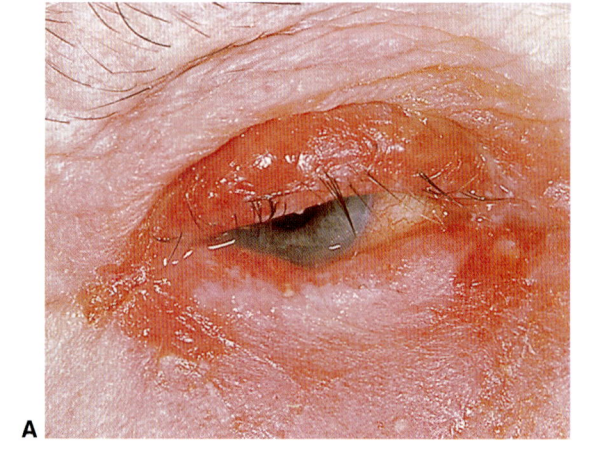

Figure 13-16 Sebaceous carcinoma. **A,** Note the eyelid erythema suggesting blepharitis. Note also the loss of eyelashes and the irregular eyelid thickening. **B,** Pagetoid invasion of the epithelium by tumor cells *(arrows)*. Tumor mass is invading the dermis *(T)*.

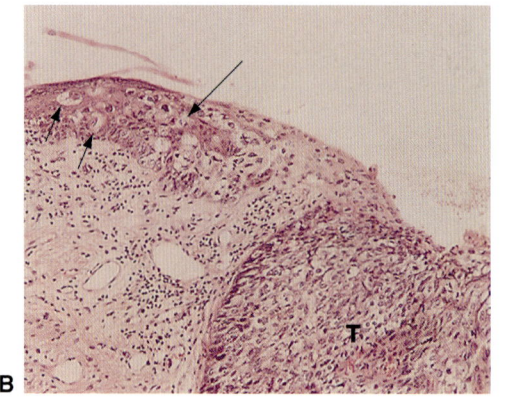

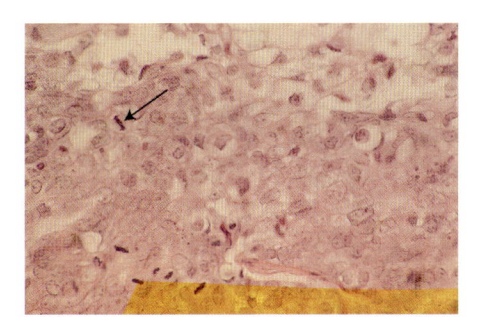

Figure 13-17 Sebaceous carcinoma. Note the mitotic figures *(arrow)* and tumor cells with foamy cytoplasm.

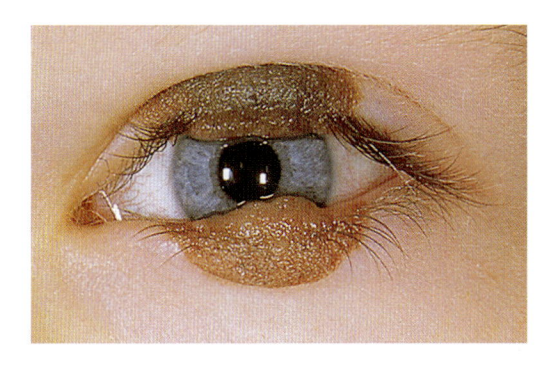

Figure 13-18 Congenital split, or "kissing," nevus of the eyelid.

the accuracy of intraoperative frozen section diagnosis of margins. Preoperative mapping by routine processing of multiple biopsies may afford a more accurate assessment of the extent of spread of the carcinoma. Survival rates for sebaceous carcinoma are worse than those for squamous cell carcinoma but have improved in recent years as a result of increased awareness, earlier detection, more accurate diagnosis, and appropriate treatment. Metastases first involve regional lymph nodes.

For American Joint Committee on Cancer definitions and staging of malignant neoplasms of the eyelid, see Table A-5 in the appendix.

> Albert DM, Jakobiec FA, eds. *Principles and Practice of Ophthalmology.* 2nd ed. Philadelphia: Saunders; 2000.

Melanocytic Neoplasms

Nevocellular nevi occur commonly on the eyelids and may be visible at birth (congenital nevi) or become apparent in adolescence or adulthood. Congenital nevi are often larger than those appearing in later years, sometimes reaching substantial size. Nevi greater than 20 cm in diameter are referred to as *giant congenital melanocytic nevi.* The risk for development of melanoma in congenital nevi is proportional to the size of the nevus; close follow-up and/or excision of congenital nevi is warranted. Congenital melanocytic nevi in the eyelid may develop in utero prior to the separation of the upper and lower eyelids and result in the clinical appearance of "kissing" nevi (Fig 13-18). Features associated with congenital nevi include the presence of nevus cells within and around adnexal structures, vessel walls, and the perineurium; extension into the deep reticular dermis or subcutaneous tissue; and a single- or double-file arrangement of nevus cells.

Melanocytic nevi appearing after childhood typically begin as small (less than 0.5 cm), round brown macules, gradually attaining increased thickness to become papules that may or may not be pigmented. This growth pattern corresponds to the histopathologic classification of melanocytic nevi. Macular (flat) nevi histopathologically show nests of melanocytes along the dermal–epidermal junction and are consequently termed *junctional nevi* (Fig 13-19). A junctional nevus is clinically indistinguishable from an ephelis, or freckle. Histopathologically, however, an ephelis is a result of increased melanization of basal keratinocytes without proliferation or aggregation of melanocytes. As the junctional nests, or theques, of the nevus begin to migrate into the superficial dermis, the nevus becomes a dome-shaped, or papillomatous, papule. When both junctional and intradermal components are present, the histopathologic classification becomes *compound nevus* (Fig 13-20). Finally, the junctional component disappears, leaving only nevus cells within the dermis, and the classification accordingly becomes *intradermal nevus* (Fig 13-21).

An evolution in the cytomorphology of the nevus cells also takes place: those in the superficial portion of the nevus are polygonal, or epithelioid, in shape (type A nevus cells). Within the midportion of the nevus, the cells become smaller, have less cytoplasm, and resemble lymphocytes (type B nevus cells). At the deepest levels, the nevus cells become spindled and appear similar to Schwann cells of peripheral nerves (type C nevus cells). Recognition of this "maturation" is useful in classifying melanocytic neoplasms as benign. Other histopathologic criteria favoring a benign melanocytic process include the following:

- absence of intraepidermal migration of nevus cells
- absence of mitotic activity in the dermal component of the mass
- absence of nuclear enlargement or prominent nucleoli
- cytoplasmic melanin pigment content greatest in superficial layers and absent in deeper layers

Multinucleated giant melanocytes and interspersed adipose tissue are common in older nevi.

Figure 13-19 Junctional nevus. Nests of nevus cells are seen at the junction between epidermis and dermis.

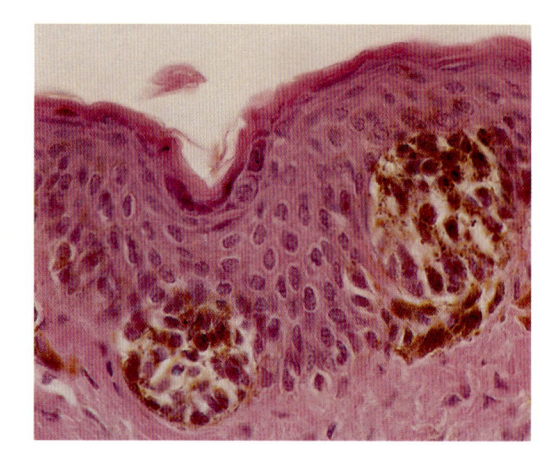

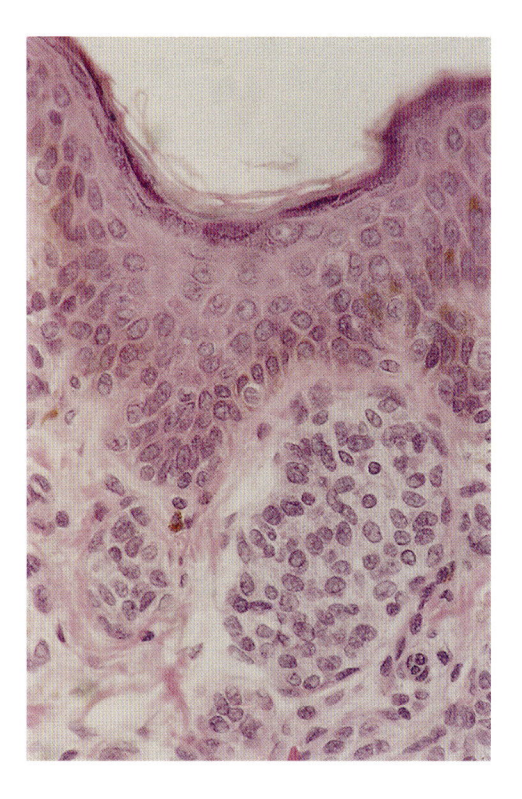

Figure 13-20 Compound nevus. Nests of nevus cells are present in the dermis as well as at the junction of epidermis and dermis.

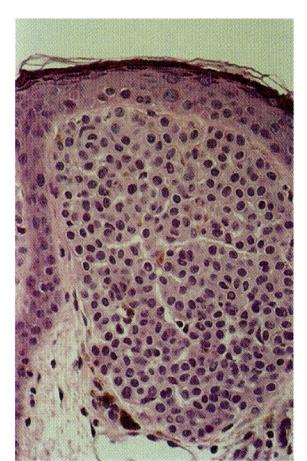

Figure 13-21 Intradermal nevus. The nests of nevus cells are confined to the dermis.

Nevi that show some clinical or pathologic atypicality include the Spitz nevus and the dysplastic nevus. *Spitz nevi* develop in late childhood or in adolescence and are uncommon after the second decade. In contrast to the clinical picture of the usual nevus, they may be larger (up to 1.0 cm) and have a pink-red color. Histopathologically, they are usually compound and exhibit nuclear and cytoplasmic enlargement and pleomorphism. Other features suggesting malignancy, however, such as atypical mitotic figures, intraepidermal migration, and lack of maturation, are generally lacking.

Clinical features suggesting a *dysplastic nevus* may include size greater than 0.5 cm, irregular margins, and irregular pigmentation. Nevi are considered dysplastic when they demonstrate certain architectural or cytomorphologic characteristics on histopathologic examination. Architectural features include lentiginous (single-cell) melanocytic hyperplasia, bridging of melanocytes across the bases of adjacent rete pegs, and lamellar fibrosis of the papillary dermis. Cytologic atypia is characterized by nuclear enlargement, hyperchromasia, and prominent nucleoli. Clinically suspicious lesions should be completely excised. Persons with multiple dysplastic nevi are at increased risk for development of melanoma and may represent a genetic susceptibility, suggesting that family members should also be examined and followed closely.

Cutaneous malignant melanoma is a rare occurrence on the eyelids. It may be associated with a preexisting nevus or it may develop de novo. Clinical features suggesting malignancy are the same as those just mentioned for dysplastic nevi; in addition, invasive melanoma is heralded by a vertical (perpendicular to the skin surface) growth phase that results in an elevated or indurated mass. There are 4 main histopathologic subtypes of malignant melanoma:

1. superficial spreading
2. lentigo maligna
3. nodular
4. acral-lentiginous

Superficial spreading is the most common type of cutaneous melanoma and demonstrates a radial (intraepidermal) growth pattern extending beyond the invasive component, distinguishing it from nodular melanoma. Lentigo maligna melanoma occurs on the face of elderly individuals, with a long preinvasive phase. Acral-lentiginous melanoma, as the name implies, involves the extremities and is not seen in the eyelid.

Histopathologic features characteristic of melanoma include pagetoid intraepidermal spread of atypical melanocytic nests and single cells, nuclear abnormalities as listed earlier, lack of maturation in the deeper portions of the mass, and atypical mitotic figures. A bandlike lymphocytic host response along the base of the mass is more common in melanoma than in benign proliferations, with the exception of a halo nevus. Prognosis is correlated with depth of invasion in stage I (localized) disease. Metastases, when they occur, typically involve regional lymph nodes first.

Font RL. Eyelids and lacrimal drainage system. In: Spencer WH, ed. *Ophthalmic Pathology: An Atlas and Textbook.* 4th ed. Philadelphia: Saunders; 1996:2263–2277.

McLean IW, Burnier MN, Zimmerman LE, Jakobiec FA. *Tumors of the Eye and Ocular Adnexa.* Washington: Armed Forces Institute of Pathology; 1995.

CHAPTER 14

Orbit

Topography

Bony Orbit and Soft Tissues

Seven bones form the boundaries of the orbit (Fig 14-1). These 7 bones are the

- frontal
- zygoma
- palatine
- lacrimal
- sphenoid
- ethmoid
- maxilla

The orbital cavity is pear-shaped and has a volume of 30 cc. Other structures and tissues occupying the cavity are the

- globe
- lacrimal gland
- muscles
- tendons
- fat
- fascia
- vessels
- nerves
- sympathetic ganglia
- cartilaginous trochlea

Inflammatory and neoplastic processes that increase the volume of the orbital contents lead to *proptosis* (protrusion) of the globe and/or *displacement* (deviation) from the horizontal or vertical position. The degree and direction of ocular displacement help to localize the position of the mass.

The *lacrimal gland* is situated anteriorly in the superotemporal quadrant of the orbit. The gland is divided into orbital and palpebral lobes by the aponeurosis of the levator palpebrae superioris muscle. The acini of the glands are composed of low cuboidal epithelium. The ducts, which lie within the fibrovascular stroma, are lined by low cuboidal epithelium with a second outer layer of low, flat myoepithelial cells.

220 • Ophthalmic Pathology and Intraocular Tumors

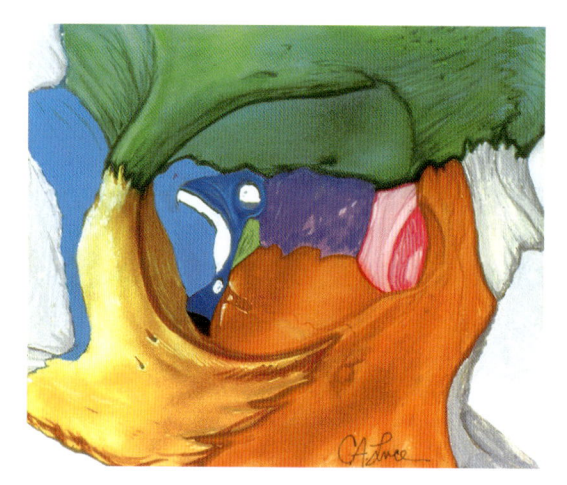

Figure 14-1 Bony components of the right orbit identified by color: maxilla *(orange)*; zygoma *(beige)*; sphenoid bone, greater wing *(light blue)*, lesser wing *(dark blue)*; palatine bone *(light green)*; ethmoid bone *(purple)*; lacrimal bone *(pink)*; frontal bone *(green)*. *(Reproduced with permission from Zide BM, Jelks GW, eds.* Surgical Anatomy of the Orbit. *New York: Raven; 1985:3.)*

BCSC Section 2, *Fundamentals and Principles of Ophthalmology,* covers orbital anatomy in Part I, Anatomy. BCSC Section 7, *Orbit, Eyelids, and Lacrimal System,* also discusses orbital anatomy, as well as the conditions covered in the following pages, in detail.

Congenital Anomalies

Dermoid and Other Epithelial Cysts

Dermoid cysts are believed to arise as embryonic epithelial nests that became entrapped during embryogenesis. They may protrude through the frontozygomatic suture to take a dumbbell shape. Most manifest in childhood as a mass in the superotemporal quadrants of the orbit. Rupture of cyst contents may produce a marked granulomatous reaction. Histologically, dermoid cysts are encapsulated, lined by keratinized stratified squamous epithelium. The cysts contain keratin and hair, and the walls of the cysts are lined with adnexal structures, including sebaceous glands, hair roots, sweat glands, and may include glandular tissue (Fig 14-2). If the wall does not bear adnexal structures, the term *epidermal cyst* is applied. Intraorbital cysts may also be lined by respiratory epithelium or conjunctival epithelium.

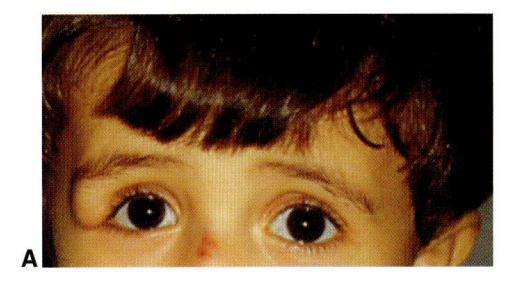

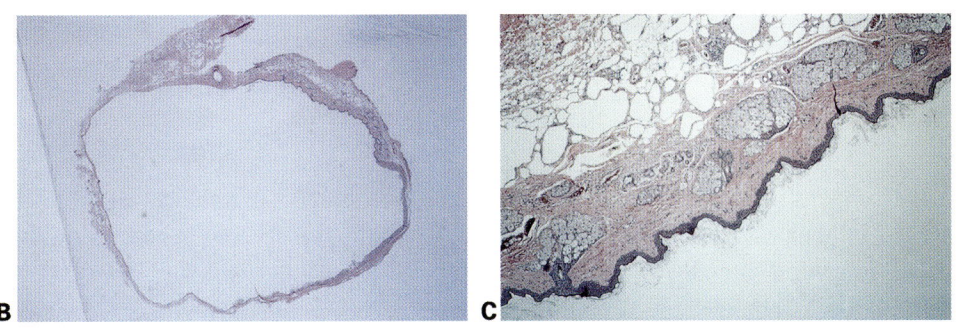

Figure 14-2 A, Clinical appearance of dermoid cyst of the orbit. Note the typical superotemporal location. **B,** Low-power photomicrograph discloses a cyst lined by stratified squamous epithelium. **C,** The wall of the cyst contains sebaceous glands and adnexal structures. *(Part A courtesy of Sander Dubovy, MD; parts B and C courtesy of Hans E. Grossniklaus, MD.)*

Inflammations

Infectious

Bacterial infections

The causes of bacterial infections of the orbit include bacteremia, trauma, retained surgical hardware, and adjacent sinus infection. Infection may involve a variety of organisms, including *Haemophilus influenzae, Streptococcus, Staphylococcus aureus, Clostridium, Bacteroides, Klebsiella,* and *Proteus*. Histologically, acute inflammation, necrosis, and abscess formation may be present. Tuberculosis, which rarely involves the orbit, produces a necrotizing granulomatous reaction.

Fungal and parasitic infections

A common fungal infection of the orbit is caused by sinus infection from mucormycosis (zygomycosis). Poorly controlled diabetes can make patients particularly prone to mucormycosis, although any immunocompromised condition may increase susceptibility. Histologically, acute and chronic inflammation appear in a background of necrosis, often with histiocytes. Broad, nonseptated hyphae may be identified in periodic acid–Schiff (PAS) and Gomori methenamine silver (GMS) stains. Diagnosis is achieved by biopsy of necrotic-appearing tissues in the nasopharynx. These fungi can invade blood vessel walls and produce a thrombosing vasculitis.

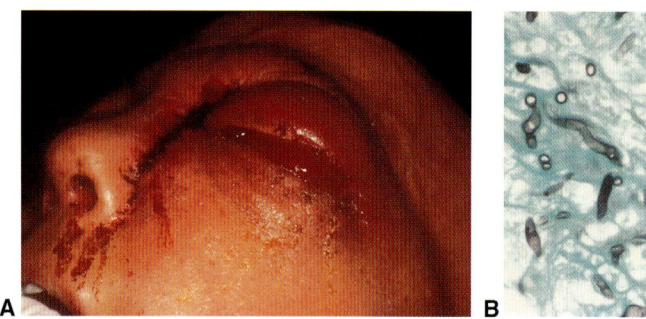

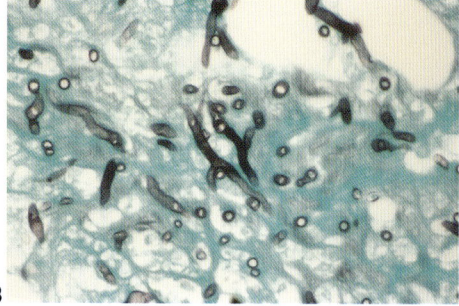

222 • Ophthalmic Pathology and Intraocular Tumors

Figure 14-3 *Aspergillus* infections of the orbit generally produce severe, insidious orbital inflammation. **A,** Clinical appearance. **B,** Microscopic section demonstrates the branching hyphal structure on silver stains. *(Courtesy of Hans E. Grossniklaus, MD.)*

Aspergillus infection of the orbit may occur in immunocompromised or otherwise healthy individuals. Often, the symptoms are slowly progressive and insidious, producing a sclerosing granulomatous disease. *Aspergillus* has often been difficult to culture but may be observed in tissue as septated hyphae with 45° angle branching (Fig 14-3). Despite aggressive surgical therapy and adjunctive therapy with amphotericin B, orbital infections with either *Aspergillus* or mucormycosis may be fatal if extension into the brain occurs. Allergic fungal sinusitis has also been noted to extend into the orbit in some instances.

Parasitic infections of the orbit are rare and may be produced by *Echinococcus, Taenia solium* (cysticercosis), *Onchocerca volvulus* (onchocerciasis), and *Loa loa* (loiasis). These infections are mostly seen in patients who come from, or have traveled to, areas where the infections are endemic.

Noninfectious

Thyroid-associated orbitopathy

Also known as *Graves disease* and *thyroid ophthalmopathy,* thyroid-associated orbitopathy is related to thyroid dysfunction and is the most common cause of unilateral or bilateral proptosis (exophthalmos) in adults. A cellular infiltrate of mononuclear cells, lymphocytes, plasma cells, mast cells, and fibroblasts involves the interstitial tissues of the extraocular muscles, most commonly the inferior and medial rectus muscles (Fig 14-4). The muscles appear firm and white, and the tendons are usually not involved. The fibroblasts produce mucopolysaccharide, leading to increased water content in the tissues. As a result of the increased bulk, the optic nerve may be compromised at the orbital apex and papilledema may result. Progressive fibrosis results in restriction of ocular movement, and exposure keratitis is also a complication. BCSC Section 1, *Update on General Medicine,* and Section 7, *Orbit, Eyelids, and Lacrimal System,* discuss thyroid disease in greater detail.

Albert DM, Jakobiec FA, eds. *Principles and Practice of Ophthalmology.* 2nd ed. Philadelphia: Saunders; 2000.

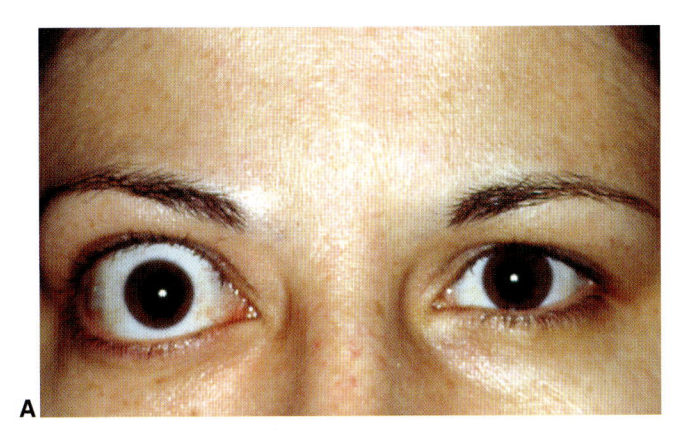

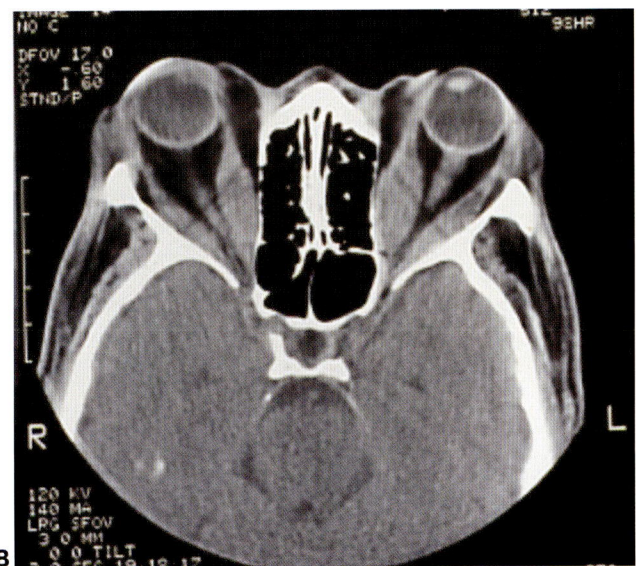

Figure 14-4 Thyroid-associated orbitopathy (Graves disease or thyroid ophthalmopathy). **A,** Clinical appearance demonstrating asymmetric proptosis and eyelid retraction. **B,** CT scan (axial view) showing fusiform enlargement of the extraocular muscles. **C,** The muscle bundles of the extraocular muscle are separated by fluid, accompanied by an infiltrate of mononuclear inflammatory cells. The inflammatory process expands the volume of the muscles, potentially causing proptosis and, in extreme cases, corneal exposure. *(Parts A and B courtesy of Sander Dubovy, MD.)*

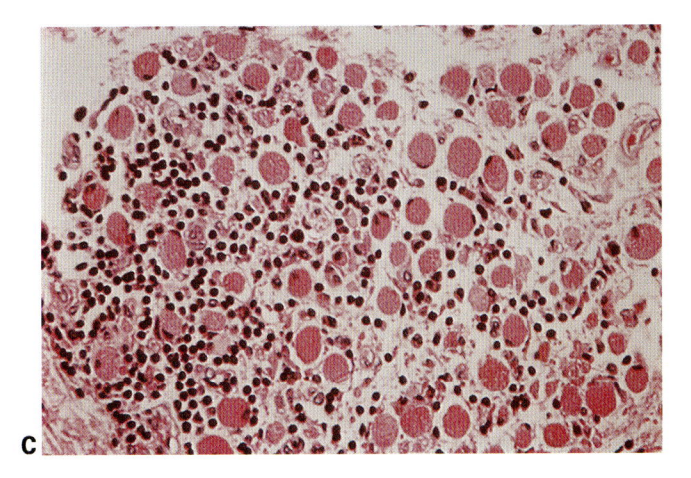

Idiopathic orbital inflammation

Idiopathic orbital inflammation, or *orbital inflammatory syndrome (sclerosing orbititis)*, refers to a space-occupying inflammatory disorder that simulates a neoplasm (thus, it is sometimes known as *orbital pseudotumor*) but has no recognizable cause, such as Graves disease or a ruptured epidermal inclusion cyst. This disorder accounts for about 5% of orbital lesions. Clinically, patients have an abrupt course and usually complain of pain. The condition may affect children as well as adults. The inflammatory response may be diffuse or compartmentalized. When localized to an extraocular muscle, the condition is called *orbital myositis* (Fig 14-5); when localized to the lacrimal gland, it is frequently called *sclerosing dacryoadenitis*.

In the early stages, inflammation predominates, with a polymorphous inflammatory response (eosinophils, neutrophils, plasma cells, lymphocytes, and macrophages) that is often perivascular and that frequently infiltrates muscle, producing fat necrosis. In later stages, fibrosis is the predominant feature, often with interspersed lymphoid follicles bearing germinal centers. The fibrosis may inexorably replace orbital fat and encase extraocular muscles and the optic nerve (Fig 14-6). The majority of patients with early idiopathic orbital inflammation respond promptly to corticosteroids; patients with the advanced stages of fibrosis may be unresponsive. See BCSC Section 7, *Orbit, Eyelids, and Lacrimal System*, for further discussion.

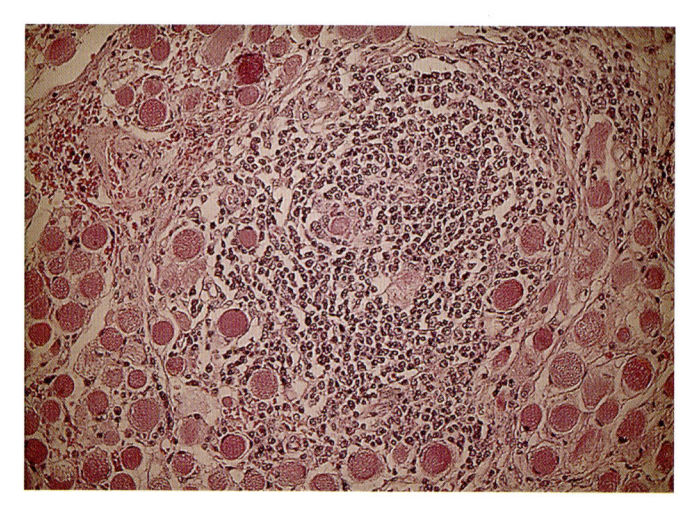

Figure 14-5 Idiopathic orbital inflammation (orbital inflammatory syndrome). In this case, an inflammatory infiltrate involves extraocular muscle. Unlike Graves disease, in which the tendons of the muscles typically are spared, this condition can affect any orbital structure, including the muscle tendons.

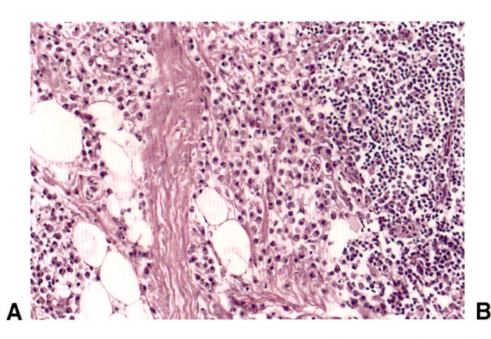

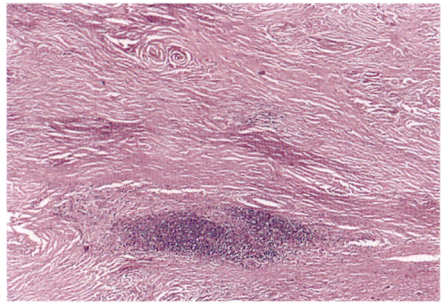

Figure 14-6 Idiopathic orbital inflammation. **A,** Note the mixture of inflammatory cells in the bundle of collagen running through the orbital fat. **B,** Diffuse fibrosis dominates the histologic picture of this fibrosing orbititis, considered by some authorities to represent a later stage of the condition illustrated in part **A**.

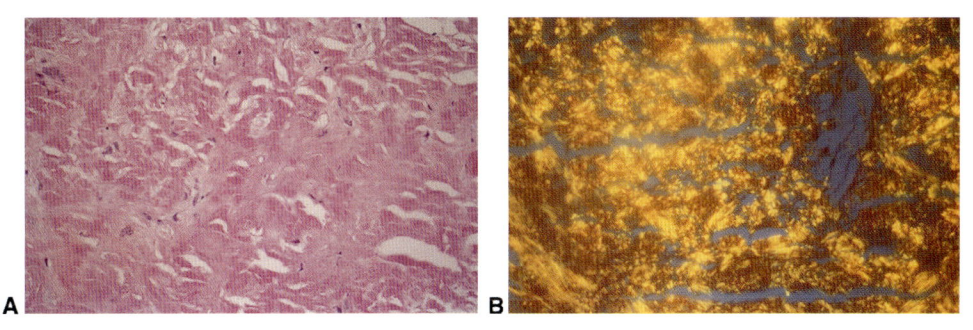

Figure 14-7 Orbital amyloidosis. **A,** Tissue infiltration by pink amorphous material. **B,** Polarized light of a Congo red–stained section demonstrates red-green dichroism. *(Courtesy of Hans E. Grossniklaus, MD.)*

Degenerations

Amyloid

Amyloid deposition in the orbit occurs in primary systemic amyloidosis; when it involves the extraocular muscles and nerves, it can produce ophthalmoplegia and ptosis. Amyloidosis may also be localized within the orbit and have no systemic manifestations. Histologic sections stained with Congo red dye show deposits of a hyalinized amorphous material that exhibits green-red dichroism with polarized light (Fig 14-7). Electron microscopy demonstrates characteristic fibrils. Amyloid deposition may be associated with a plasma cell dyscrasia or atypical lymphomatous proliferation. BCSC Section 8, *External Disease and Cornea,* discusses both systemic and localized amyloidosis in greater detail.

Neoplasia

Neoplasms of the orbit may be primary, secondary from adjacent structures, or metastatic. The incidence of primary neoplasms is low, with hemangioma and lymphoma being the most common. Secondary tumors from adjacent sinuses are slightly more common than primary tumors.

In children, approximately 90% of orbital tumors are benign. Most benign lesions are cystic (dermoid or epidermoid cysts), and most malignant tumors are rhabdomyosarcomas. The orbit may be involved secondarily by retinoblastoma, neuroblastoma, or leukemia/lymphoma.

The various tumors discussed in the following sections are covered at greater length in BCSC Section 7, *Orbit, Eyelids, and Lacrimal System*.

Lacrimal Gland Neoplasia

Pleomorphic adenoma

Pleomorphic adenoma (benign mixed tumor) describes the most common epithelial tumor of the lacrimal gland. Initially, the tumor is encapsulated; it grows slowly by expansion. This progressive expansive growth may indent the bone of the lacrimal fossa, producing excavation of the area. Tumor growth stimulates the periosteum to deposit a thin layer of new bone (cortication). The adjacent orbital bone is not eroded. Typically, the patient experiences no pain. This tumor is more common in men than in women, and the median age at presentation is approximately 35 years.

The histologic appearance of pleomorphic adenoma is a mixture of epithelial and stromal elements. The epithelial component may form nests or tubules lined by 2 layers of cells, the outermost layer blending imperceptibly with the stroma (Fig 14-8). The stroma may appear myxoid and may contain heterologous elements, including cartilage and bone. Although the tumor may appear to be encapsulated, microscopic lobules can prolapse through the capsule, which is formed by the compression of adjacent normal orbital tissue and is not an anatomical barrier cleanly separating the tumor from the adjacent orbit.

Although pleomorphic adenoma is a benign neoplasm, tumor left behind in the orbit after incomplete surgical removal may produce clinically significant recurrences that are difficult to extirpate surgically. The possibility of orbital recurrence leads to 2 important surgical principles. The surgeon should

1. try to excise the tumor with a rim of normal orbital tissue and not merely shell it out
2. avoid incisional biopsies into this tumor to prevent seeding of the orbit

Transformation into a malignant mixed tumor may take place in a long-standing pleomorphic adenoma with relatively rapid growth after a period of relative quiescence. Carcinomas, including adenocarcinoma and adenoid cystic carcinoma, may also arise in recurrent pleomorphic adenomas.

> Spencer WH, ed. *Ophthalmic Pathology: An Atlas and Textbook.* 4th ed. Philadelphia: Saunders; 1996:2484–2494.

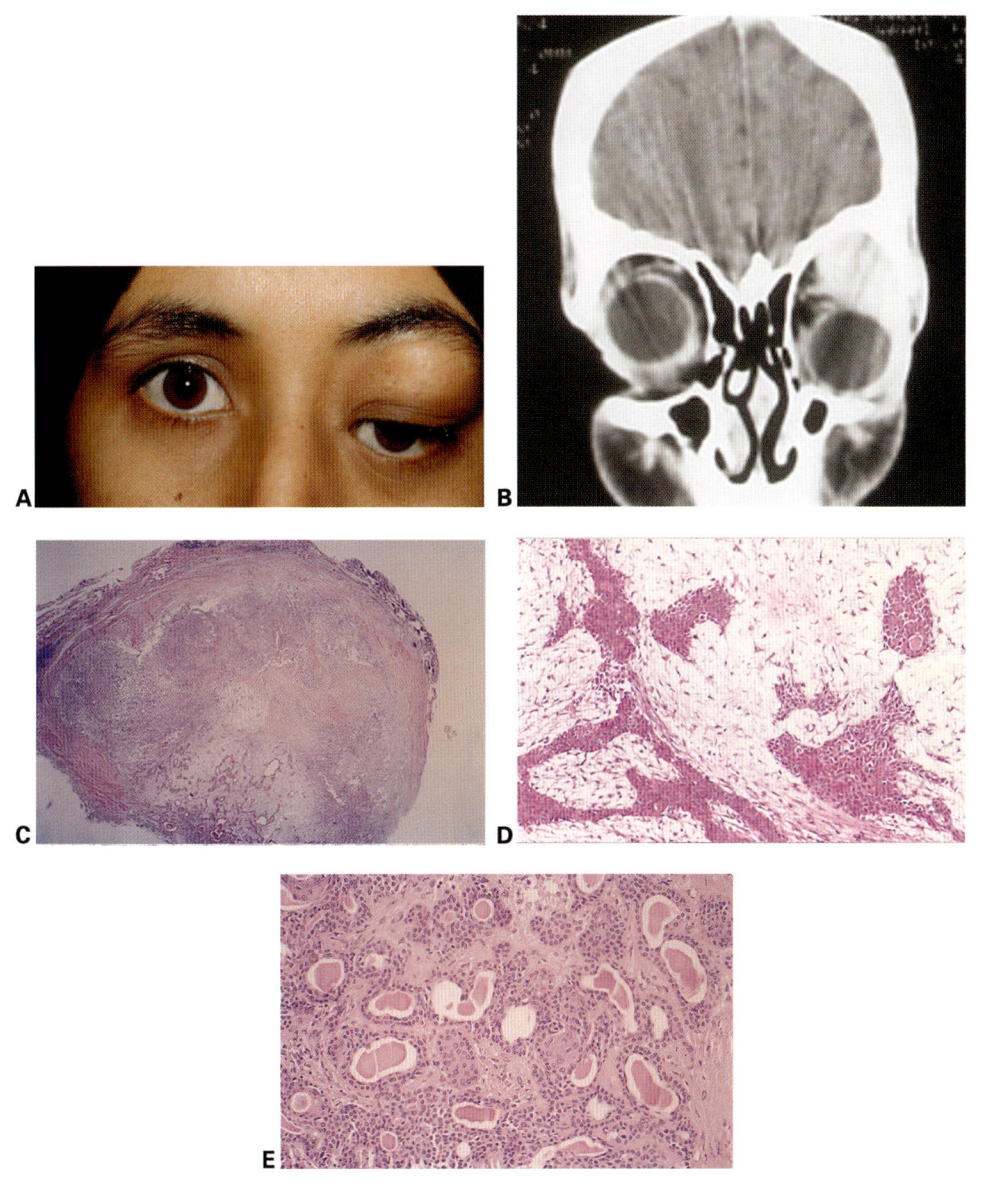

Figure 14-8 Pleomorphic adenoma (benign mixed tumor) of the lacrimal gland. **A,** Clinical appearance. A superotemporal orbital mass is present, causing proptosis and downward displacement of the left globe. **B,** CT scan (coronal view) demonstrating left orbit tumor. **C,** Low power shows the circumscribed nature of this pleomorphic adenoma. **D,** Note both the epithelial and the mesenchymal elements. **E,** Well-differentiated glandular structures (epithelial component). *(Parts A and B courtesy of Sander Dubovy, MD; parts C–E courtesy of Hans E. Grossniklaus, MD.)*

Adenoid cystic carcinoma

As mentioned in the previous section, adenoid cystic carcinoma can arise in a pleomorphic adenoma or de novo in the lacrimal gland. The tumor is slightly more common in women than in men, and the median age of presentation is about 40. Unlike pleomorphic adenoma, adenoid cystic carcinoma is not encapsulated; it tends to erode the adjacent bone and invade orbital nerves, accounting for the pain that is a frequent presenting complaint. Grossly, the appearance is grayish white, firm, and nodular. Histologically, a variety of patterns may appear, including the Swiss cheese (cribriform) pattern (Fig 14-9). Other histologic patterns include basaloid (solid), comedo, sclerosing, and tubular. Presence of the basaloid pattern has been associated with a worse prognosis (5-year survival of 21%) than those tumors without a basaloid component (5-year survival of 71%). Because of the diffuse infiltration of this tumor, exenteration may be recommended, often with removal of adjacent bone. Despite aggressive surgical intervention, the long-term prognosis is poor.

For American Joint Committee on Cancer (AJCC) definitions and staging of lacrimal gland carcinomas, see Table A-6 in the appendix.

> Font RL, Smith SL, Bryan RG. Malignant epithelial tumors of the lacrimal gland: a clinicopathologic study of 21 cases. *Arch Ophthalmol.* 1998;116:613–616.

Lymphoproliferative Lesions

Most classifications of lymphoid lesions have been based on lymph node architecture, and such nodal classifications have been difficult to apply to so-called extranodal lymphoid lesions. Because there are no lymph nodes in the orbit, it is problematic to classify these lesions according to the criteria used for lymph nodes. The development of classification schemes for lymphomas is, thus, an ongoing and controversial process. The most recent classification schemes, which incorporate data from morphology, immunophenotyping, and gene rearrangement studies, have attempted to include orbital lymphomas. Data that reveal the prognosis of patients with orbital lymphomas using these classifications are just beginning to emerge. Many lymphoid masses in the orbit that were previously classified as reactive would now be considered neoplastic.

Malignant lymphoma

Malignant lymphomas of the orbit may be a presenting manifestation of systemic lymphomas, or they may arise primarily from the orbit. The incidence of orbital involvement in systemic lymphomas is 1.3%. Hodgkin disease is exceedingly rare in the orbit, and the majority of primary malignant orbital lymphomas are non–Hodgkin lymphomas of diffuse architecture that mark immunophenotypically as B cells (Fig 14-10). The classification of non–Hodgkin lymphomas is controversial and continues to evolve. The current Revised European-American Lymphoma (REAL) classification includes extranodal lymphomas.

Figure 14-9 Adenoid cystic carcinoma of the lacrimal gland. Note the characteristic Swiss cheese (cribriform) pattern of tumor cells. *(Courtesy of Ben J. Glasgow, MD.)*

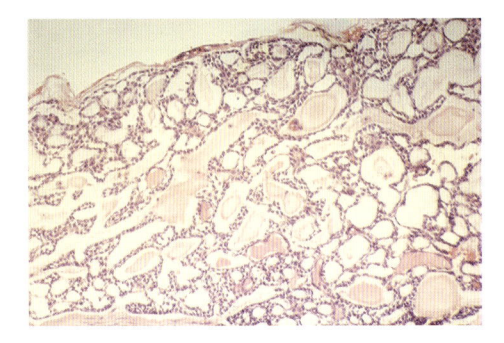

Harris NL, Jaffe ES, Stein H, et al. A revised European-American classification of lymphoid neoplasms: a proposal from the International Lymphoma Study Group. *Blood.* 1994;84:1361–1392.

The most commonly encountered low-grade orbital lymphoma in the REAL classification is an extranodal marginal zone, or mucosa-associated lymphoid tissue (MALT), lymphoma. The MALT lymphoma often shows poorly formed follicles with heterogeneous cellular composition, including small atypical cells with cleaved nuclei, monocytoid cells, small lymphocytes, and plasma cells. The neoplastic monocytoid B-cell population may expand the marginal zone and infiltrate follicles (follicular colonization). MALT lymphomas are characterized by a B-cell immunophenotype that is generally CD5- and CD10-negative (Fig 14-11).

The lymphomas of the chronic lymphocytic leukemia (CLL) type are also low grade and are composed of homogeneous sheets of small, mature-appearing lymphocytes.

In some studies, follicular center lymphoma is the most common secondary type of lymphoma to involve the orbit. In this low-grade B-cell lymphoma, follicles are well formed and dominated by cleaved cells (centrocytes), with fewer noncleaved cells (centroblasts).

High-grade lymphomas of the orbit in the REAL classification include large cell lymphoma, lymphoblastic lymphoma, and Burkitt lymphoma. With the exception of Burkitt

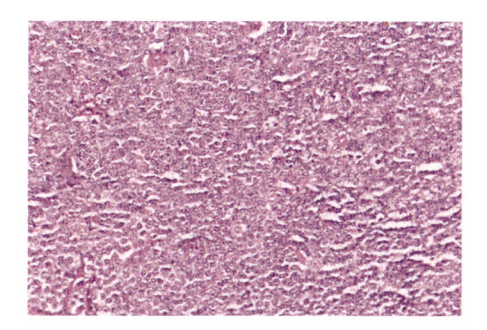

Figure 14-10 B-cell lymphoma of the orbit. Orbital soft tissues are diffusely replaced by sheets of cytologically malignant lymphocytes.

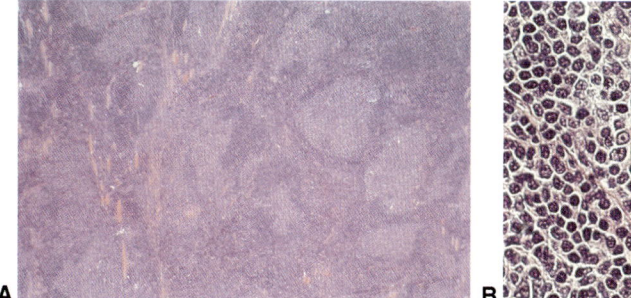

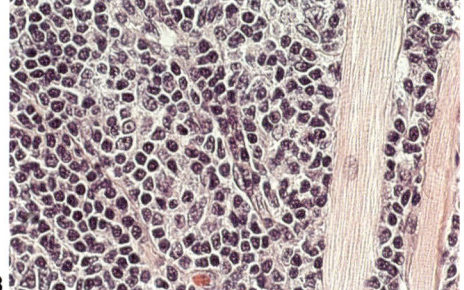

Figure 14-11 MALT. **A,** Low power shows a hint of follicular architecture in a dense lymphoid infiltrate with infiltration of muscle. **B,** Higher magnification demonstrates a heterogeneous infiltrate that includes small lymphocytes, plasma cells, and cleaved and noncleaved cells, as well as atypical lymphocytes with cytoplasmic clearing (monocytoid B cells). *(Courtesy of Ben J. Glasgow, MD.)*

lymphoma, orbital lymphoma is not likely to occur in children, although leukemic infiltrates and so-called granulocytic sarcomas are encountered in children.

Neither immunophenotypic nor gene rearrangement studies to identify clonal lymphocyte populations have thus far proven helpful in predicting the development of systemic disease. Location is 1 factor that may have a bearing on prognosis; conjunctival lesions have a better prognosis than orbital lesions, for example. Eyelid lesions may have the highest association with systemic involvement (67%).

It is important for the ophthalmologist to distinguish orbital lymphoproliferative lesions from orbital inflammatory syndrome. Unlike patients with orbital inflammatory syndrome, those with orbital lymphoproliferative lesions present with a gradual, painless progression of proptosis. Every patient with an orbital lymphoproliferative lesion must be investigated for evidence of systemic lymphoma, including examination for lymphadenopathy, a complete blood count (CBC) and differential, and imaging of the thoracic and abdominal viscera. In general, biopsy of an accessible lymph node is preferred over an orbital biopsy because nodal architecture is helpful in diagnosis and the procedure may be safer. A bone marrow biopsy is preferred to an aspirate because it includes bone spicules; the presence of a paratrabecular lymphoid infiltrate may indicate systemic lymphoma. In contrast to most cases of idiopathic orbital inflammation, which are treated with corticosteroids, lymphoproliferative lesions confined to the orbit are treated with radiation.

The ophthalmologist taking a biopsy of an orbital or conjunctival lymphoproliferative lesion should consult with the pathologist to determine the optimal method for handling the tissue. Fresh (unfixed) tissue is preferred for touch preparations, immunohistochemistry, flow cytometry, and gene rearrangement studies. The type of fixative used for permanent sections varies from one laboratory to another. Exposure of the biopsy specimen to air for long periods of time should be avoided. Tissue samples may be wrapped in saline-moistened gauze and transported on ice. It is very important that the tissue be handled gently; crush artifact can prevent the pathologist from rendering a diagnosis.

Albert DM, Jakobiec FA, eds. *Principles and Practice of Ophthalmology.* 2nd ed. Philadelphia: Saunders; 2000.

Vascular Tumors

Lymphangiomas occur in children and are characterized by fluctuation in proptosis. Lymphangiomas of the orbit are unencapsulated, diffusely infiltrating tumors that feature lymphatic vascular spaces and well-formed lymphoid aggregates in a fibrotic interstitium (Fig 14-12).

Hemangioma in the adult is encapsulated and consists of cavernous spaces *(cavernous hemangioma)* with thick, fibrosed walls (Fig 14-13). Vessels may show thrombosis and calcification. Hemangioma in the child is unencapsulated, more cellular, and composed of capillary-sized vessels *(capillary hemangioma)* (Fig 14-14).

Hemangiopericytoma occurs mainly in adults (median age is 42 years) and manifests with proptosis, pain, diplopia, and decreased visual acuity. Histologically, a staghorn vascular pattern is displayed with densely packed oval to spindle-shaped cells. The reticulin stain is useful in demonstrating tumor cells that are individually wrapped in a network of collagenous material (Fig 14-15). Hemangiopericytomas include a spectrum of benign,

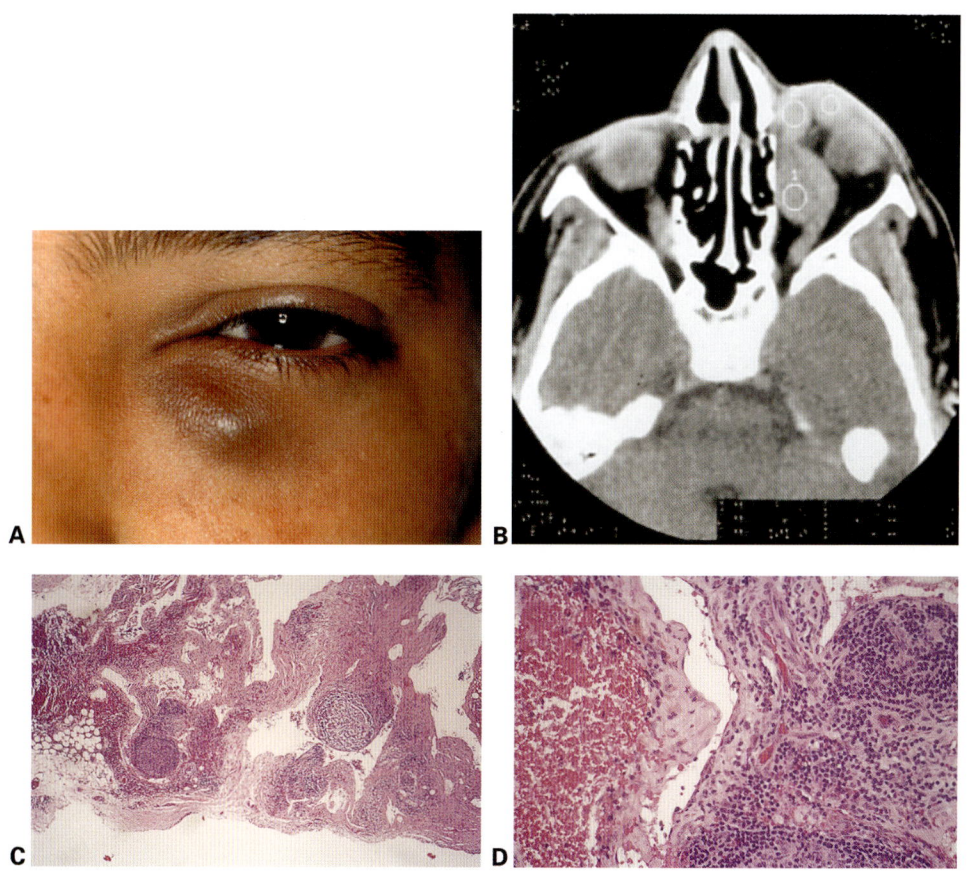

Figure 14-12 Lymphangioma. **A,** Clinical appearance. A young boy with an inferior orbital lesion extending anteriorly to the right lower lid. **B,** CT scan (axial view) showing a multilobulated mass within the left orbit. **C,** Photomicrograph shows numerous vascular channels with a fibrotic interstitium. **D,** Higher magnification demonstrates the lymphocytes and plasma cells within the fibrous walls. *(Parts A and B courtesy of Sander Dubovy, MD; parts C and D courtesy of Ben J. Glasgow, MD.)*

intermediate, and malignant lesions. Features of malignancy include an infiltrating border, anaplasia, mitotic figures, and necrosis. However, these features may be absent in tumors that eventually metastasize.

Tumors With Muscle Differentiation

Rhabdomyosarcoma
Rhabdomyosarcoma is the most common primary malignant orbital tumor of childhood (average age of onset is 7–8 years). Proptosis is often sudden and rapidly progressive, and it requires emergency treatment. Reddish discoloration of the eyelids is *not* accompanied by local heat or systemic fever, as it is in cellulitis. Orbital rhabdomyosarcomas are classified slightly differently and have a better prognosis (overall 5-year survival of 92%) than do their extraorbital counterparts.

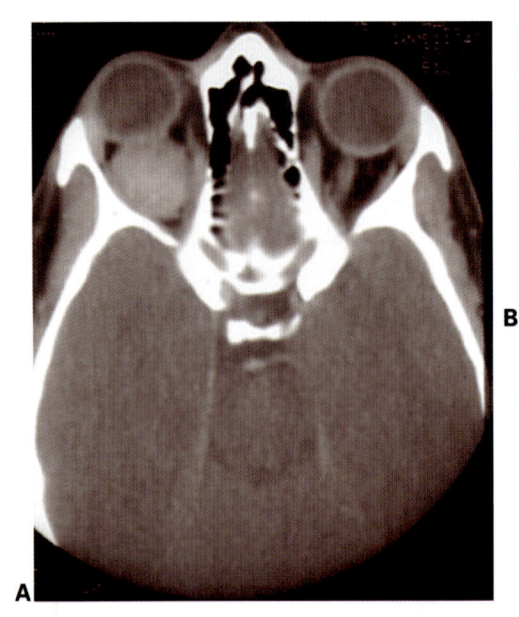

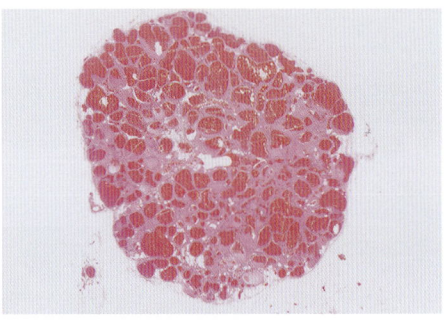

232 • Ophthalmic Pathology and Intraocular Tumors

Figure 14-13 Cavernous hemangioma. **A,** CT scan (axial view) showing a well-circumscribed retrobulbar mass. **B,** Large spaces of blood are separated by thick septa. *(Part A courtesy of Sander Dubovy, MD; part B courtesy of Hans E. Grossniklaus, MD.)*

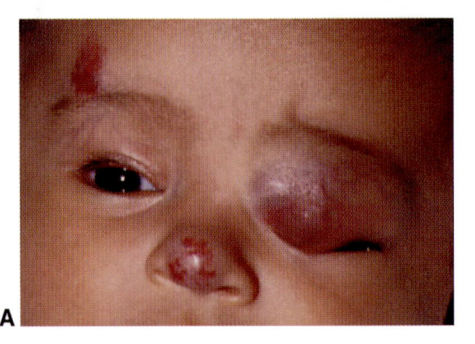

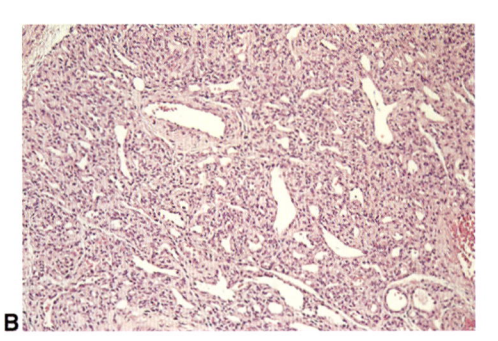

Figure 14-14 Capillary hemangioma. **A,** Infant with multiple capillary hemangiomas. **B,** Note the small capillary-sized vessels and the proliferation of benign endothelial cells. *(Part A courtesy of Sander Dubovy, MD.)*

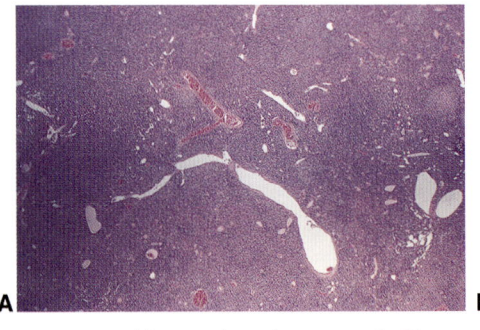

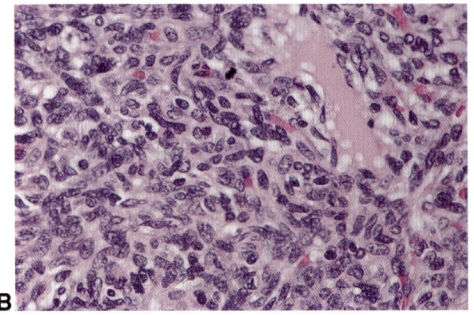

Figure 14-15 Hemangiopericytoma. **A,** Photomicrograph demonstrates a dense spindle-cell tumor with a characteristic branching vascular pattern. **B,** Higher magnification demonstrates closely packed, round to oval cells with vesicular nuclei. *(Courtesy of Ben J. Glasgow, MD.)*

CHAPTER 14: Orbit • 233

Three histologic types of orbital rhabdomyosarcoma are recognized (Fig 14-16):

1. embryonal (the most common)
2. alveolar
3. differentiated (pleomorphic)

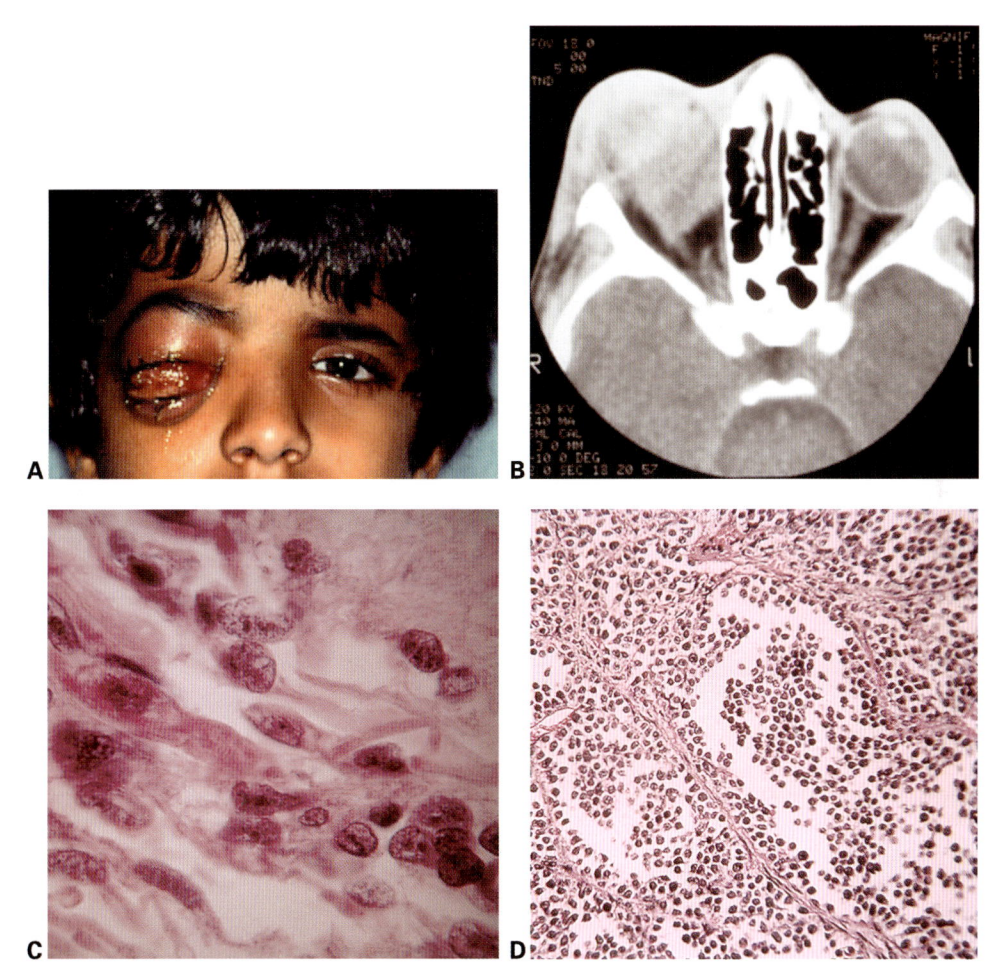

Figure 14-16 Rhabdomyosarcoma. **A,** Child with a large orbital mass. **B,** CT scan (axial view) showing a large, poorly circumscribed orbital tumor. **C,** The neoplastic cells tend to differentiate toward muscle cells. In this moderately differentiated embryonal example, cross-striations representing Z-bands of actin–myosin complexes within the cytoplasm can be easily identified. It is common for these cells to be more primitive, with a featureless abundant cytoplasm. In the less-differentiated cases, electron microscopy and immunohistochemistry may be necessary to correctly identify this neoplasm. **D,** Poorly cohesive rhabdomyoblasts separated by fibrous septa into "alveoli" are low-magnification histologic features of the alveolar variant of rhabdomyosarcoma. This variant may have a less favorable natural history than the more common embryonal type. *(Parts A and B courtesy of Sander Dubovy, MD.)*

Embryonal rhabdomyosarcoma may develop in the conjunctiva and may present as grape-like submucosal clusters *(botryoid variant)*. Histologically, spindle cells are arranged in a loose syncytium with occasional cells bearing cross-striations, which are found in about 60% of embryonal rhabdomyosarcomas. Well-differentiated rhabdomyosarcomas feature numerous cells with striking cross-striations. Immunohistochemical reactivity for desmin and muscle-specific actin may be identified. Electron microscopy is often helpful, especially in the less well-differentiated cases of embryonal rhabdomyosarcoma, to demonstrate the typical sarcomeric banding pattern.

Leiomyomas and leiomyosarcomas

Tumors with smooth-muscle differentiation are rare. *Leiomyomas* are benign tumors that typically manifest with slowly progressive proptosis in patients in the fourth and fifth decades. Histologically, these spindle-cell tumors show blunt-ended, cigar-shaped nuclei and trichrome-positive filamentous cytoplasm. *Leiomyosarcomas* are malignant lesions that typically occur in patients in the seventh decade. Histologically, more cellularity, necrosis, pleomorphism, and mitotic figures appear in leiomyosarcomas than in leiomyomas.

Tumors With Fibrous Differentiation

Fibrous histiocytoma (fibroxanthoma) is one of the most common mesenchymal tumors of the orbit in adults. The median age at presentation is 43 years (with a range of 6 months to 85 years), and the upper nasal orbit is the most common site. Most fibrous histiocytomas are benign. The tumor is composed of an admixture of histiocytes and fibroblasts, some of which form a storiform (matlike) pattern (Fig 14-17). Although most are benign, intermediate and malignant varieties do exist. Malignant tumors are identified by a high rate of mitotic activity (more than 1 mitotic figure per high-power field), pleomorphism, and necrosis. Other primary tumors of fibrous connective tissue include nodular fasciitis, fibroma, solitary fibrous tumor, and fibrosarcoma.

Bony Lesions of the Orbit

Fibrous dysplasia of bone may be monostotic or polyostotic. When the orbit is affected, the condition is usually monostotic, and the patient often presents during the first 3 decades of life. The tumor may cross suture lines to involve multiple orbital bones. Narrowing of the optic canal and lacrimal drainage system can occur. Plain radiographic studies show a ground-glass appearance with lytic foci. Cysts containing fluid also appear. As a result of

Figure 14-17 Fibrous histiocytoma. This photomicrograph illustrates the storiform (matlike) pattern.

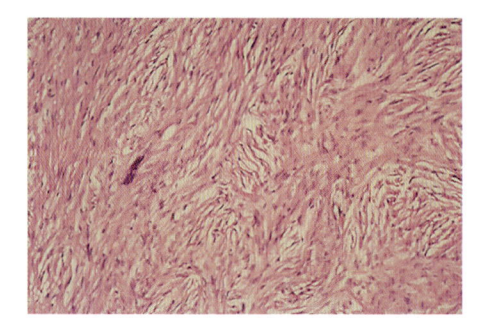

arrest in the maturation of bone, trabeculae are composed of woven bone with a fibrous stroma that is highly vascularized rather than lamellar bone. The bony trabeculae often have a C-shaped appearance.

> Katz BJ, Nerad JA. Ophthalmic manifestations of fibrous dysplasia: a disease of children and adults. *Ophthalmology.* 1998;105:2207–2215.

Juvenile ossifying fibroma, a variant of fibrous dysplasia, is characterized histologically by spicules of bone rimmed by osteoblasts. At low magnification, ossifying fibroma may be confused with a psammomatous meningioma. The inexperienced histologist can find the correct identification difficult.

Osseous and cartilaginous tumors are rare; of these, *osteoma* is the most common. It is slow growing, well circumscribed, and composed of mature bone. Most commonly, an osteoma arises from the frontal sinus. Other primary tumors in this group include

- osteoblastoma
- giant cell tumor
- chondroma
- Ewing sarcoma
- osteogenic sarcoma
- chondrosarcoma

For AJCC definitions and staging of orbital sarcomas, see Table A-7 in the appendix.

Nerve Sheath Tumors

Neurofibromas are the most common nerve sheath tumor. This slow-growing tumor includes an admixture of endoneural fibroblasts, Schwann cells, and axons. Neurofibromas may be circumscribed but are not encapsulated. The consistency is firm and rubbery. Microscopically, the spindle-shaped cells are arranged in ribbons and cords in a matrix of myxoid tissue and collagen that contains axons.

Isolated neurofibromas do not necessarily indicate systemic involvement, but the plexiform type of neurofibroma is associated with neurofibromatosis type 1, also called von Recklinghausen disease (Fig 14-18).

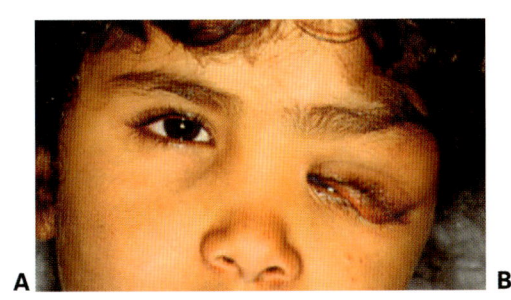

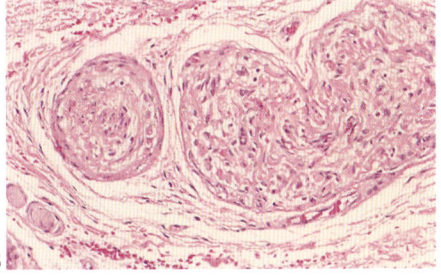

Figure 14-18 Plexiform neurofibroma. **A,** Clinical photograph depicting a typical S-shaped deformity of the upper eyelid. **B,** The trunk of the nerve is enlarged by proliferation of endoneural fibroblasts and Schwann cells. Axons may be demonstrated within the lesion. *(Part A courtesy of Sander Dubovy, MD.)*

The *neurilemoma* (also called *schwannoma*) arises from Schwann cells. Slow growing and encapsulated, this yellowish tumor may show cysts and areas of hemorrhagic necrosis. It may be solitary or associated with neurofibromatosis. Two histologic patterns appear microscopically: Antoni A spindle cells are arranged in interlacing cords, whorls, or palisades that may form Verocay bodies, or collections of fibrils resembling sensory corpuscles. Antoni B tissue is made up of stellate cells with a mucoid stroma. Vessels are usually prominent and thick-walled, and no axons are present (Fig 14-19).

Adipose Tumors

Lipomas are rare in the orbit. Pathologic characteristics include encapsulation and a distinctive lobular appearance. Because lipomas are histologically difficult to distinguish from normal or prolapsed fat, their incidence might have been previously overestimated.

Liposarcomas are malignant tumors that are extremely rare in the orbit. Histologic criteria depend on the type of liposarcoma, but the unifying diagnostic feature is the presence of lipoblasts. These tumors tend to recur before they metastasize.

Metastatic Tumors

Secondary tumors are those that invade the orbit by direct extension from adjacent structures such as sinus, bone, or eye. *Metastatic* tumors are those that spread from a primary site such as the breast in women and the prostate in men. In children, neuroblastoma is the most common primary origin.

McLean IW, Burnier MN, Zimmerman LE, Jakobiec FA. *Tumors of the Eye and Ocular Adnexa.* Washington: Armed Forces Institute of Pathology; 1995:215–298.

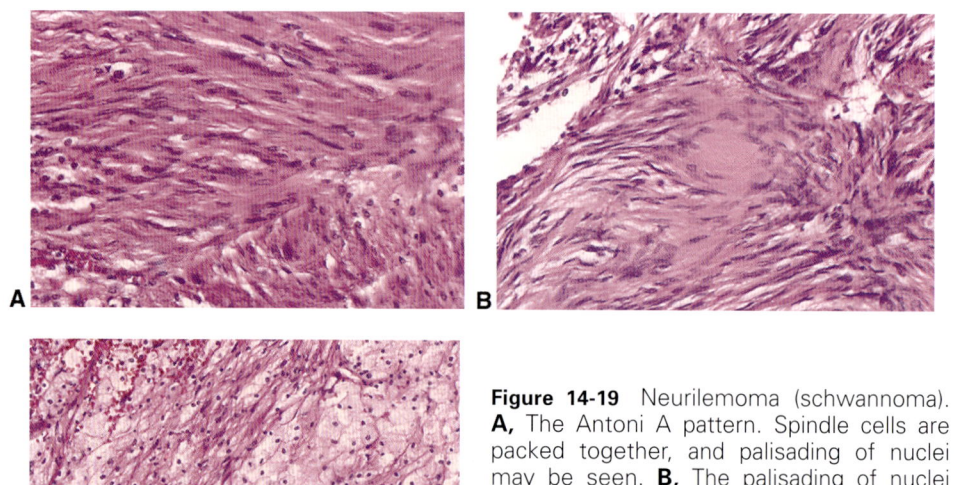

Figure 14-19 Neurilemoma (schwannoma). **A,** The Antoni A pattern. Spindle cells are packed together, and palisading of nuclei may be seen. **B,** The palisading of nuclei may form a Verocay body. **C,** The Antoni B pattern represents degeneration within the tumor. The histologic structures are loosely teased apart.

CHAPTER 15

Optic Nerve

Topography

The optic nerve, embryologically derived from the optic stalk, is a continuation of the optic tract; thus, the pathology of the optic nerve reflects that of the central nervous system (CNS). The optic nerve is 35–55 mm in length and extends from the eye to the optic chiasm (Fig 15-1). Its axons originate from the retinal ganglion cell layer and have a myelin coat posterior to the lamina cribrosa. The intraocular portion is 0.7–1.0 mm in length, the intraorbital portion 25–30 mm, and the intracanalicular portion 4–10 mm. The length of the intracranial portion varies according to the position of the chiasm but averages 10 mm. The diameter is 3.0–3.5 mm, tapering to 1.5 mm in the scleral canal.

Oligodendrocytes, astrocytes, and microglial cells are glial cells (*glia* = glue). Oligodendrocytes produce and maintain the myelin that sheaths the optic nerve. Myelination stops at the lamina cribrosa (Fig 15-2). Occasionally, aberrant patches of myelin are seen in the nerve fiber layer of the retina as discrete, flat, feathery white patches. Astrocytes are involved with support and nutrition. Microglial cells (CNS histiocytes) have a phagocytic function.

The coat of meninges includes the dura mater (which merges with the sclera), the cellular arachnoid layer, and the vascular pia. Arachnoid cells may lie in nests that can contain corpora arenacea; these nests are most obvious in young patients. The pial vessels extend into the optic nerve and subdivide the nerve fibers into fascicles. The subarachnoid space, which contains cerebrospinal fluid (CSF), ends blindly at the termination of the meninges (Fig 15-3).

Blood supply to different portions of the optic nerve comes from a variety of sources. The ophthalmic artery comes through the pia and supplies the intraorbital and intraocular portion. In general, the periaxial fibers are supplied by the pial vessels, and the axial fibers by the central retinal artery, which passes directly through the subarachnoid space to the nerve. The vein, however, is oblique and has a variable course.

BCSC Section 2, *Fundamentals and Principles of Ophthalmology*, discusses and illustrates the anatomy of the optic nerve. Section 5, *Neuro-Ophthalmology*, also covers the physiology and pathology of the optic disc and optic nerve.

238 • Ophthalmic Pathology and Intraocular Tumors

Figure 15-1 Low-power photomicrograph shows the relationship of the optic nerve to the eye and extraocular muscle. *(Courtesy of Hans E. Grossniklaus, MD.)*

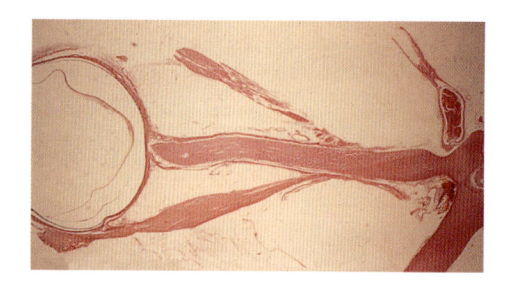

Figure 15-2 Photomicrograph shows the termination of myelinated axons at the lamina cribrosa *(arrows)*.

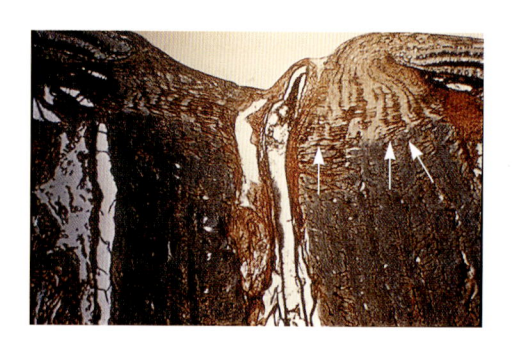

Figure 15-3 Normal optic nerve. The dura mater *(D)* is continuous with the sclera anteriorly. Note the arachnoid *(A)* and the pia *(P)*.

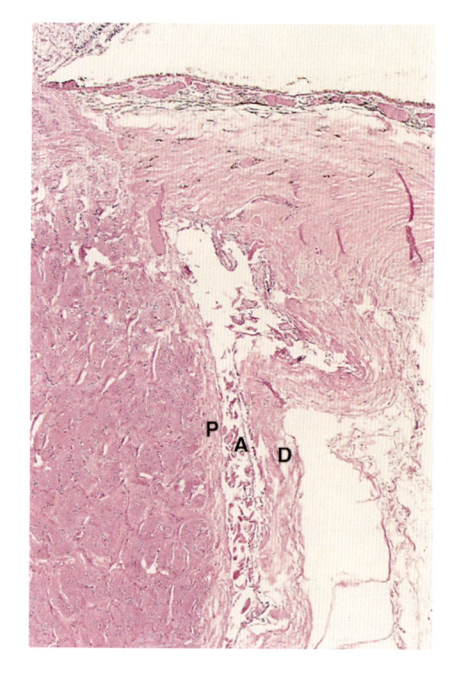

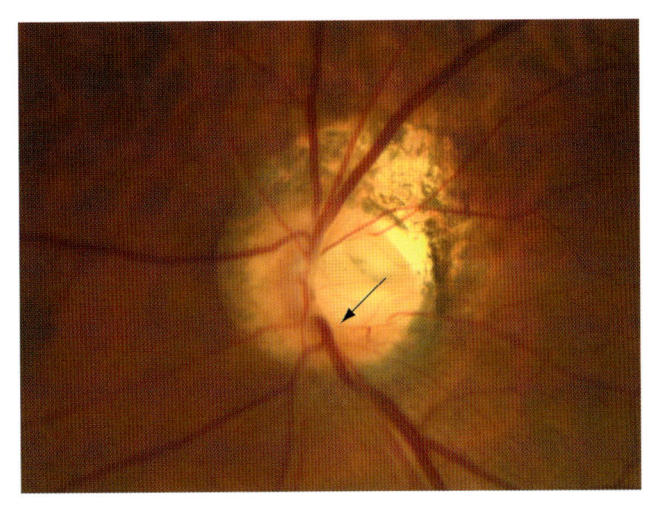

Figure 15-4 Clinical appearance of optic nerve head pit *(arrow)*. *(Courtesy of Debra J. Shetlar, MD.)*

Congenital Anomalies

Pits
Optic nerve head pits presumably arise as defects in closure of the fetal fissure. Pits usually appear temporally and are associated with visual field defects, serous retinal detachments, and occasionally colobomas in the fellow eye. Loss of retinal ganglion cells and nerve fibers occurs in the region of the pit, and meningeal cysts have been described in association with closed pits (Fig 15-4).

Colobomas
Colobomas of the optic nerve head result from failure of closure of the fetal fissure. Optic nerve head colobomas are located inferior to the nerve head and are associated with colobomas of the retina, choroid, ciliary body, and iris. Cystic outpouchings in the sclera may produce a cyst lined by degenerated choroid and gliotic retina (microphthalmos with cyst). (See BCSC Section 6, *Pediatric Ophthalmology and Strabismus,* Chapter 25, Fig 25-2.)

Inflammations

Infectious
Infections of the optic nerve may be secondary to bacterial and mycotic infections of adjacent anatomical structures, such as the eye, brain, or sinus, or they may occur as part of a systemic infection, particularly in the immunosuppressed patient. Fungal infections include mucormycosis, cryptococcosis, and coccidioidomycosis. Mucormycosis generally results from contiguous sinus infection. Cryptococcosis results from direct extension of the infection from the CNS and often produces multiple foci of necrosis with little inflammatory reaction. Coccidioidomycosis produces necrotizing granulomas.

Viral infections of the optic nerve are usually associated with other CNS lesions. Multiple sclerosis and acute disseminated myelitis produce loss of myelin early, but initially the axons are undamaged, and visual function may return. The damaged myelin is removed by macrophages (Fig 15-5). Astrocytic proliferation then occurs to produce a glial scar, which is known as a *plaque*.

Noninfectious

Noninfectious inflammatory disorders of the optic nerve include giant cell arteritis and sarcoidosis. *Giant cell arteritis* may produce granulomatous mural inflammation and occlusion of posterior ciliary vessels with liquefactive necrosis of the optic nerve.

Sarcoidosis of the optic nerve is often associated with retinal, vitreal, and uveitic lesions (Fig 15-6; see also Fig 12-8). Unlike the characteristic noncaseating granulomas in the eye, optic nerve lesions may feature necrosis.

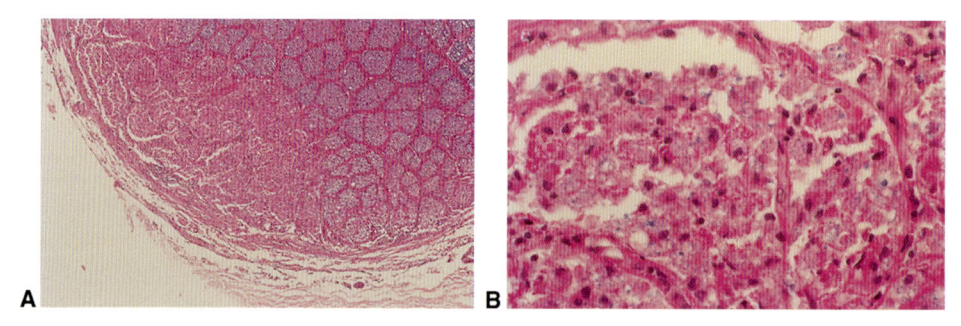

Figure 15-5 Multiple sclerosis, optic nerve. **A,** Luxol-fast blue stain, counterstained with H&E. The blue-staining area indicates normal myelin. Note the absence of myelin in the lower left corner of the optic nerve, corresponding to a focal lesion. **B,** Higher magnification. The blue material (myelin) is engulfed by macrophages.

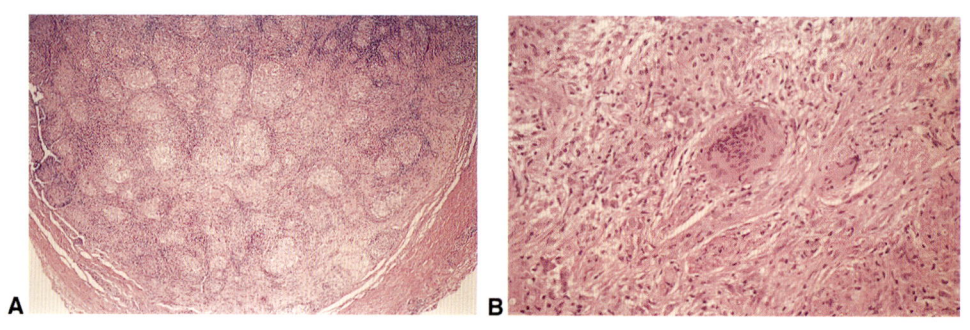

Figure 15-6 Sarcoidosis. **A,** Low-magnification photomicrograph of the optic nerve with discrete noncaseating granuloma. **B,** Higher magnification shows multinucleated giant cells in the granulomas. *(Courtesy of Hans E. Grossniklaus, MD.)*

Degenerations

Optic Atrophy

Loss of retinal ganglion cells because of glaucoma or infarction results in degeneration of their axons and is known as *ascending atrophy*. (See BCSC Section 5, *Neuro-Ophthalmology*, Chapter 3, Fig 3-2.) Pathologic processes within the cranial cavity or orbit result in *descending atrophy*. Axonal degeneration is accompanied by loss of myelin and oligodendrocytes. The optic nerve shrinks despite the proliferation of astrocytes, and thickened pial strands result from proliferation of connective tissue (Fig 15-7).

The portion of the optic nerve nearer the lateral geniculate body is described as *central*, and the portion nearer the retina is described as *peripheral*. Injury to the retina or to any peripheral portion of the optic nerve results in rapid ascending atrophy of the central portion. Initially, the axons at the peripheral portion swell. Retrograde degeneration of the axons then occurs with loss of retinal ganglion cells.

Cavernous optic atrophy of Schnabel is characterized microscopically by large cystic spaces containing mucopolysaccharide material, which stains with alcian blue, posterior to the lamina cribrosa (Fig 15-8). The intracystic material that penetrates into the parenchyma

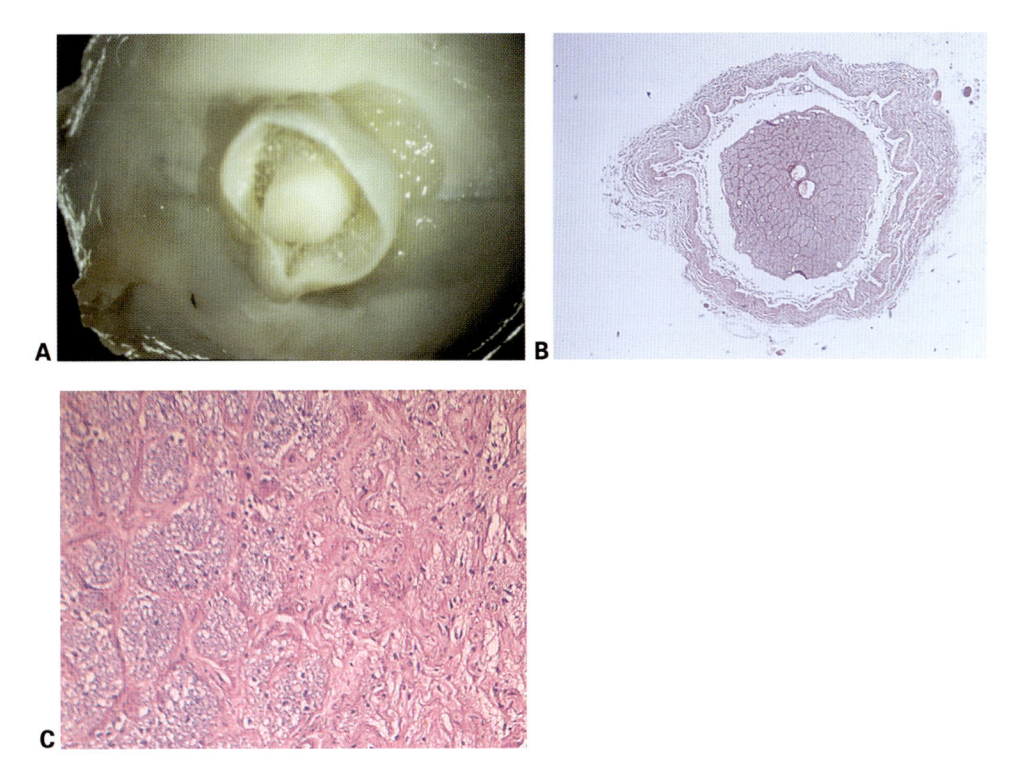

Figure 15-7 Atrophic optic nerve. **A,** Gross appearance of atrophic optic nerve. **B,** Low magnification. Note the widened subdural space. **C,** Higher magnification shows changes in the dura mater, arachnoid, and pia. *(Part A courtesy of Debra J. Shetlar, MD.)*

through the internal limiting membrane of the optic nerve head is thought to be vitreous. These changes occur most commonly in patients with glaucoma after acute IOP elevation, but they have also been seen in nonglaucomatous elderly patients with generalized arteriosclerotic disease

> Albert DM, Jakobiec FA, eds. *Principles and Practice of Ophthalmology.* 2nd ed. Philadelphia: Saunders; 2000:3875–3877.

Drusen

Drusen of the optic disc consist of hyaline-like calcified material within the nerve substance (Fig 15-9). They are usually bilateral and may be complicated by neovascularization and hemorrhage. They are thought to result from intracellular mitochondrial calcification within the axons. Optic disc drusen may produce field defects, and their presence can cause enlargement of the papilla that may be mistaken for papilledema (pseudopapilledema).

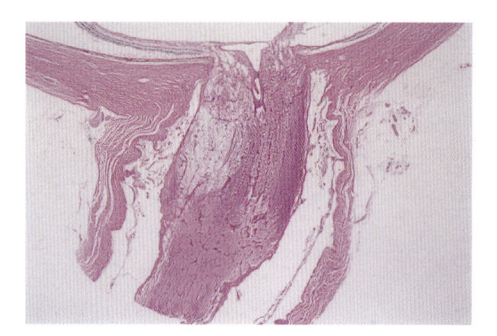

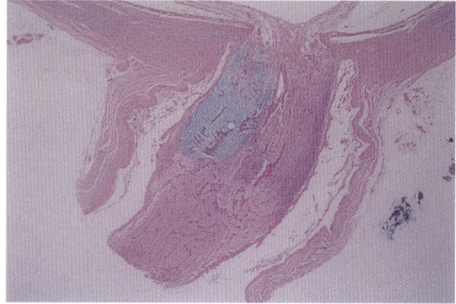

Figure 15-8 Cavernous optic atrophy of Schnabel. Photomicrographs show cystic atrophy within the optic nerve. The cystic space is filled with alcian blue–staining material. *(Courtesy of Hans E. Grossniklaus, MD.)*

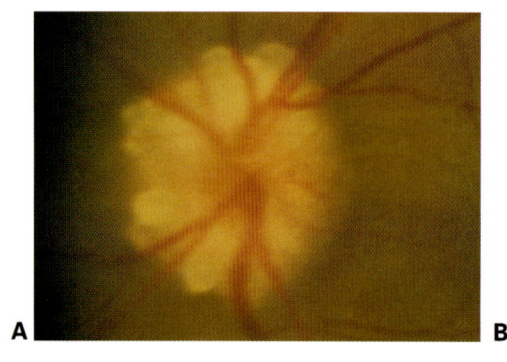

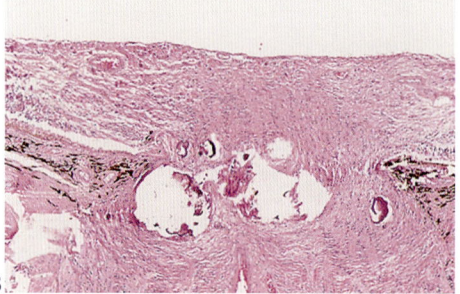

Figure 15-9 Drusen of the optic nerve head. **A,** Clinical appearance of optic disc drusen. **B,** Note the local zones of calcification just anterior to the lamina cribrosa. *(Part A courtesy of Debra J. Shetlar, MD.)*

Giant drusen are associated with the phakomatoses such as tuberous sclerosis and neurofibromatosis, which are considered to be hamartomatous proliferations of astrocytes with secondary calcification. (See BCSC Section 6, *Pediatric Ophthalmology and Strabismus,* for further discussion of the phakomatoses.) Giant drusen lie anterior to the lamina cribrosa.

Optic disc drusen may be associated with acquired disease such as angioid streaks, papillitis, optic atrophy, chronic glaucoma, and vascular occlusions. They may occur in otherwise normal eyes and are occasionally dominantly inherited. They can be diagnosed using B-scan echography, ultrasound, or fundus photography with a fluorescein filter in place (autofluorescence).

> Spencer WH, ed. *Ophthalmic Pathology: An Atlas and Textbook.* 4th ed. Philadelphia: Saunders; 1996:537–541.

Neoplasia

Tumors may affect the optic nerve head (eg, melanocytoma, peripapillary choroidal melanoma, pigment epithelium proliferation, and hemangioma) or the retrobulbar portion of the optic nerve (eg, glioma and meningioma).

Melanocytoma

A melanocytoma is a benign, deeply pigmented melanocytic tumor situated eccentrically on the disc, projecting less than 2 mm into the vitreous and extending into the lower temporal retina and posteriorly beyond the lamina (Fig 15-10). Slow growth may occur. A bleached section shows closely apposed plump cells of uniform character with abundant cytoplasm and small nuclei with little chromatin. Nucleoli are small and regular. See also Chapter 17.

Glioma

A glioma may arise in any part of the visual pathway, including the optic disc and optic nerve. The most common cell of origin is the spindle-shaped or hairlike (pilocytic) astrocyte (juvenile pilocytic astrocytoma) (Fig 15-11A and B). Optic nerve gliomas are frequently associated with neurofibromatosis (NF1), an autosomal dominant disorder, with

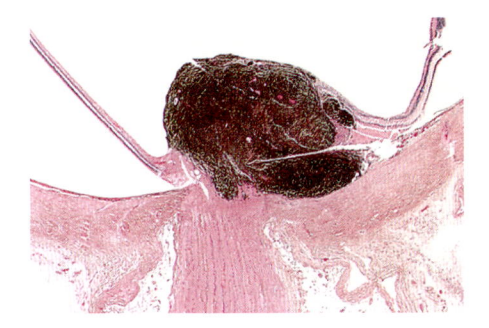

Figure 15-10 Melanocytoma of the optic nerve. The choroid adjacent to the optic nerve is also involved by this tumor. The cells of the tumor are so densely packed with melanin that the cytologic detail is not visible without higher magnification and melanin bleaching.

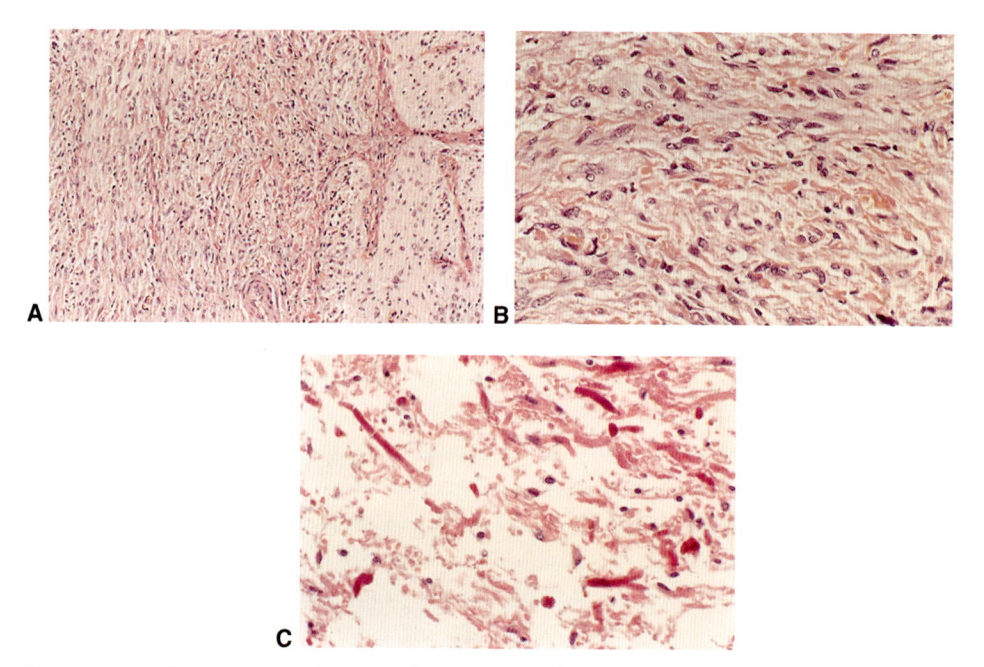

Figure 15-11 Astrocytoma of the optic nerve. **A,** The right side of this photograph demonstrates normal optic nerve, and the left side shows a pilocytic astrocytoma. **B,** The neoplastic glial cells are elongated to resemble hairs (hence the term *pilocytic*). **C,** Degenerating eosinophilic filaments, known as *Rosenthal fibers,* are not unique to astrocytoma of the optic nerve.

the gene, a tumor suppressor, located on the long arm of chromosome 17q11. The tumors most commonly present in the first decade and are of low grade.

Enlarged, deeply eosinophilic filaments, representing degenerating cell processes known as *Rosenthal fibers,* may be found in these low-grade tumors (Fig 15-11C). Foci of microcystic degeneration and calcification may occur, and the pial septa are thickened. The meninges show a reactive hyperplasia with proliferation of spindle-shaped meningeal cells and infiltration with astrocytes. The dura mater remains intact, so the nerve appears tubular or sausage-shaped. Some evidence indicates that these tumors may undergo slow, progressive growth.

High-grade tumors (grade 4 astrocytomas, glioblastoma multiforme) rarely involve the optic nerve. When this does occur, the optic nerve is usually involved secondarily from a brain tumor.

Meningioma

Primary optic nerve sheath meningiomas occur much less frequently than secondary orbital meningiomas. Optic nerve meningiomas arise within the arachnoid of the optic nerve, whereas secondary orbital meningiomas extend from an intracranial primary site (Fig 15-12A and B). Extradural tumors that arise from ectopic meningothelial cells, within the muscle cone or at the roof or orbital floor, are rare.

The mean age at presentation of primary meningioma is lower than that of the secondary type (20% of patients are less than 10 years of age). Tumor growth is slow. Primary

CHAPTER 15: Optic Nerve • 245

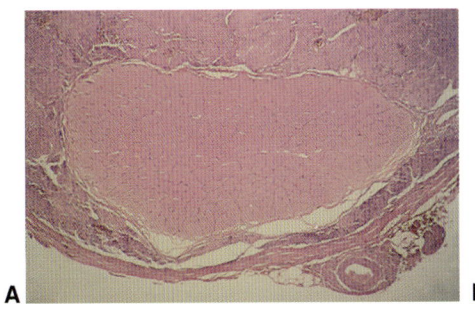

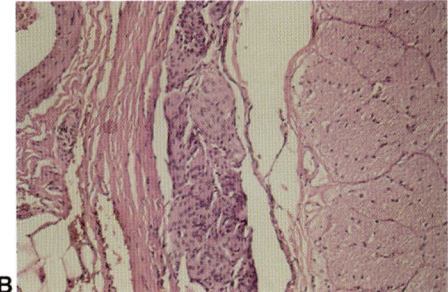

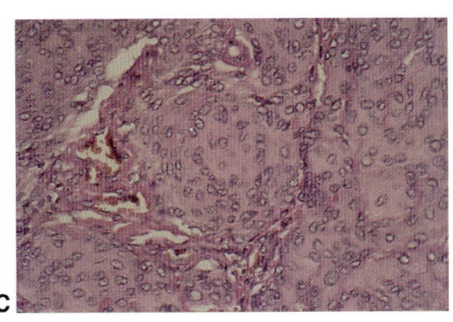

Figure 15-12 Optic nerve meningioma. **A,** This meningioma has grown circumferentially around the optic nerve and has compressed the nerve. **B,** Meningioma of the optic nerve originates from the arachnoid. **C,** Note the whorls of tumor cells, characteristic of the meningothelial type of meningioma, the most common histologic variant arising from the optic nerve.

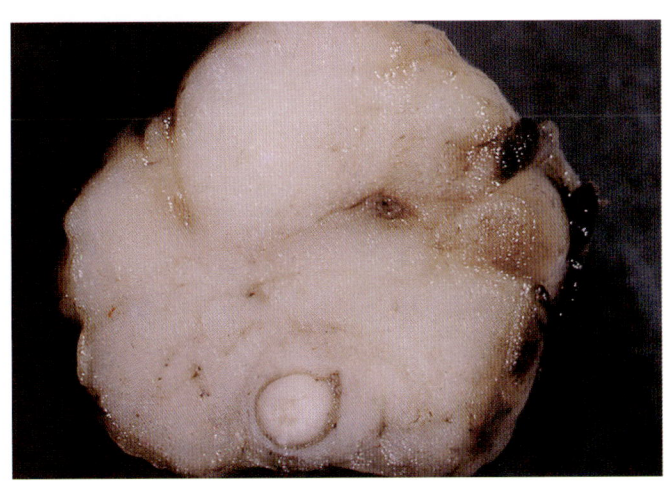

Figure 15-13 Optic nerve meningioma. The shaggy border of this gross specimen emphasizes the tendency of the perioptic meningioma to invade surrounding orbital tissues.

optic nerve meningiomas may invade the nerve and the eye and may extend through the dura mater to invade muscle (Fig 15-13).

Microscopically, the tumor (primary or secondary) is usually of the meningotheliomatous type, with plump cells arranged in whorls (Fig 15-12C). Psammoma bodies tend to be sparse. Patient survival is longer (up to 19 years) with primary orbital meningiomas than with those of secondary type (up to 15 years). Although meningioma may rarely be associated with neurofibromatosis in the younger age group, it is a less frequent hallmark of NF1 than is optic nerve glioma.

Albert DM, Jakobiec FA, eds. *Principles and Practice of Ophthalmology.* 2nd ed. Philadelphia: Saunders; 2000:3881–3883.

PART II

Intraocular Tumors: Clinical Aspects

CHAPTER 16

Introduction to Part II

Intraocular tumors comprise a broad spectrum of benign and malignant lesions that can lead to loss of vision and loss of life. Effective management of these lesions depends on accurate diagnosis. In most cases, experienced ophthalmologists diagnose intraocular neoplasms by clinical examination and ancillary diagnostic tests, and investigators in the Collaborative Ocular Melanoma Study (COMS) reported a misdiagnosis rate of less than 0.2%. One diagnostic aid that may be used to evaluate intraocular tumors is fine-needle aspiration biopsy (FNAB), although the indications for this technique are limited. FNAB may help to confirm the presence of choroidal metastases or provide tumor for cytogenetic studies in patients with choroidal melanoma, but FNAB of tumors suspected to be retinoblastoma is strongly discouraged, as it may result in extraocular dissemination of the disease. (FNAB is discussed in greater detail in Chapter 4.)

Important information concerning the most common primary intraocular malignancy in adults, choroidal melanoma, was gathered in the COMS. The COMS, which was funded in 1985, incorporated both randomized clinical trials for patients with medium and large choroidal melanomas and an observational study for patients with small choroidal melanomas. The COMS reported outcomes for enucleation versus brachytherapy for the treatment of medium tumors and for enucleation alone versus pre-enucleation external-beam radiotherapy for large melanomas. Survival data from the large, medium, and small treatment arms of the COMS are available. In addition to the study's primary objectives, the COMS has provided data regarding local tumor failure rates after iodine 125 brachytherapy as well as visual acuity outcomes following this globe-conserving treatment. These findings have shifted the primary treatment of choroidal melanoma from enucleation toward globe-conserving brachytherapy. (See Chapter 17.)

The predisposing gene for retinoblastoma has been isolated, cloned, and sequenced. As with choroidal melanoma, retinoblastoma therapy is also undergoing a transition toward globe-conserving therapy, with a renewed interest in combined-modality therapy focused particularly on systemic chemotherapy coupled with focal therapy. This trend toward chemotherapy has been fueled by our growing understanding of the potential risks of primary external-beam radiotherapy for increasing the incidence of secondary (radiation-induced) malignancies in children with a germline mutation of the retinoblastoma gene. Advances in our understanding of the molecular genetics of retinoblastoma continue to enhance our ability to screen and treat this pediatric ocular malignancy. (See Chapter 19.)

CHAPTER 17

Melanocytic Tumors

Iris Nevus

An iris nevus generally appears as a darkly pigmented lesion of the iris stroma with minimal distortion of the iris architecture (Fig 17-1). The true incidence of iris nevi remains uncertain because many of these lesions produce no symptoms and are recognized incidentally during routine ophthalmic examination. Iris nevi may present in 2 forms:

1. *circumscribed iris nevus:* typically nodular, involving a discrete portion of the iris
2. *diffuse iris nevus:* may involve an entire sector or, rarely, the entire iris

In some cases, the lesion causes slight ectropion iridis and sectoral cataract. The incidence of iris nevi may be higher in the eyes of patients with neurofibromatosis.

Iris nevi are best evaluated by slit-lamp biomicroscopy coupled with gonioscopic evaluation of the angle structures. Specific attention should be given to lesions involving the angle structures to rule out a previously unrecognized ciliary body tumor. The most important possibility in the differential diagnosis of iris nevi is iris melanoma. When iris melanoma is included within the differential diagnosis, close observation with scheduled serial reevaluation is indicated. Clinical evaluation of suspicious iris nevi should include slit-lamp photography and high-frequency ultrasound biomicroscopy. Iris nevi usually require no treatment once they are diagnosed, but, when suspected, they should be followed closely and photographed to evaluate for growth.

Nevus of the Ciliary Body or Choroid

Nevi of the ciliary body are occasionally incidental findings in histopathologic examination of globes that are enucleated for other reasons. Choroidal nevi may occur in up to 7% of the population. In most cases, they have no clinical symptoms and are recognized on routine ophthalmic examination. The typical choroidal nevus appears ophthalmoscopically as a flat or minimally elevated pigmented (gray-brown) choroidal lesion with indistinct margins (Fig 17-2). Some nevi are amelanotic and may be less apparent. Choroidal nevi may be associated with overlying RPE disturbance, serous detachment, drusen, choroidal neovascular membranes, and orange pigment; and they may produce visual field defects. On fluorescein angiography, choroidal nevi may either hypofluoresce or hyperfluoresce, depending on the associated findings. Ocular and oculodermal

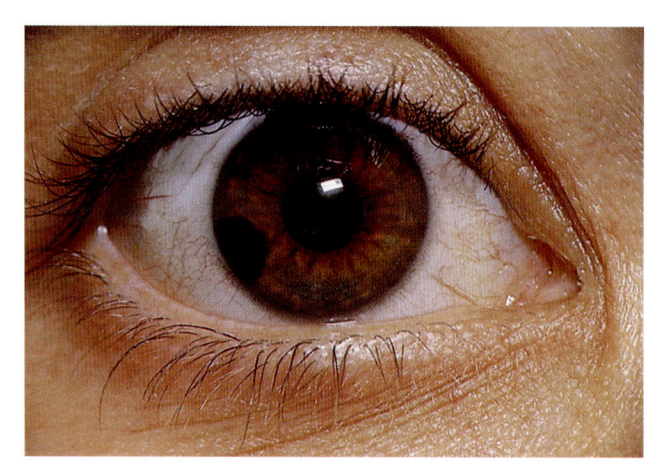

Figure 17-1 Iris nevus, clinical appearance. The lesion is only slightly raised from the iris surface, and lesion color is homogeneous brown.

melanocytosis may predispose to uveal malignancy, with an estimated lifetime risk of 1 in 400 in the white population. Choroidal nevi are distinguished from choroidal melanomas by clinical evaluation and ancillary testing. No single clinical factor is pathognomonic for benign versus malignant choroidal melanocytic lesions. The differential diagnosis for pigmented lesions in the ocular fundus most commonly includes the following:

- choroidal nevus
- malignant melanoma
- atypical disciform scar associated with age-related macular degeneration (AMD)
- suprachoroidal hemorrhage
- RPE hyperplasia
- congenital hypertrophy of the retinal pigment epithelium (CHRPE)
- choroidal hemangioma with RPE hyperpigmentation
- melanocytoma
- metastatic carcinoma with RPE hyperpigmentation
- choroidal osteoma

Virtually all choroidal melanocytic tumors thicker than 3 mm are melanomas, and virtually all choroidal melanocytic lesions thinner than 1 mm are nevi. Many lesions 1–2 mm in thickness (apical height) may be benign, although the risk of malignancy increases with height. It is difficult to classify with certainty tumors that are 1–2 mm in thickness. Flat lesions with a basal diameter of 10 mm or less are almost always benign. The risk of malignancy increases for lesions that are larger than 10 mm in basal diameter.

Clinical risk factors for enlargement of choroidal melanocytic lesions have been well characterized and include

- subjective clinical symptoms such as metamorphopsia, photopsia, visual field loss
- presence of orange pigmentation
- associated subretinal fluid

CHAPTER 17: Melanocytic Tumors • 253

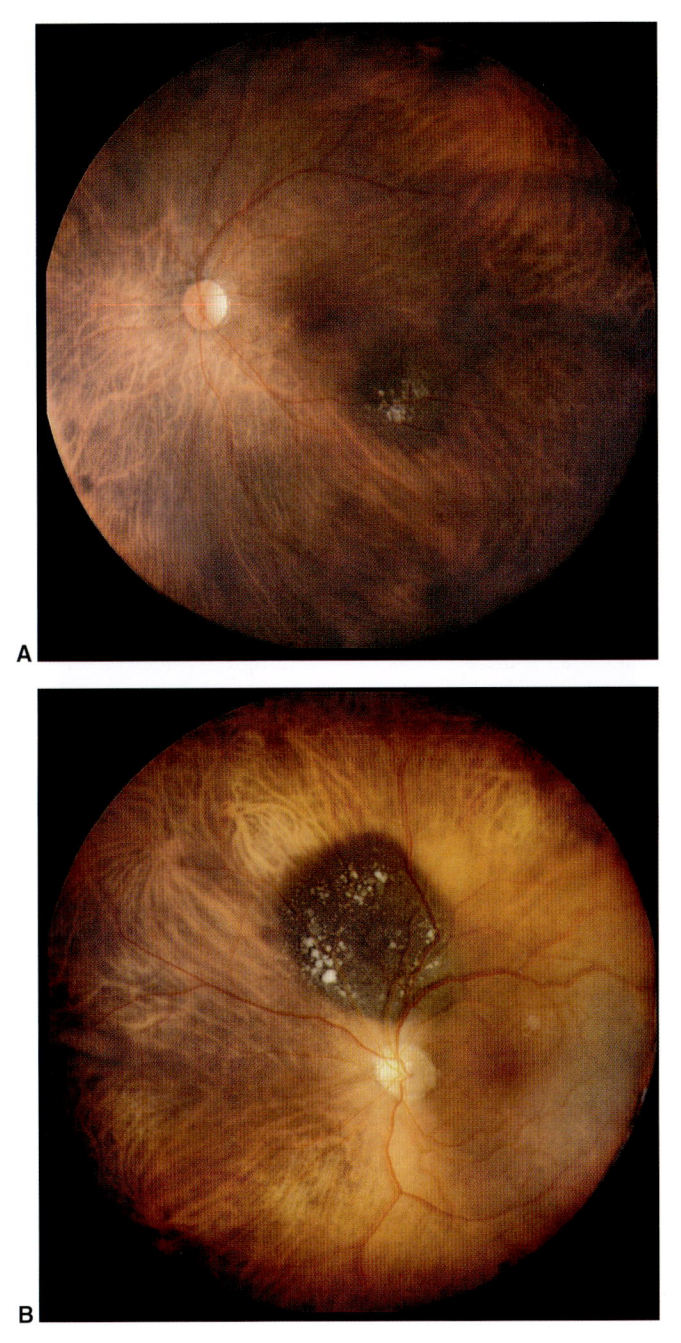

Figure 17-2 Choroidal nevi, clinical appearance. **A,** Choroidal nevus with overlying drusen, under the lower temporal retinovascular arcade. **B,** Medium-sized choroidal nevus with overlying drusen, superior to the optic nerve head. *(Courtesy of Jacob Pe'er, MD.)*

- larger size at presentation
- juxtapapillary location
- absence of drusen or RPE changes
- hot spots on fluorescein photography
- homogeneity on ultrasonography

If definite enlargement is documented, malignant change should be suspected.

The recommended management of choroidal nevi is photographic documentation for lesions less than 1 mm in thickness and photographic and ultrasonographic documentation for lesions greater than 1 mm in thickness, coupled with regular, periodic reassessment for signs of growth.

Melanocytoma of the Iris, Ciliary Body, or Choroid

Melanocytomas are rare tumors with a characteristic large, polyhedral shape; small nuclei; and cytoplasm filled with melanin granules (see Fig 15-10). Cells from iris melanocytomas may seed to the anterior chamber angle, causing glaucoma. Melanocytomas of the ciliary body are usually not seen clinically due to their peripheral location. In some cases, extrascleral extension of the tumor along an emissary canal appears as a darkly pigmented, fixed subconjunctival mass. Melanocytomas of the choroid appear as elevated, pigmented tumors, simulating a nevus or melanoma. Melanocytomas have been reported to undergo malignant change in some instances. When a melanocytoma is suspected, photographic and echographic studies are appropriate. If growth is documented, the lesion should be treated as a malignancy.

Iris Melanoma

Iris melanomas account for 3%–10% of all uveal melanomas. Small malignant melanomas of the iris may be impossible to differentiate clinically from benign iris nevi and other simulating lesions. The following conditions may be included in a differential diagnosis of iris melanoma:

- iris nevus
- primary iris cyst (pigment epithelial and stromal)
- iridocorneal endothelial syndrome
- iris foreign body
- peripheral anterior synechiae
- metastatic carcinoma to iris
- aphakic iris cyst
- iris atrophy, miscellaneous
- pigment epithelial hyperplasia or migration

- juvenile xanthogranuloma
- medulloepithelioma
- retained lens material simulating iris nodule

Signs suggesting malignancy include extensive ectropion iridis, prominent vascularity, sectoral cataract, secondary glaucoma, seeding of the peripheral angle structures, extrascleral extension, lesion size, and documented progressive growth. Iris melanomas range in appearance from amelanotic to dark brown lesions, and three quarters of them involve the inferior iris (Fig 17-3). In rare instances, they assume a diffuse growth pattern, producing a syndrome of unilateral acquired hyperchromic heterochromia and secondary glaucoma. Clinical evaluation is identical to that for iris nevi. The differential diagnosis of iris nodules is listed in Table 17-1; Figure 17-4 illustrates the various iris nodules. See also Figure 12-10 in Chapter 12.

Recent advances in high-frequency ultrasonography allow for excellent characterization of tumor size and anatomical relationship to normal ocular structures (Fig 17-5). Fluorescein angiography may document intrinsic vascularity, although this finding is of limited value in establishing a differential diagnosis. In rare instances, biopsy may be considered when the management of the lesion is in question. In most cases, when growth or severe glaucoma occurs, diagnostic and therapeutic excisional treatment is indicated. Brachytherapy using custom-designed plaques may be used in selected cases. Specifically designed proton-beam radiotherapy has also been reported for iris melanoma. The prognosis for most patients with iris melanomas is excellent, with a lower mortality rate (1%–4%) than that for ciliary body and choroidal melanomas, possibly because the biological behavior of most of these iris tumors appears distinctly different from that of ciliary or choroidal melanoma.

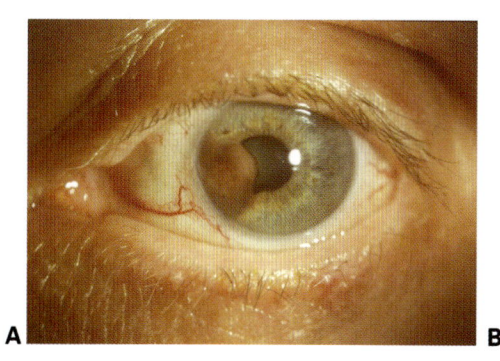

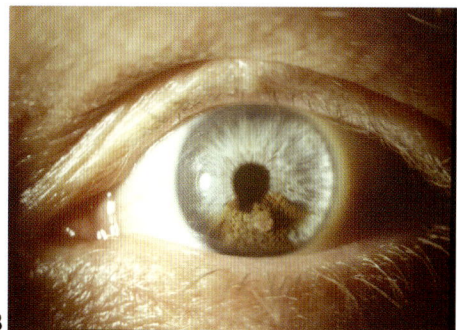

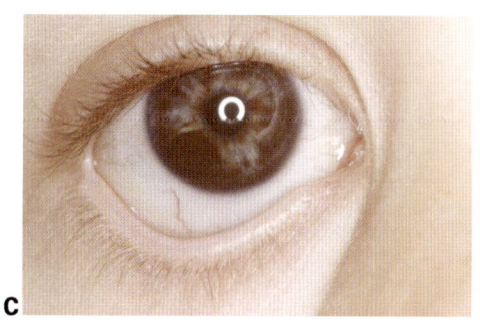

Figure 17-3 Iris melanoma, clinical appearance. **A,** Mildly pigmented iris melanoma on the nasal side, involving also the anterior chamber angle. A sentinel vessel is growing toward the area of the melanoma. **B,** Melanoma in the lower part of the iris. **C,** Melanoma in the lower temporal area, spreading to other parts of the iris. *(Photographs courtesy of Jacob Pe'er, MD.)*

Table 17-1 Differential Diagnostic Features of Iris Nodules (alphabetical list)

Lesion	Features
Brushfield spots (Down syndrome) (Fig 17-4A)	Elevated white to light yellow spots in periphery of iris, 10–20 per eye. Incidence in Down syndrome is 85%; otherwise, 24%. Histopathologically, the spots are areas of relatively normal iris stroma surrounded by a ring of mild iris hypoplasia. Anterior border layer slightly increased in density.
Epithelial invasion, serous cyst, solid or pearl cyst, implantation membrane	Each follows surgery or injury. Appears as serous or solid cysts in continuity with the wound or as implantation cysts or membranes on the anterior iris surface.
Foreign body, retained	Usually becomes secondarily pigmented and may be associated with chronic iridocyclitis and peripheral anterior synechiae.
Fungal endophthalmitis	Irregular yellow-white mass on iris. May be accompanied by hypopyon or only mild inflammatory signs.
Iridocyclitis	The iris nodules of classic granulomatous anterior uveitis occur either superficially or deeply within the iris. Koeppe nodules occur at the papillary border, and Busacca nodules lie on the anterior iris surface. Microscopically, they are composed of large and small mononuclear cells.
Iris freckle (Fig 17-4B)	Stationary, lightly to darkly pigmented flat areas on anterior iris surface composed of anterior border layer melanocytes containing increased pigmentation without increase in number of melanocytes.
Iris nevus (Fig 17-1)	Discrete mass(es) or nodule(s) on anterior iris surface and in the iris stroma. Variable pigmentation. Composed of benign nevus cells. Increased incidence of iris nevi in patients with neurofibromatosis.
Iris nevus syndrome (Cogan-Reese)	Acquired diffuse nevus of iris associated with unilateral glaucoma, heterochromia, peripheral anterior synechiae, and extension of endothelium and Descemet's membrane over trabecular meshwork. Obliteration of normal iris architecture. (See ICE syndrome, Chapter 7.)
Iris pigment epithelial cysts (Fig 17-4C)	Cysts encompassing both layers of neuroepithelium. Produce a localized elevation of stroma and may be pigmented. May transilluminate. May be better seen after dilation. B-scan ultrasonography of value in diagnosis.
Iris pigment epithelial proliferation	Congenital or acquired (trauma or surgery) plaques of pigment epithelium displaying a black, velvety appearance.
Juvenile xanthogranuloma	Yellowish to gray, poorly demarcated iris lesions associated with raised orange skin lesion(s) (single or multiple) appearing in the first year of life. May be associated with spontaneous hyphema and secondary glaucoma. Histopathologically, there is a diffuse granulomatous infiltrate with lipid-containing histiocytes and Touton giant cells. The lesions regress spontaneously. May also be found in ciliary body, anterior choroid, episclera, cornea, eyelids, and orbit.
Leiomyoma	May be well localized and even pedunculated, often diffuse and flat, and usually lightly pigmented. Electron microscopy required for clear differentiation between leiomyoma and amelanotic spindle cell melanoma.
Leukemia (Fig 17-4D)	Very rare nodular or diffuse milky lesions with intense hyperemia. Often, the iris loses its architecture, becomes thickened, and develops heterochromia. Pseudohypopyon is common.

(Continued)

Table 17-1 *(continued)*

Lesion	Features
Lisch nodules (neurofibromatosis) (Fig 17-4E)	One of the diagnostic criteria for neurofibromatosis. Multiple lesions varying from tan to dark brown and about the size of a pinhead. May be flat or project from the surface. Histopathologically, they are composed of collections of nevus cells.
Malignant melanoma (Fig 17-3)	Occurs as nodular or flat growths, usually in the periphery, especially inferiorly or inferotemporally. Variably pigmented, often with satellite pigmentation and pigmentation in the anterior chamber angle and nutrient vessels. Pupil may dilate irregularly, and elevated IOP may be present.
Melanocytosis, congenital ocular and oculodermal	Generally unilateral with diffuse uveal nevus causing heterochromia iridis associated with blue or slate gray patches of sclera and episclera. In oculodermal melanocytosis, eyelid and brow are also involved. Malignant potential exists.
Metastatic carcinoma	Gelatinous to white vascularized nodules on the iris surface and in the anterior chamber angle. May be associated with anterior uveitis, hyphema, rubeosis, and glaucoma.
Retinoblastoma	White foci on the anterior iris surface or in the anterior chamber angle, or a pseudohypopyon.
Tapioca melanoma	Tapioca-like nodules lying over a portion or all of the iris. May be translucent to lightly pigmented in color. Often associated with unilateral glaucoma.

Butler P, Char DH, Zarbin M, Kroll S. Natural history of indeterminate pigmented choroidal tumors. *Ophthalmology.* 1994;101:710–716.

Demirci H, Shields CL, Shields JA, Eagle RC Jr, Honavar SG. Diffuse iris melanoma: a report of 25 cases. *Ophthalmology.* 2002;109:1553–1560.

Girkin CA, Goldberg I, Mansberger SL, Shields JA, Shields CL. Management of iris melanoma with secondary glaucoma. *J Glaucoma.* 2002;11:71–74.

Jakobiec FA, Silbert G. Are most iris "melanomas" really nevi? A clinicopathologic study of 189 lesions. *Arch Ophthalmol.* 1981;99:2117–2132.

Marigo FA, Finger PT, McCormick SA, et al. Iris and ciliary body melanomas: ultrasound biomicroscopy with histopathologic correlation. *Arch Ophthalmol.* 2000;118:1515–1521.

Shields CL, Shields JA, Kiratli H, De Potter P, Cater JR. Risk factors for growth and metastasis of small choroidal melanocytic lesions. *Ophthalmology.* 1995;102:1351–1361.

Singh AD, De Potter P, Fijal BA, Shields CL, Shields JA, Elston RC. Lifetime prevalence of uveal melanoma in white patients with oculo(dermal) melanocytosis. *Ophthalmology.* 1998;105:195–198.

Singh AD, Kalyani P, Topham A. Estimating the risk of malignant transformation of a choroidal nevus. *Ophthalmology.* 2005;112:1784–1789.

Sumich P, Mitchell P, Wang JJ. Choroidal nevi in a white population: the Blue Mountains Eye Study. *Arch Ophthalmol.* 1998;116:645–650.

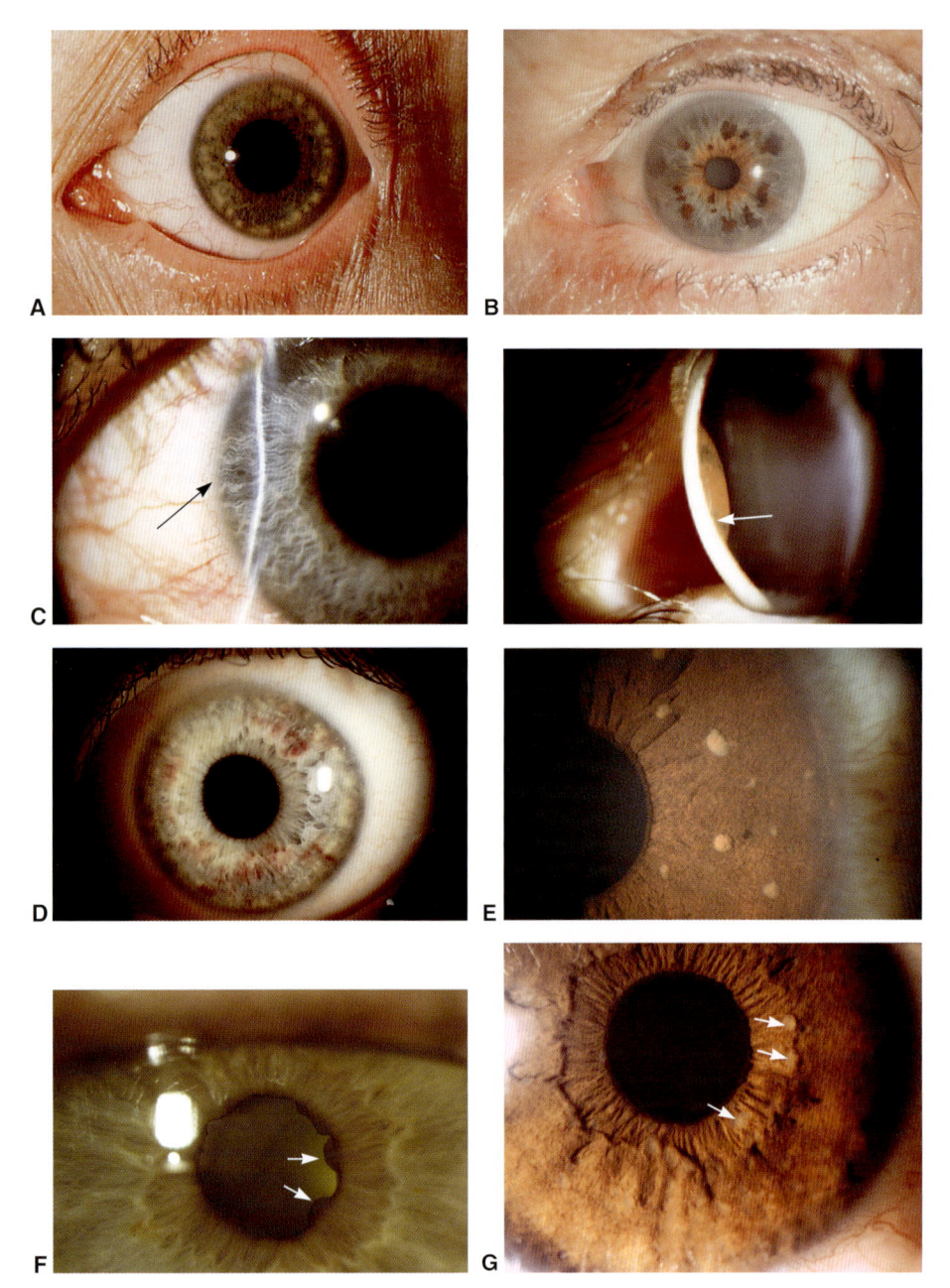

Figure 17-4 **A–G,** Iris nodules. **A,** Brushfields spots in Down syndrome. **B,** Iris freckles. **C,** Pigment epithelial cyst. Prior to dilation *(left),* the iris stroma is bowed forward *(arrow)* in the area of the cyst, which is invisible posteriorly. After dilation *(right),* the cyst of the posterior iris epithelium can be seen *(arrow)* with eye adduction. **D,** Leukemic infiltration of the iris. Note heterochromia, prominent vascularity, and stromal thickening. **E,** Multiple Lisch nodules in neurofibromatosis. **F,** Koeppe nodules at pupil margin *(arrows)* in sarcoidosis. **G,** Busacca nodules in mid-iris *(arrows)* in sarcoidosis. *(Part A courtesy of W.R. Green, MD; parts B and E courtesy of Timothy G. Murray, MD; parts F and G courtesy of R. Christopher Walton, MD.)*

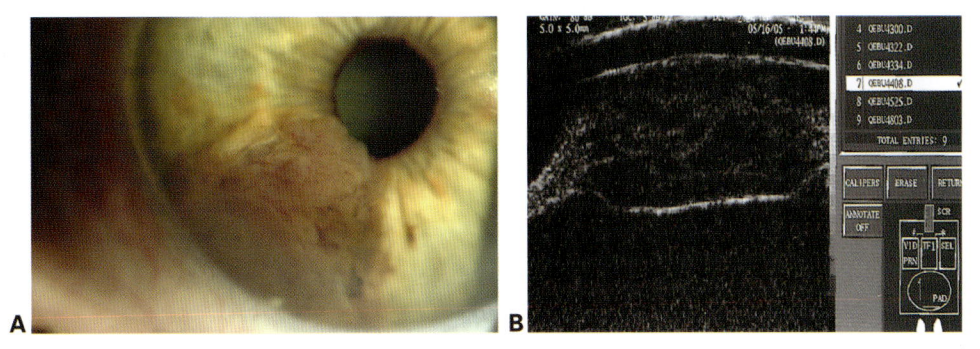

Figure 17-5 A, Iris melanoma, clinical appearance. **B,** High-resolution ultrasound, showing replacement of the normal iris stroma by a melanoma. *(Courtesy of Matthew W. Wilson, MD.)*

Melanoma of the Ciliary Body or Choroid

Ciliary body and choroidal melanomas are the most common primary intraocular malignancies in adults. The incidence in the United States is approximately 6–7 cases per million. The tumor, extremely rare in children, primarily affects patients in their 50s and early 60s; it has a predilection for lightly pigmented individuals. Risk factors have not been conclusively identified but may include

- light-colored complexion (white skin, blue eyes, blond hair)
- ocular melanocytic conditions such as melanosis oculi and oculodermal melanocytosis
- genetic predisposition (dysplastic nevus syndrome)
- cigarette smoking

Ciliary body melanomas can be asymptomatic in the early stages. Because of their location behind the iris, ciliary body melanomas may be rather large by the time they are detected. Patients who have symptoms most commonly note visual loss, photopsias, or visual field alterations. Ciliary body melanomas are not usually visible unless the pupil is widely dilated (Fig 17-6A). Some erode through the iris root into the anterior chamber and eventually become visible on external examination or with gonioscopy. Rarely, tumors extend directly through the sclera in the ciliary region, producing a dark epibulbar mass. The initial sign of a ciliary body melanoma may be dilated episcleral sentinel vessels in the quadrant of the tumor (Fig 17-6B). The tumor may eventually become quite large, producing a sectoral or diffuse cataract, subluxated lens (Fig 17-6C), secondary glaucoma, retinal detachment, and even iris neovascularization. Rarely, a ciliary body melanoma assumes a diffuse growth pattern that extends 180°–360° around the ciliary body. This type of melanoma is called a *ring melanoma* (see Fig 12-20 in Chapter 12).

The typical *choroidal melanoma* is a pigmented, elevated, dome-shaped subretinal mass (Fig 17-7A, B). The degree of pigmentation ranges from totally amelanotic to dark brown. With time, many tumors erupt through Bruch's membrane to assume a mushroom-like shape (Fig 17-7C, D). Prominent clumps of orange pigment at the RPE level may appear over the surface of the tumor, and serous detachment of the neurosensory

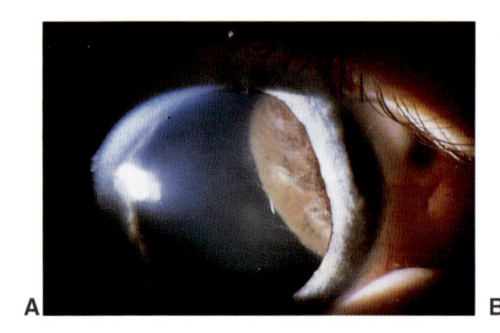

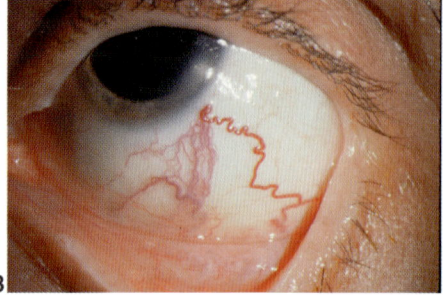

Figure 17-6 **A,** Ciliary body melanoma, clinical appearance. Such tumors may not be evident unless the pupil is widely dilated. **B,** Sentinel vessels. **C,** Ciliary body melanoma, gross pathology. Note mostly amelanotic appearance of this tumor, which is subluxing the lens and causing secondary angle closure. *(Part B courtesy of Timothy G. Murray, MD.)*

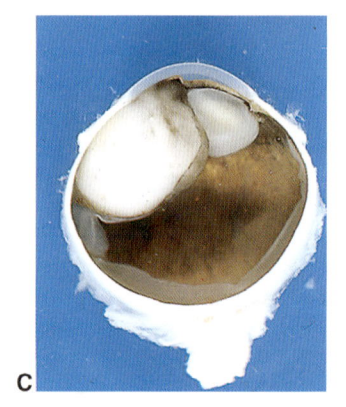

retina is common. If an extensive retinal detachment develops, anterior displacement of the lens–iris diaphragm and secondary angle-closure glaucoma occasionally occur. Neovascularization of the iris may also appear in such eyes, and there may be spontaneous hemorrhage into the subretinal space. Vitreous hemorrhage is usually seen only in cases when the melanoma has erupted through Bruch's membrane.

> Accuracy of diagnosis of choroidal melanomas in the Collaborative Ocular Melanoma Study. COMS report no. 1. *Arch Ophthalmol.* 1990;108:1268–1273.
>
> Gallagher RP, Elwood JM, Rootman J, et al. Risk factors for ocular melanoma: Western Canada Melanoma Study. *J Natl Cancer Inst.* 1985;74:775–778.
>
> Hu DN, Yu GP, McCormick SA, Schneider S, Finger PT. Population-based incidence of uveal melanoma in various races and ethnic groups. *Am J Ophthalmol.* 2005;140:612–617.
>
> Seddon JM, Gragoudas ES, Glynn RJ, Egan KM, Albert DM, Blitzer PH. Host factors, UV radiation, and risk of uveal melanoma: a case-control study. *Arch Ophthalmol.* 1990;108:1274–1280.

Diagnostic Evaluation

Clinical evaluation of all suspected posterior uveal melanomas of the ciliary body and the choroid should include a history, ophthalmoscopic evaluation, and ancillary testing to definitively establish the diagnosis. When used appropriately, the tests described here enable accurate diagnosis of melanocytic tumors in almost all cases. Atypical lesions may be characterized by several other testing modalities, such as FNAB; or, when appropriate,

CHAPTER 17: Melanocytic Tumors • 261

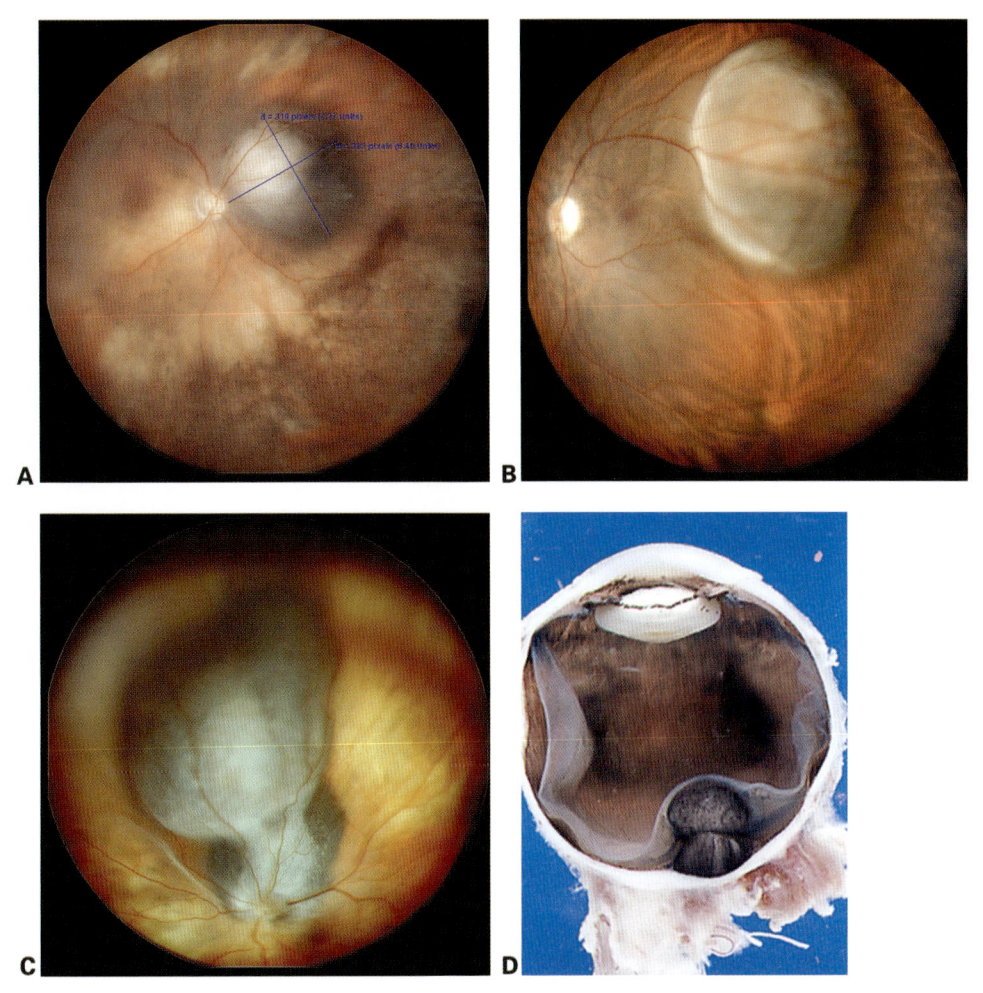

Figure 17-7 Choroidal melanoma. **A,** Small choroidal melanoma touching the nasal border of the optic nerve head, with digital measurement of the tumor diameter. **B,** Medium-sized choroidal melanoma temporal to the macula. **C,** A large choroidal melanoma surrounding the optic nerve head and extending upward to the ora serrata. Note the retinal detachment in the lower half of the retina. **D,** Gross pathology. Note the mushroom-shaped cross section of this darkly pigmented tumor and the associated retinal detachment. *(Parts A–C courtesy of Jacob Pe'er, MD.)*

lesions may be observed for characteristic changes in clinical behavior that will establish a correct diagnosis.

Indirect ophthalmoscopic viewing of the tumor remains the gold standard. It is the single most important diagnostic technique for evaluating patients with intraocular tumors, as it provides stereopsis and a wide field of view and facilitates visualization of the peripheral fundus, particularly when performed with scleral depression. Indirect ophthalmoscopy allows for clinical assessment of tumor basal dimension and apical height. However, it is not useful in eyes with opaque media, which require other diagnostic methods, such as ultrasonography, computed tomography (CT), and/or magnetic resonance imaging (MRI).

Slit-lamp biomicroscopy used in combination with *gonioscopy* offers the best method for establishing the presence and extent of anterior involvement of ciliary body tumors. The use of high-frequency ultrasonography (biomicroscopy) enables excellent visualization of anterior ocular structures and is a significant adjunct to slit-lamp photography for the evaluation and documentation of anterior segment pathology.

In addition, the presence of sectoral cataract, secondary angle involvement, or sentinel vessel formation may be a clue to the diagnosis of ciliary body tumor. Hruby, Goldmann, and other wide-field fundus lenses can be used with the slit lamp to evaluate lesions of the posterior fundus under high magnification. High-magnification fundus evaluation can delineate neurosensory retinal detachment, orange pigmentation, rupture of Bruch's membrane, intraretinal tumor invasion, and vitreous involvement. Fundus biomicroscopy with the 3-mirror contact lens is useful in assessing lesions of the peripheral fundus.

Ultrasonography is the most important ancillary study for evaluating ciliary body and choroidal melanomas (Fig 17-8). It also remains the ancillary test of choice for detection of orbital extension associated with intraocular malignancy. Standardized A-scan ultrasonography provides an accurate assessment of a lesion's internal reflectivity, vascularity, and measurement. Serial examination with A-scan ultrasonography can be used to document growth or regression of an intraocular tumor.

A-scan ultrasonography usually demonstrates a solid tumor pattern with high-amplitude initial echoes and low-amplitude internal reflections (low internal reflectivity). Spontaneous vascular pulsations can also be demonstrated in most cases. B-scan examination provides information about the relative size (height and basal diameters), general shape, and position of intraocular tumors. Occasionally, cross-sectional tumor shape and

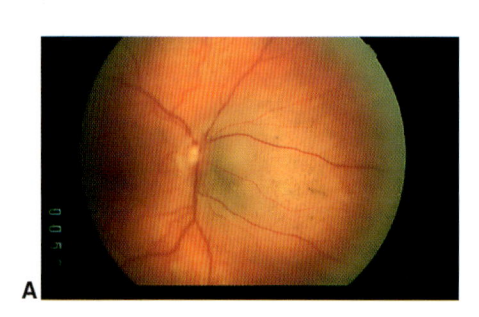

Figure 17-8 **A,** Peripapillary choroidal melanoma. **B,** The peripapillary tumor is seen nasal to the optic nerve. B-scan ultrasonography is used primarily to show the tumor location and its topography. **C,** The A-scan ultrasonogram shows characteristic low internal reflectivity. The pattern of the A scan is used to differentiate tumor types more reliably than does the B-scan pattern.

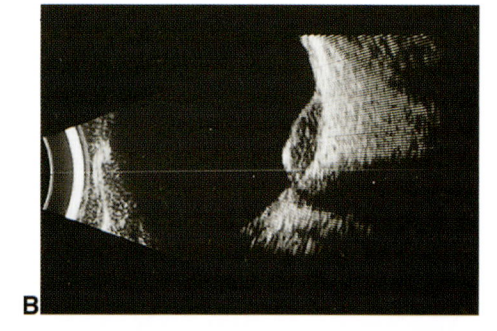

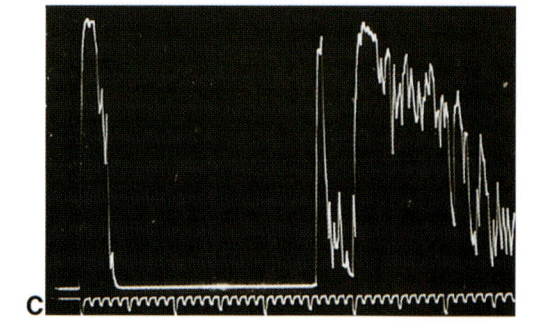

associated retinal detachment can be detected more easily by ultrasonography than by ophthalmoscopy. B-scan ultrasonography usually shows a dome- or mushroom-shaped choroidal mass with a highly reflective anterior border, acoustic hollowness, choroidal excavation, and occasional orbital shadowing. B-scan ultrasonography can be used to detect intraocular tumors in eyes with either clear or opaque media.

Ultrasonography for ciliary body melanomas is more difficult to interpret because the peripheral location of these tumors makes the test technically more demanding to perform. High-frequency ultrasonography is not limited by the technical difficulties associated with standard B-scan testing and enables excellent imaging of the anterior segment and ciliary body.

Although ultrasonography is generally considered highly reliable in the differential diagnosis of posterior uveal malignant melanoma, it may be difficult or impossible to differentiate a necrotic melanoma from a small subretinal hematoma or a metastatic carcinoma. Advances in 3-dimensional ultrasound imaging may allow for better evaluation of tumor volume, and advances in high-resolution imaging may be able to determine tumor microvasculature patterns predictive of tumor biology (see Chapter 12).

Transillumination may be helpful in evaluating suspected ciliary body or anterior choroidal melanomas. It is valuable in assessing the degree of pigmentation within a lesion and in determining basal diameters of anterior tumors. The shadow of a tumor is visible with a transilluminating light source, preferably a high-intensity fiberoptic device, placed either on the surface of the topically anesthetized eye in a quadrant opposite the lesion or directly on the cornea with a smooth, dark, specially designed corneal cap (Fig 17-9). Fiberoptic transillumination is used during surgery for radioactive applicator insertion to locate the uveal melanoma and delineate its borders.

Fundus photography is valuable for documenting the ophthalmoscopic appearance of choroidal melanoma and for identifying interval changes in the basal size of a lesion in follow-up examinations. Wide-angle fundus photographs (60°–180°) of intraocular tumors can reveal the full extent of most lesions and can document the relationship between lesions and other intraocular structures. The relative positions of retinal blood vessels can be helpful markers of changes in the size of a lesion. New wide-angle fundus cameras enable accurate measurement of the basal diameter of a choroidal melanoma as well as changes in its size, using intrinsic scales. No patterns of *fluorescein angiography* are pathognomonic for choroidal melanoma.

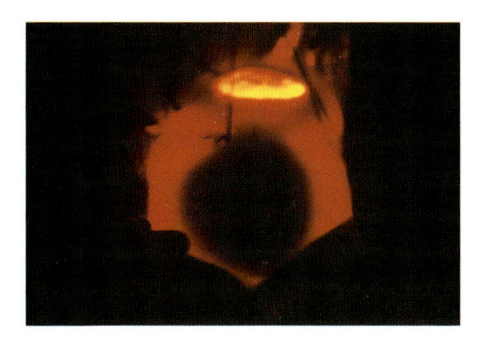

Figure 17-9 Choroidal melanoma, transillumination shadow.

Although *CT* and *MRI* are not widely used in the assessment of uncomplicated intraocular melanocytic tumors, these modalities are useful in identifying tumors in eyes with opaque media and in determining extrascleral extension and involvement of other organs. MRI may be helpful in differentiating atypical vascular lesions from melanocytic tumors.

Differential Diagnosis

The most common lesions that should be considered in the differential diagnosis of posterior uveal malignant melanoma include suspicious choroidal nevus, disciform macular and extramacular lesions, congenital hypertrophy of the RPE (CHRPE), choroidal hemangioma (see Chapter 18), melanocytoma, hemorrhagic detachment of the choroid or RPE, metastatic carcinoma (see Chapter 20 and later in this chapter), and choroidal osteoma. Table 17-2 offers a more complete list to be considered in cases with *amelanotic* choroidal masses.

Choroidal nevus has been discussed previously, but it should be reemphasized that no single clinical characteristic is pathognomonic of choroidal melanoma. Diagnostic accuracy is associated with clinical experience and outstanding ancillary testing facilities. Evaluation and management of these complex cases within regional ocular oncology referral centers appears to enhance patient outcome.

Age-related macular degeneration (AMD) may present with extramacular or macular subretinal neovascularization and fibrosis accompanied by varying degrees and patterns of pigmentation. Hemorrhage, a common finding associated with disciform lesions, is not commonly seen with melanomas unless the tumor extends through Bruch's membrane. Clinical evaluation of the fellow eye is important in documenting the presence of degenerative changes in AMD. Fluorescein angiography results are virtually pathognomonic, revealing early hypofluorescence secondary to blockage from the hemorrhage, often followed by late hyperfluorescence in the distribution of the choroidal neovascular

Table 17-2 Differential Diagnosis of Amelanotic Choroidal Mass

Amelanotic melanoma
Choroidal metastasis
Choroidal hemangioma
Choroidal osteoma
Age-related macular or extramacular degeneration
Choroidal detachment
Uveal effusion syndrome
Posterior scleritis
Chorioretinal granuloma
Toxoplasmic retinochoroiditis
Rhegmatogenous retinal detachment
Degenerative retinoschisis
Presumed acquired retinal hemangioma
Neurilemoma
Leiomyoma
Retinal cavernous hemangioma
Combined hamartoma of the retinal pigment epithelium

Modified from Shields JA, Shields CL. Differential diagnosis of posterior uveal melanoma. In: Shields JA, Shields CL. *Intraocular Tumors: A Text and Atlas*. Philadelphia: Saunders; 1992:137–153.

membrane. Ultrasound testing may reveal increased heterogeneity and a lack of intrinsic vascularity on standardized A scan. Serial observation will document involutional alterations of the evolving disciform lesion.

Congenital hypertrophy of the RPE (CHRPE) is a well-defined, flat, darkly pigmented lesion ranging in size from 1 mm to greater than 10 mm in diameter. Patients are asymptomatic, and the lesion is noted during ophthalmic examination, typically in patients in their teens or twenties. In younger patients, CHRPE often appears homogeneously black; in older individuals, foci of depigmentation (lacunae) often develop (Fig 17-10).

Histologically, CHRPE consists of tall, melanin-containing pigment epithelial cells with large spherical pigment granules. The histology is identical to a condition known as *grouped pigmentation of the retina,* or *bear tracks* (Fig 17-11). The presence of multiple patches of congenital hypertrophy in family members of patients with Gardner syndrome, a familial polyposis, appears to be a marker for the development of colon carcinoma. Fundus findings enable the ophthalmologist to help the gastroenterologist determine the recommended frequency of colon carcinoma screening in family members (see Chapter 11).

Melanocytoma (magnocellular nevus) of the optic disc typically appears as a dark brown to black epipapillary lesion, often with fibrillar margins as a result of extension into the nerve fiber layer (Fig 17-12; see also Fig 15-10 in Chapter 15). It is usually located

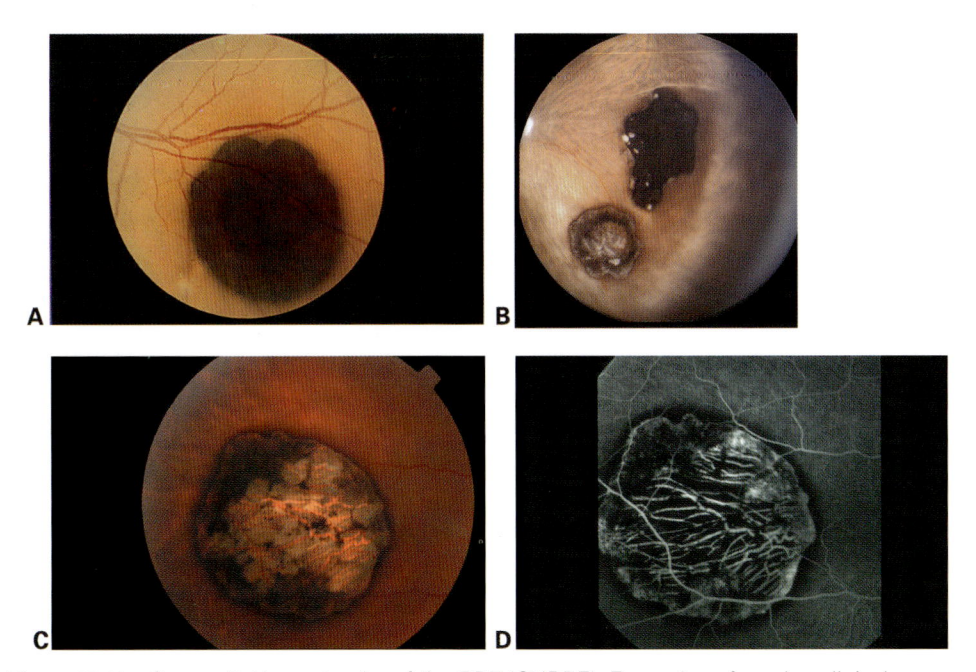

Figure 17-10 Congenital hypertrophy of the RPE (CHRPE). Examples of varying clinical appearances. **A,** CHRPE. Note the homogeneous black color and well-defined margins of the nummular lesion. **B,** Two lesions of CHRPE in the nasal periphery of the fundus. **C, D,** Color fundus photograph and corresponding fluorescein angiogram of a large CHRPE. Note loss of RPE architecture and highlighted choroidal vasculature. *(Part B courtesy of Jacob Pe'er, MD; parts C and D courtesy of Timothy G. Murray, MD.)*

Figure 17-11 Bear tracks. Grouped pigmentation of the retina/RPE represents a form fruste of CHRPE. Note the distinct bear track configuration and heavy pigmentation.

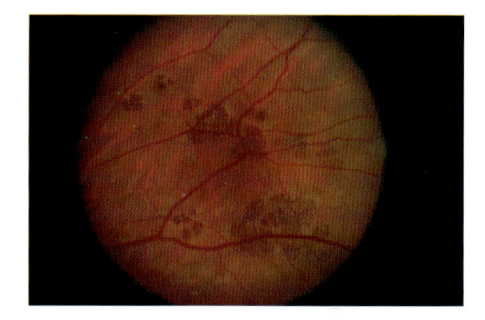

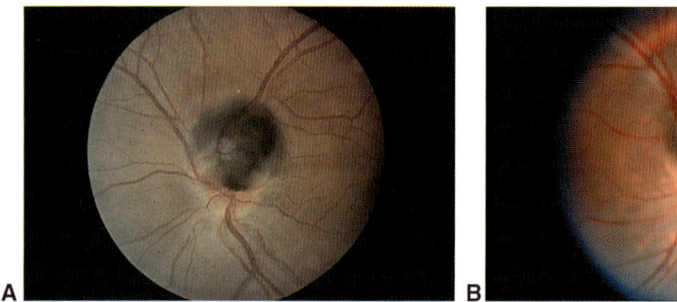

Figure 17-12 Melanocytoma of the optic disc. Note varying clinical appearance in these 2 examples based on degree of choroidal pigmentation: lesion in **(A)** darkly pigmented fundus and **(B)** lightly pigmented fundus. *(Part B courtesy of Timothy G. Murray, MD.)*

eccentrically over the optic disc and may be elevated. It is important to differentiate this lesion from melanoma, because a melanocytoma has minimal malignant potential.

Recent studies have shown that about one third of optic disc melanocytomas have a peripapillary nevus component and that 10% of cases will show minimal but definite growth over a 5-year period. In addition, these lesions can produce an afferent pupillary defect and a variety of visual field abnormalities, ranging from an enlarged blind spot to extensive nerve fiber layer defects.

Suprachoroidal detachments present in 2 forms: *hemorrhagic* and *serous.* These lesions are often associated with hypotony and may present in the immediate period after ophthalmic surgery. Clinically, hemorrhagic detachments are often dome-shaped, involve multiple quadrants, and are associated with breakthrough vitreous bleeding. A- and B-scan ultrasonography readings may closely resemble melanoma but show an absence of intrinsic vascularity and an evolution of the hemorrhage over time. Observational management is indicated in the majority of cases. MRI with gadolinium enhancement may be of benefit in selected cases to document characteristic alterations.

Choroidal osteomas are benign bony tumors that typically arise from the juxtapapillary choroid in adolescent to young adult patients (more commonly in women than men) and are bilateral in 20%–25% of cases. The characteristic lesion appears yellow to orange, and it has well-defined pseudopod margins (Fig 17-13). Ultrasonography reveals a high-amplitude echo corresponding to the plate of bone and loss of the normal orbital echoes

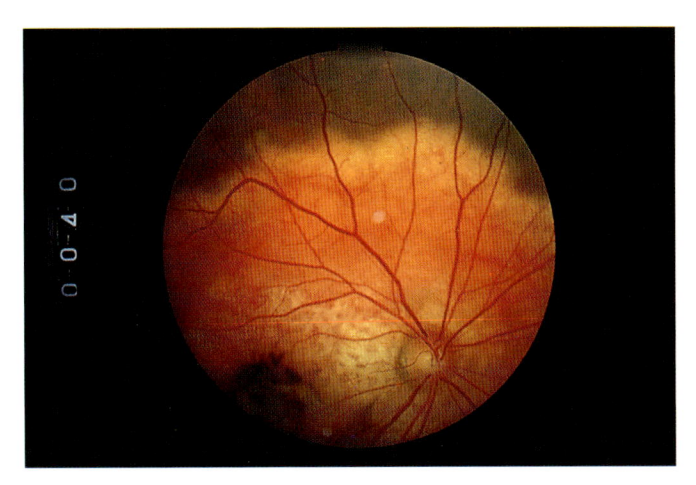

Figure 17-13 Choroidal osteoma, clinical appearance. Note the yellow-orange color, well-defined pseudopod-like margins, and characteristic spotted pigmentation on the surface of this circumpapillary tumor.

behind the lesion. These tumors can also be seen on CT; their hallmark is calcification. Choroidal osteomas typically enlarge slowly over many years. If these lesions involve the macula, vision is generally impaired. Subretinal neovascularization is a common complication of macular choroidal osteomas. The etiology of these lesions is unknown, but chronic low-grade choroidal inflammation has been suspected in some cases (see Chapter 12).

> Accuracy of diagnosis of choroidal melanomas in the Collaborative Ocular Melanoma Study. COMS report no. 1. *Arch Ophthalmol.* 1990;108:1268–1273.
>
> Byrne SF, Marsh MJ, Boldt HC, Green RL, Johnson RN, Wilson DJ. Consistency of observations from echograms made centrally in the Collaborative Ocular Melanoma Study. COMS report no. 13. *Ophthalmic Epidemiol.* 2002;9:11–27.
>
> Mukai S, Reinke MH, Gragoudas ES. Diagnosis of choroidal melanoma. In: Albert DM, Jakobiec FA, eds. *Principles and Practice of Ophthalmology.* 2nd ed. Philadelphia: Saunders; 2000:5017–5027.
>
> Scott IU, Murray TG, Hughes JR. Evaluation of imaging techniques for detection of extraocular extension of choroidal melanoma. *Arch Ophthalmol.* 1998;116:897–899.
>
> Shields CL, Shields JA, Augsburger JJ. Choroidal osteoma. *Surv Ophthalmol.* 1988;33:17–27.

Classification

Melanomas of the ciliary body and choroid have been categorized by size in a number of different ways. Although a size classification based on tumor volume is logical, no simple and reliable method for assessing tumor volume is currently available. The common practice of estimating tumor volume by multiplying maximal basal diameter, minimal basal diameter, and thickness yields only a crude assessment of actual tumor size. Most commonly, posterior uveal melanomas are classified as small, medium, or large based on maximal thickness and basal diameter (Table 17-3). See also Table A-4 in the appendix for the American Joint Committee on Cancer definitions and staging.

Table 17-3 **Classification of Posterior Uveal Melanoma by Tumor Dimension**

	Basal Diameter (mm)	Thickness (mm)
Nevus	<5	<2
Small	5–10	2–3
Medium	10–15	3–5
Large	15–20	5–10
Extra large	>20	>10

Modified from Shields JA, Shields CL. *Intraocular Tumors: A Text and Atlas.* Philadelphia: Saunders; 1992.

Metastatic Evaluation

In a study by Kujala and colleagues, the incidence of metastatic uveal melanoma was observed to be as high as 50% at 25 years after treatment for choroidal melanoma. The Collaborative Ocular Melanoma Study (COMS) reported an incidence of metastatic disease of 25% at 5 years after initial treatment and 34% at 10 years. Nevertheless, clinically evident metastatic disease at the time of initial presentation can be detected in less than 2% of patients. Currently, it is hypothesized that many patients have undetectable micrometastatic disease at the time of their primary treatment. Despite achieving great accuracy in correctly diagnosing uveal melanoma, mortality owing to this tumor has not changed significantly for many years. In general, survival with metastatic uveal melanoma is poor, with a median survival of less than 6 months, although early detection and prompt treatment of liver metastases can increase survival time significantly.

The liver is the predominant organ involved in metastatic uveal melanoma. Liver involvement also tends to be the first manifestation of metastatic disease. In the presence of liver involvement, lung, bone, and skin are other sites that may be affected. An assessment of metastatic disease patterns in COMS revealed liver involvement in 89% of patients, lung involvement in 24%, bone involvement in 17%, and skin and subcutaneous tissue involvement in 12%. In cases that were autopsied, liver involvement was found in 100% and lung involvement in 50% of the patients with metastatic disease.

All patients require metastatic evaluation prior to definitive treatment of the intraocular melanoma (Table 17-4). The purpose of this evaluation is twofold:

1. To determine whether the patient has any other medical conditions that contraindicate surgical treatment or need to be ameliorated before surgery. For example, in one small series, 15% of the patients had a second malignancy at the time of presentation or during the course of a 10-year follow-up; the COMS found preexisting independent primary cancers in about 10% of patients. If there is any question whether the lesion in the eye is a metastatic tumor, this possibility must be ruled out with a thorough medical evaluation directed at determining the site of primary malignancy.

Table 17-4	Clinical Evaluation of Metastatic Uveal Melanoma
	• Liver imaging—ultrasound in routine evaluation
	• Liver function test
	• Chest x-ray
	If any of the above are abnormal:
	• Triphasic liver CT
	• CT-PET of the abdomen/chest
	• MRI of the abdomen/chest

2. To rule out the possibility of detectable metastatic melanoma from the eye. Only rarely is metastatic disease from uveal melanoma detectable at the time of initial presentation. If metastatic disease is clinically present during the pretreatment evaluation of the eye tumor, enucleation is inappropriate unless the eye is painful.

In order to detect metastatic disease of uveal melanoma at an early stage, metastatic evaluation should be performed on all patients on a yearly follow-up basis, and some centers will do so every 6 months. Metastatic evaluation should include a comprehensive physical examination and liver function tests. Chest x-ray is also usually performed, although its yield was found to be low. Recently, research has been performed in several centers investigating possible blood markers for early detection of metastatic uveal melanoma.

Liver imaging studies are included in the metastatic evaluation at some centers. Ultrasound of the abdomen is usually sufficient, but when a suspicion of metastatic disease is raised, triphasic CT or PET-CT is usually recommended in order to evaluate the extent of the disease. A liver or other organ site biopsy may be confirmatory of metastatic disease and is appropriate prior to institution of any treatment for metastatic disease.

The interval between the diagnosis of primary uveal melanoma and its metastasis depends on various clinical, histopathologic, cytogenetic, and molecular genetic factors. It varies from 1–2 years to over 15–20 years. When metastatic disease is diagnosed early enough, before developing miliary spread, the options for treatment of the metastasis, mainly liver metastasis, include surgical resection; chemotherapy, including intra-arterial hepatic chemotherapy and chemoembolization; and immunotherapy.

Development of metastatic disease after enrollment in the COMS trials for treatment of choroidal melanoma: Collaborative Ocular Melanoma Study Group report no. 26. *Arch Ophthalmol.* 2005;123:1639–1643.

Eskelin S, Pyrhonen S, Summanen P, Prause JU, Kivela T. Screening for metastatic malignant melanoma of the uvea revisited. *Cancer.* 1999;85:1151–1159.

Kaiserman I, Amer R, and Pe'er J. Liver function tests in metastatic uveal melanoma. *Am J Ophthalmol.* 2004;137:236–243.

Kujala E, Makitie T, Kivela T. Very long term prognosis of patients with malignant uveal melanoma. *Invest Ophthalmol Vis Sci.* 2003;44:4651–4659.

Singh AD, Topham A. Survival rate with uveal melanoma in the United States: 1973–1997. *Ophthalmology.* 2003;110:962–965.

Treatment

Management of posterior uveal melanomas has long been the subject of considerable controversy. Two factors lie at the heart of this controversy:

1. the limited amount of data on the natural history of untreated patients with posterior uveal malignant melanoma
2. the lack of groups of patients matched for known and for unknown risk factors and managed by different therapeutic techniques to assess the comparative effectiveness of those treatments

In 1882, Fuchs wrote that all intraocular melanomas were treated by enucleation and the only untreated cases were in the "older literature." Presently, both surgical and radiotherapeutic management are used for intraocular melanoma. The COMS has reported randomized, prospectively administered treatment outcomes for patients with medium and large choroidal melanomas. The methods of patient management currently in use depend on several factors:

- size, location, and extent of the tumor
- visual status of the affected eye and of the fellow eye
- age and general health of the patient

Observation

In certain instances, serial observation without treatment of an intraocular tumor is indicated. Most types of benign retinal and choroidal tumors, such as choroidal nevi, choroidal osteoma, or hyperplasia of the RPE, can be managed with observation. Growth of small melanocytic lesions of the posterior uvea that are less than 1.0 mm in thickness can be documented periodically by fundus photography and ultrasonography. Significant controversy persists regarding the management of small choroidal melanomas. Lesions greater than 1.0 mm in thickness, with documented growth, should be evaluated for indications for definitive treatment. Observation of active larger tumors may be appropriate in very elderly and systemically ill patients who are not candidates for any sort of therapeutic intervention.

Enucleation

Historically, enucleation has been the gold standard in the treatment of malignant intraocular tumors. Although some authors in the past hypothesized that surgical manipulation of eyes containing malignant melanoma leads to tumor dissemination and increased mortality, this hypothesis is no longer accepted, and enucleation remains appropriate for some medium-sized, many large, and all extra-large choroidal melanomas. The COMS compared the application of pre-enucleation external-beam radiation therapy followed by enucleation with enucleation alone for patients with large choroidal melanomas and found no statistically significant survival difference in 5-year mortality rates. Enucleation remains one of the most common primary treatments for choroidal melanoma.

Radioactive plaque (brachytherapy)

The application of a radioactive plaque to the sclera overlying an intraocular tumor is probably the most common method of treating uveal melanoma. It allows the delivery of a high dose of radiation to the tumor and a relatively low dose to the surrounding normal structures of the eye. The technique has been available for 50 years. Although various isotopes have been used, the most common today are iodine 125 and ruthenium 106. Cobalt 60 plaques, which were the main source for brachytherapy in the past, are rarely used today. Other isotopes that have been used are strontium 90, iridium 192, and palladium 103. In the United States, iodine 125 is the isotope most frequently used in the treatment of ciliary body and choroidal melanomas. Advances in intraoperative localization, especially the use of ultrasound, have increased local tumor control rates to as high as 96%. In most patients, the tumor decreases in size (Fig 17-14); in others, the result is total flattening of the tumor with scar formation or no change in tumor size, although clinical and ultrasound changes can be seen. Regrowth is diagnosed in only 4%–5% of the treated tumors. Late radiation complications, especially optic neuropathy and retinopathy, are visually limiting in as many as 50% of patients undergoing treatment. Radiation complications appear dose-dependent, and they increase for tumors involving, or adjacent to, the macula or optic nerve.

Charged-particle radiation

High-linear-energy transfer radiation with charged particles (protons and helium ions) has been used effectively in managing ciliary body and choroidal melanomas. The technique requires surgical attachment of tantalum clips to the sclera to mark the basal margins of the tumor prior to the first radiation fraction. The charged-particle beams deliver a more

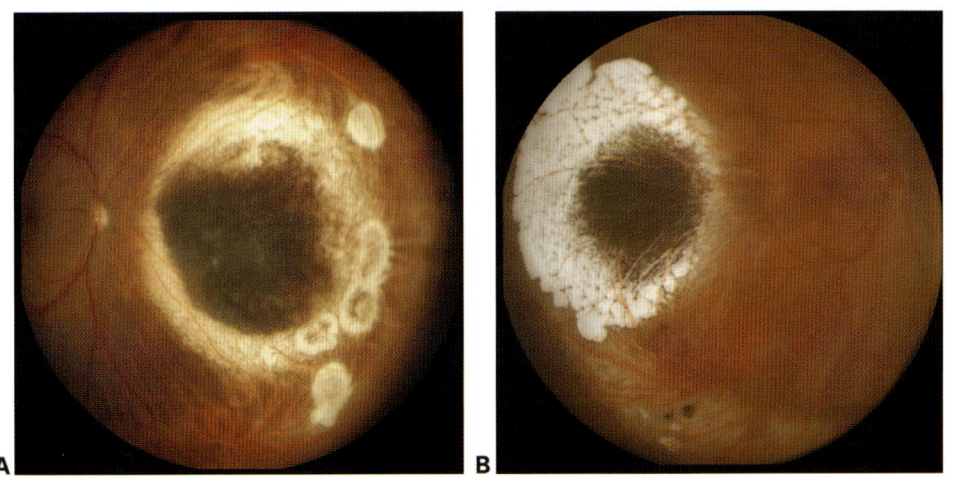

Figure 17-14 Choroidal melanoma treated by radioactive brachytherapy. **A,** Mildly elevated remnants of melanoma surrounded by atrophic chorioretinal scarring, nasal to the optic nerve head. **B,** Flat remnants of melanoma pigmentation surrounded by chorioretinal scarring located temporal to the macula. *(Parts A and B courtesy of Jacob Pe'er, MD.)*

homogeneous dose of radiation energy to a tumor than does a radioactive plaque, and the lateral spread of radiation energy from such beams is less extensive (Bragg peak effect). Local tumor control rates of up to 98% have been reported. The response is similar to that seen after brachytherapy.

Unfortunately, charged-particle radiation often delivers a higher dose to anterior segment structures. Radiation complications, most commonly anterior, lead to uncontrolled neovascular glaucoma in 10% of treated eyes and vision loss in approximately 50%.

External-beam radiation

Conventional external-beam radiation therapy is ineffective as a single-modality treatment for malignant melanoma. Pre-enucleation external-beam radiotherapy combined with enucleation appears to limit orbital recurrence in large melanomas and showed a non–statistically significant reduction in 5-year mortality in the COMS large-tumor trial. In recent years, several centers have used fractionated stereotactic radiotherapy and gamma knife radiosurgery, reporting good results.

Cataract may develop following all types of radiotherapy. Surgical removal of radiation-induced cataract is indicated if the intraocular tumor is nonviable and the patient appears to have visual limitations attributable to the cataract. No increase in mortality after cataract extraction has been documented.

Alternative treatments

Photoablation and hyperthermia Photocoagulation has played a limited role in the treatment of melanocytic tumors. Reports of focal/grid treatment to eradicate active subretinal fluid in choroidal melanoma have documented a propensity for accelerated tumor growth with rupture of Bruch's membrane. Recently, advances in the delivery of hyperthermia (heat) using transpupillary thermotherapy (TTT) have been reported. Direct diode laser treatment using long duration, large spot size, and relatively low-energy laser have been associated with a reduction in tumor volume. Some reports have suggested that TTT is associated with an increased rate of local tumor recurrence compared with brachytherapy.

Cryotherapy Although cryotherapy using a triple freeze-thaw technique has been tried in the treatment of small choroidal melanomas, it is not considered standard therapy and is not currently undergoing further evaluation for efficacy.

Transscleral diathermy Diathermy is *contraindicated* in the treatment of malignant intraocular tumors because the induced scleral damage may provide a route for extrascleral extension of tumor cells.

Surgical excision of tumor Surgical excision has been performed successfully in many eyes with malignant and benign intraocular tumors. Concerns regarding surgical excision include the inability to evaluate tumor margins for residual disease and the high incidence of pathologically recognized scleral, retinal, and vitreous involvement in medium and large choroidal melanomas. When this treatment is used, the surgical techniques are generally quite difficult, requiring an experienced surgeon. In some instances, local excision of uveal melanoma has been coupled with globe-conserving radiotherapy, such as brachytherapy.

Chemotherapy Currently, chemotherapy is not effective in the treatment of primary or metastatic uveal melanoma. Various regimens have been used, however, for palliative treatment of patients with metastatic disease.

Immunotherapy Presently, immunotherapy is under investigation in the treatment of gross and microscopic metastatic disease. Immunotherapy uses systemic cytokines, immunomodulatory agents, or local vaccine therapy to try to activate a tumor-directed T-cell immune response.

Exenteration Exenteration, traditionally advocated for patients with extrascleral extension of a posterior uveal melanoma, is rarely employed today. The current trend is toward more conservative treatment for these patients, with enucleation plus a limited tenonectomy. The addition of local radiotherapy appears to achieve survival outcomes similar to those of exenteration.

> Bergman L, Nilsson B, Lundell G, Lundell M, Seregard S. Ruthenium brachytherapy for uveal melanoma, 1979–2003: survival and functional outcomes in the Swedish population. *Ophthalmology.* 2005;112:834–840.
>
> The Collaborative Ocular Melanoma Study (COMS) randomized trial of pre-enucleation radiation of large choroidal melanoma, II: initial mortality findings. COMS report no. 10. *Am J Ophthalmol.* 1998;125:779–796.
>
> Damato B, Jones AG. Uveal melanoma: resection techniques. *Ophthalmol Clin North Am.* 2005;18:119–128.
>
> Diener-West M, Earle JD, Fine SL, et al. The COMS randomized trial of iodine 125 brachytherapy for choroidal melanoma, III: initial mortality findings. COMS report no. 18. *Arch Ophthalmol.* 2001;119:969–982.
>
> Gragoudas ES, Marie Lane A. Uveal melanoma: proton beam irradiation. *Ophthalmol Clin North Am.* 2005;18:111–118.
>
> Harbour JW, Murray TG, Byrne SF, et al. Intraoperative echographic localization of iodine 125 episcleral radioactive plaques for posterior uveal melanoma. *Retina.* 1996;16:129–134.
>
> Shields JA, Shields CL. Current management of posterior uveal melanoma. *Mayo Clin Proc.* 1993;68:1196–1200.

Prognosis and Prognostic Factors

A meta-analysis from the published literature of tumor mortality after treatment documented a 5-year mortality rate of 50% for large choroidal melanoma and 30% for medium-sized choroidal melanoma; 5-year melanoma-related mortality in treated patients with small choroidal melanoma has been reported to be as high as 12%. Retrospective analysis among patients with melanoma suggests that clinical risk factors for mortality are

- larger tumor size at time of treatment
- tumor growth
- anterior tumor location
- extraocular extension
- older age
- tumor regrowth after globe-conserving therapy
- rapid decrease in tumor size after globe-conserving therapy
- juxtapapillary tumors

274 • Ophthalmic Pathology and Intraocular Tumors

Histopathologic features associated with a higher rate of metastases include

- epithelioid cells
- high mitotic index and high cell proliferation indices
- complex microvascular patterns (loops, networks of loops, and parallel with cross-linking)
- mean of 10 largest nuclei
- tumor-infiltrating lymphocytes
- monosomy 3
- trisomy 8

A more in-depth discussion is provided in Chapter 12.

> Coleman DJ, Rondeau MJ, Silverman RH, et al. Correlation of microcirculation architecture with ultrasound backscatter parameters of uveal melanoma. *Eur J Ophthalmol.* 1995;5:96–106.
> Folberg R, Pe'er J, Gruman LM, et al. The morphologic characteristics of tumor blood vessels as a marker of tumor progression in primary human uveal melanoma: a matched case-control study. *Hum Pathol.* 1992;23:1298–1305.
> Mueller AJ, Freeman WR, Folberg R, et al. Evaluation of microvascular pattern visibility in human choroidal melanomas: comparison of confocal fluorescein with indocyanine green angiography. *Graefes Arch Clin Exp Ophthalmol.* 1999;237:448–456.
> Sisley K, Rennie IG, Parsons MA, et al. Abnormalities of chromosomes 3 and 8 in posterior uveal melanoma correlate with prognosis. *Genes Chromosomes Cancer.* 1997;19:22–28.

Collaborative Ocular Melanoma Study (COMS)

Survival data from the COMS have now been reported for the randomized clinical trials of large and medium choroidal melanoma and for the observational study of small choroidal melanoma. These results provide the framework for patient discussions concerning treatment-related long-term survival, rates of globe conservation with iodine 125 brachytherapy, and predictors of small-tumor growth.

- COMS Large Choroidal Melanoma Trial
    - evaluated 1003 patients with choroidal melanomas >16 mm in basal diameter and/or >10 mm in apical height
    - compared enucleation alone with enucleation preceded by external-beam radiotherapy
    - reported a 5-year survival rate of 57% and 62%, respectively, between cohorts
    - concluded that adjunctive radiotherapy did not improve overall survival
    - established the appropriateness of primary enucleation alone in managing large choroidal melanomas that are not amenable to globe-conserving therapy
- COMS Medium Choroidal Melanoma Trial
    - evaluated 1317 patients with choroidal melanomas ranging in size from 6 mm to 16 mm in basal diameter and/or 2.5 mm to 10 mm in apical height
    - compared standardized enucleation and iodine 125 brachytherapy
    - all-cause mortality at 5 years: 18% and 19%, respectively
    - histologically confirmed metastases at 5 years found in 9% of patients treated with brachytherapy as opposed to 11% in patients who underwent enucleation

- secondary finding in enucleated eyes:
    - —only 2/660 (0.3%) enucleated eyes misdiagnosed as having a choroidal melanoma
- secondary findings in patients undergoing brachytherapy:
    - —10.3% local tumor recurrence at 5 years
    - —12.5% risk of enucleation after brachytherapy at 5 years
    - —local tumor recurrence weakly associated with a reduced survival, with an adjusted risk ratio of 1.5
    - —decline in visual acuity to 20/200 in 43% of patients at 3 years
    - —quadrupling of the visual angle (6 lines of visual loss) in 49% of patients at 3 years

- COMS Small Choroidal Tumor Trial
    - observational study of 204 patients with tumors measuring 4.0–8.0 mm in basal diameter and/or 1.0–2.4 mm in apical height
    - melanoma-specific mortality 1% at 5 years
    - clinical growth factors included
        - —greater initial thickness and basal diameter
        - —presence of orange pigmentation
        - —absence of drusen and/or retinal pigment epithelial changes
        - —presence of tumor pinpoint hyperfluorescence on angiography

Detailed findings of the COMS can be found at www.jhu.edu/wctb/coms.

Pigmented Epithelial Tumors of the Uvea and Retina

Adenoma and Adenocarcinoma

Benign adenomas of the nonpigmented and pigmented ciliary epithelium may appear indistinguishable clinically from melanomas arising in the ciliary body. Benign adenomas of the RPE are very rare. These lesions occur as oval, deeply melanotic tumors arising abruptly from the RPE. Adenomas rarely enlarge and seldom undergo malignant change. Adenocarcinomas of the RPE are also very rare; only a few cases have ever been reported in the literature. Although these lesions have malignant features histologically, their metastatic potential appears to be minimal.

Rare benign asymptomatic cysts of the ciliary epithelium may occur. Opacified ciliary epithelial cysts are formed in myeloma and macroglobulinemia.

Fuchs adenoma (pseudoadenomatous hyperplasia) is usually an incidental finding at autopsy and rarely becomes apparent clinically. It appears as a glistening, white, irregular tumor arising from a ciliary crest. Histologically, it consists of benign proliferation of the nonpigmented ciliary epithelium with accumulation of basement membrane–like material.

Green WR. Retina. In: Spencer WH, ed. *Ophthalmic Pathology: An Atlas and Textbook.* 4th ed. Philadelphia: Saunders; 1996:1291–1313.

Acquired Hyperplasia

Hyperplasia of the pigmented ciliary epithelium or the retinal pigment epithelium usually occurs in response to trauma, inflammation, or other ocular insults. Ciliary body lesions, because of their location, often do not become evident clinically. Occasionally, however, they may reach a large size and simulate a ciliary body melanoma. Posteriorly located lesions may be more commonly recognized and can lead to diagnostic uncertainty. In the early management of these atypical lesions, observation is often appropriate to document stability of the lesion. Adenomatous hyperplasia, which has been reported only rarely, may clinically mimic a choroidal melanoma.

Combined Hamartoma

Combined hamartoma of the RPE and retina is a rare disorder that occurs most frequently at the disc margin. Typically, it appears as a darkly pigmented, minimally elevated lesion with retinal traction and tortuous retinal vessels (Fig 17-15). Histologically, it consists of a proliferation of RPE cells, glial cells, and retinal blood vessels. The glial cells may contract, producing the traction lines seen clinically in the retina. This lesion has been mistaken for malignant melanoma because of its dark pigmentation and slight elevation. In rare cases, a combined hamartoma may be situated in the peripheral fundus.

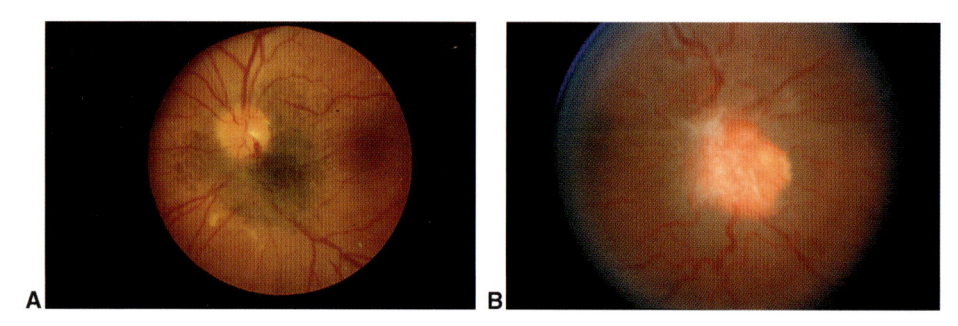

Figure 17-15 **A,** Peripapillary combined hamartoma of the retina and RPE. Note the radiating traction lines through the fovea. **B,** Example of medium-sized combined hamartoma. *(Part B courtesy of Timothy G. Murray, MD.)*

CHAPTER 18

Angiomatous Tumors

Hemangiomas

Choroidal Hemangiomas

Hemangiomas of the choroid occur in 2 specific forms: circumscribed and diffuse. The *circumscribed choroidal hemangioma* typically occurs in patients with no other systemic disorders. It generally appears as a red or orange tumor located in the postequatorial zone of the fundus, often in the macular area (Fig 18-1). Such tumors commonly produce a secondary retinal detachment that extends into the foveal region, resulting in visual blurring, metamorphopsia, and micropsia. These benign vascular tumors characteristically affect the overlying RPE and cause cystoid degeneration of the outer retinal layers.

The principal entities in the differential diagnosis of circumscribed choroidal hemangioma include

- amelanotic choroidal melanoma
- choroidal osteoma
- metastatic carcinoma to the choroid
- granuloma of the choroid

The *diffuse choroidal hemangioma* is generally seen in patients with Sturge-Weber syndrome (encephalofacial angiomatosis). This choroidal tumor produces diffuse reddish orange thickening of the entire fundus, resulting in an ophthalmoscopic pattern commonly referred to as *tomato catsup fundus* (Fig 18-2). Retinal detachment and glaucoma often occur in eyes with this lesion. See BCSC Section 12, *Retina and Vitreous,* for a discussion of choroidal hemangioma, and BCSC Section 6, *Pediatric Ophthalmology and Strabismus,* for a discussion of intraocular vascular tumors and Sturge-Weber syndrome.

Ancillary diagnostic studies may be of considerable help in evaluating choroidal hemangiomas. Fluorescein angiography reveals the large choroidal vessels in the prearterial or arterial phases with late staining of the tumor and the overlying cystoid retina. This pattern is not pathognomonic of choroidal hemangiomas. Ultrasonography has been helpful in differentiating choroidal hemangiomas from amelanotic melanomas and other simulating lesions. A-scan ultrasonography generally shows a high-amplitude initial echo and high-amplitude broad internal echoes ("high internal reflectivity"; see Fig 18-1B). B-scan ultrasonography demonstrates localized or diffuse choroidal thickening with prominent internal reflections (acoustic heterogeneity) without choroidal excavation or orbital shadowing (see

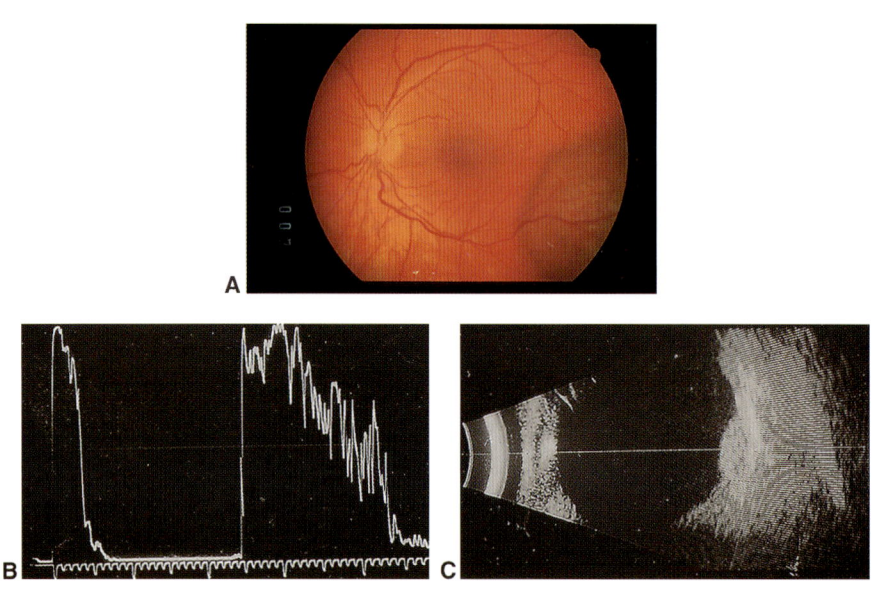

Figure 18-1 A, Circumscribed choroidal hemangioma. **B,** A-scan ultrasound study shows characteristic high internal reflectivity. **C,** B-scan ultrasound study shows a highly reflective tumor.

Fig 18-1C). Radiographic studies, particularly CT scanning, can be helpful in differentiating a choroidal hemangioma from a choroidal osteoma.

Asymptomatic choroidal hemangiomas require no treatment. The most common complication is serous detachment of the retina involving the fovea, with resultant visual loss. Traditionally, this has been managed by laser photocoagulation. The surface of the tumor is treated lightly with laser photocoagulation in an effort not to destroy the tumor but rather to create a chorioretinal adhesion that prevents further accumulation of fluid. Often, repeated treatments are necessary to eliminate active exudation of subretinal fluid. If the retinal detachment is extensive, this type of photocoagulation is usually unsuccessful. Recurrent detachments are common, and the long-term visual prognosis in patients with macular detachment or edema is guarded.

Photodynamic therapy (PDT) has recently been used to treat patients with circumscribed choroidal hemangioma and associated decreased visual function. PDT applied over the entire surface of the lesion appears to be effective in the resolution of subretinal fluid and in the involution of the vascular tumor. Further clinical experience is needed to better define the therapeutic indications and parameters for this evolving laser therapy.

Radiation, in the forms of brachytherapy, charged-particle, and external-beam, has been used to treat choroidal hemangiomas. Brachytherapy and charged-particle therapy have been used to treat patients with circumscribed choroidal hemangiomas, and external-beam radiotherapy (low dose, fractionated) has been used to treat patients with diffuse choroidal hemangioma. Each modality has been reported to cause involution of the hemangiomas, with subsequent resolution of the associated serous retinal detachment. Complications from the radiation and the serous retinal detachment may limit vision in patients who are irradiated.

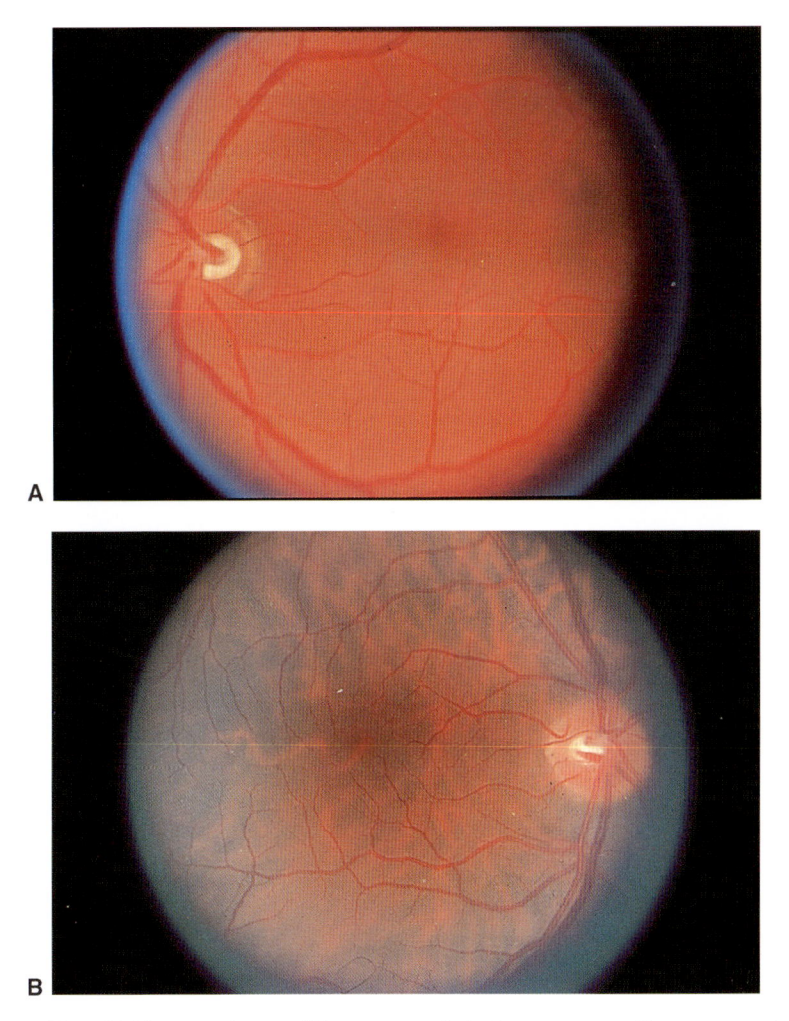

Figure 18-2 Choroidal hemangioma, diffuse type, clinical appearance. The saturated red color of the affected fundus **(A)** contrasts markedly with the color of the unaffected fundus **(B)** of the same patient.

New horizons in the treatment of choroidal hemangiomas may involve the periocular or intraocular use of antiangiogenic agents.

See Chapter 12 for further discussion of choroidal hemangiomas.

Augsburger JJ, Freire J, Brady LW. Radiation therapy for choroidal and retinal hemangiomas. *Front Radiat Ther Oncol.* 1997;30:265–280.

Chao AN, Shields CL, Shields JA, Krema H. Plaque radiotherapy for choroidal hemangioma with total retinal detachment and iris neovascularization. *Retina.* 2001;21:682–684.

Lee V, Hungerford JL. Proton beam therapy for posterior pole circumscribed choroidal haemangioma. *Eye.* 1998;12:925–928.

Madreperla SA, Hungerford JL, Plowman PN, Laganowski HC, Gregory PT. Choroidal hemangiomas: visual and anatomic results of treatment by photocoagulation or radiation therapy. *Ophthalmology.* 1997;104:1773–1778.

Meyer K, Augsburger JJ. Independent diagnostic value of fluorescein angiography in the evaluation of intraocular tumors. *Graefes Arch Clin Exp Ophthalmol.* 1999;237:489–494.

Porrini G, Giovannini A, Amato G, Ioni A, Pantanetti M. Photodynamic therapy of circumscribed choroidal hemangioma. *Ophthalmology.* 2003;110:674–680.

Schilling H, Bornfeld N. Long-term results after low-dose ocular irradiation for choroidal hemangiomas. *Curr Opin Ophthalmol.* 1998;9:51–55.

Singh AD, Kaiser PK, Sears JE, Gupta M, Rundle PA, Rennie IG. Photodynamic therapy of circumscribed choroidal haemangioma. *Br J Ophthalmol.* 2004;88:1414–1418.

Retinal Angiomas

Capillary hemangioma

Retinal capillary hemangioma (angiomatosis retinae) is a rare autosomal dominant condition with a reported incidence of 1 in 40,000. Typically, patients are diagnosed in the second to third decades of life, although retinal lesions may be present at birth. The retinal capillary hemangioma *(hemangioblastoma)* appears as a red to orange tumor arising within the retina with large-caliber, tortuous afferent and efferent retinal blood vessels (Fig 18-3). Associated yellow-white retinal and subretinal exudates that seem to have a predilection for foveal involvement may appear. Exudative detachments often occur in eyes with hemangioblastomas. Atypical variations include hemangiomas arising from the optic disc, which may appear as encapsulated lesions with or without pseudopapilledema, and in the retinal periphery, where vitreous traction may elevate the tumor from the surface of the retina, giving the appearance of a free-floating vitreous mass.

When a capillary hemangioma of the retina occurs as a solitary finding, the condition is generally known as *von Hippel disease.* This condition is familial in about 20% of cases and bilateral in about 50%. The lesions may be multiple in 1 or both eyes. If retinal capillary hemangiomatosis is associated with a cerebellar hemangioblastoma, the term *von Hippel–Lindau syndrome* is applied. The gene for von Hippel–Lindau syndrome has been isolated on chromosome 3. A number of other tumors and cysts may occur in patients with von Hippel–Lindau syndrome. The most important of these lesions are cerebellar hemangioblastomas, renal cell carcinomas, and pheochromocytomas. Genetic screening now allows for subtyping of patients with von Hippel–Lindau to determine risk for systemic

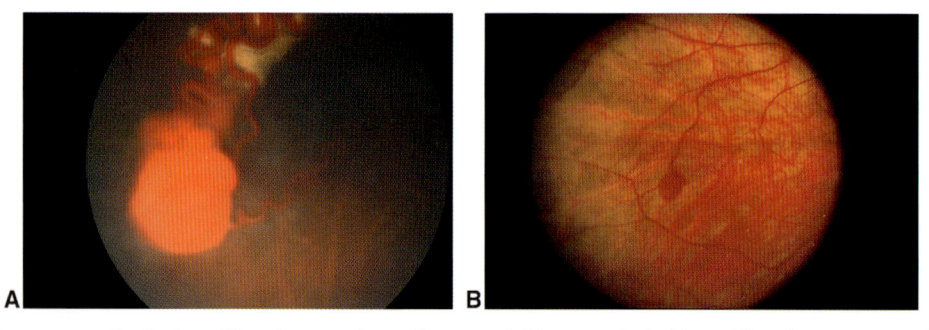

Figure 18-3 Retinal capillary hemangioma (hemangioblastoma). **A,** Note dilated, tortuous retinal vessels supplying this vascular tumor. **B,** Retinal capillary hemangiomas may be small and difficult to observe clinically. *(Part A courtesy of Timothy G. Murray, MD.)*

manifestations of the disease. When this diagnosis is suspected, appropriate consultation and screening are critical for long-term follow-up of ocular manifestations and the associated systemic complications.

Fluorescein angiography of retinal capillary hemangiomas demonstrates a rapid arteriovenous transit, with immediate filling of the feeding arteriole, subsequent filling of the numerous fine blood vessels that constitute the tumor, and drainage by the dilated venule. Massive leakage of dye into the tumor and vitreous can occur.

Treatment of retinal capillary hemangiomas includes photocoagulation for smaller lesions, cryotherapy for larger and more peripheral lesions, and scleral buckling with cryotherapy or penetrating diathermy for extremely large lesions with extensive retinal detachment. Cryotherapy, and to a lesser extent laser photocoagulation, however, may be associated with vascular decompensation leading to massive exudative retinal detachment. Eye-wall resection as well as external-beam and charged-particle radiotherapy have also been used. Recent case reports have suggested the utility of targeted antiangiogenic therapy in the management of retinal capillary hemangiomas that are unresponsive to standard treatment. The efficacy of antiangiogenic agents in the treatment of these vascular lesions is of compelling interest to von Hippel–Lindau patients, who have a lifelong risk of developing retinal angiomas. Visual prognosis remains guarded for patients with large retinal lesions. Aggressive screening and early treatment may reduce the late complications of total exudative retinal detachment. Screening for systemic vascular anomalies (eg, cerebellar hemangioblastomas) and malignancies (eg, renal cell carcinoma) may reduce mortality.

> Aiello LP, George DJ, Cahill MT, et al. Rapid and durable recovery of visual function in a patient with von Hippel–Lindau syndrome after systemic therapy with vascular endothelial growth factor receptor inhibitor su5416. *Ophthalmology.* 2002;109:1745–1751.

Cavernous hemangioma

Cavernous hemangioma of the retina is an uncommon lesion that resembles a cluster of grapes (Fig 18-4). In contrast to the lesions in Coats disease and retinal capillary hemangiomatosis, cavernous hemangiomas are generally not associated with exudates. However, small hemorrhages as well as areas of gliosis and fibrosis may appear on the surface of the lesion. Within the vascular spaces of the cavernous hemangioma, a plasma–erythrocyte separation may appear that can best be demonstrated on fluorescein angiography. Cavernous hemangiomas may occur on the optic disc, where their appearance resembles that in the extrapapillary retina. Cavernous hemangiomas of the retina are sometimes associated with similar skin and CNS lesions, and patients with intracranial lesions may have seizures.

Fluorescein angiography is virtually diagnostic of cavernous hemangiomas of the retina. In contrast to a retinal capillary hemangioma, a retinal cavernous hemangioma fills very slowly, and the fluorescein often pools in the upper part of the vascular space, while the cellular elements (erythrocytes) pool in the lower part. The fluorescein remains in the vascular spaces for an extended period of time. Unlike tumors in Coats disease and retinal capillary hemangiomatosis, cavernous hemangiomas generally show no leakage of fluorescein into the vitreous.

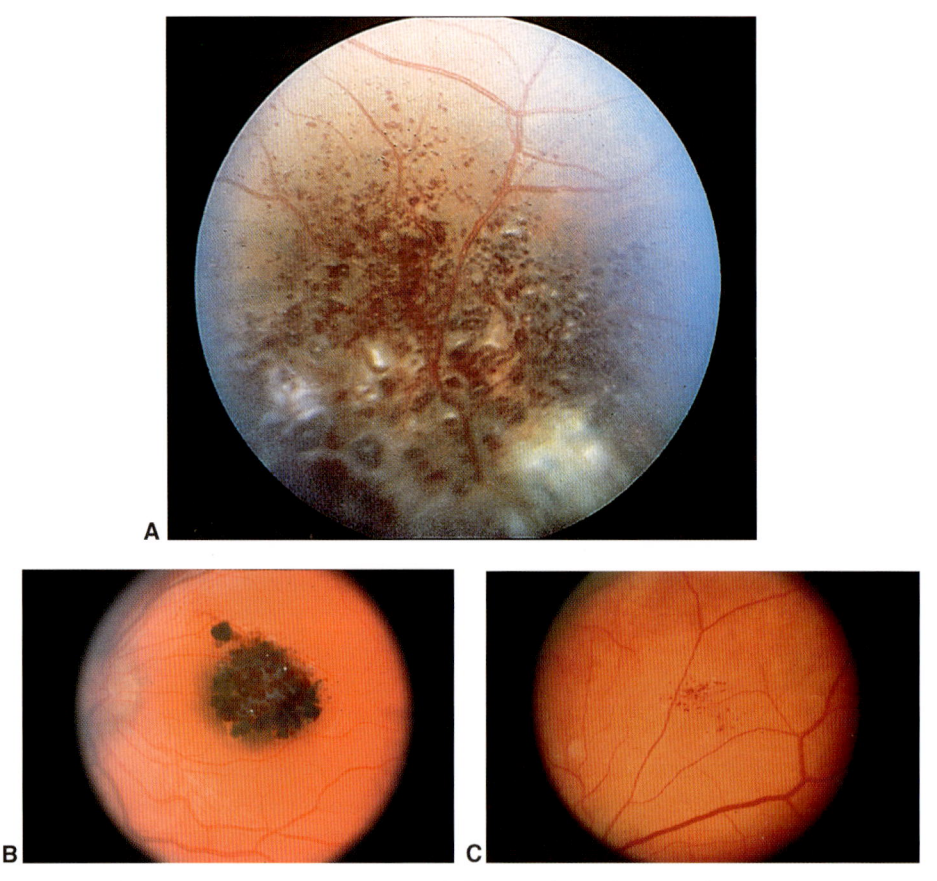

282 • Ophthalmic Pathology and Intraocular Tumors

Figure 18-4 Retinal cavernous hemangioma. **A,** Note multiple tiny vascular saccules and associated white fibrovascular tissue. **B,** Note clumped vascular saccules (grape cluster configuration). **C,** When lesions are small, findings may be subtle. *(Part B courtesy of Timothy G. Murray, MD.)*

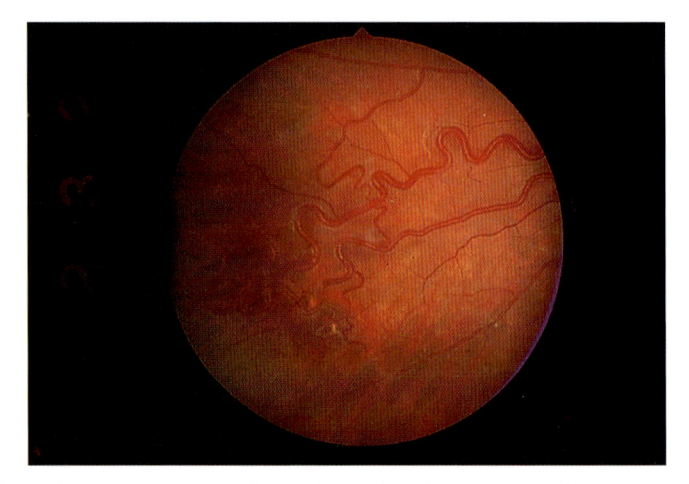

Figure 18-5 Retinal arteriovenous malformation, clinical appearance. Note the absence of capillary bed between the afferent and efferent arms of this retinal arteriovenous communication.

Histologically, a cavernous retinal hemangioma consists of dilated, thin-walled vascular channels that are interconnected by small orifices. The dilated vessels may protrude upward beneath the internal limiting membrane, and associated gliosis and hemorrhage may be seen. Treatment is rarely required.

Arteriovenous Malformation

Congenital retinal arteriovenous malformation (racemose hemangioma) is an anomalous artery-to-vein anastomosis ranging from a small, localized vascular communication near the disc or in the periphery to a prominent tangle of large, tortuous blood vessels throughout most of the fundus (Fig 18-5). When associated with an arteriovenous malformation of the midbrain region, this condition is generally referred to as *Wyburn- Mason syndrome* (see also discussions of phakomatoses in BCSC Section 5, *Neuro-Ophthalmology,* and Section 6, *Pediatric Ophthalmology and Strabismus*). Associated similar arteriovenous malformations may appear in the orbit and mandible.

CHAPTER 19

Retinoblastoma

Retinoblastoma is the most common primary intraocular malignancy of childhood, second only to uveal malignant melanoma as the most common primary intraocular malignancy in all age groups (Table 19-1). The frequency of retinoblastoma ranges from 1 in 14,000 to 1 in 20,000 live births, depending on the country. It is estimated that approximately 250–300 new cases occur in the United States each year. In Mexico, 6.8 cases per million population have been reported compared to 4 cases per million in the United States. In Central America, there has been an increased incidence in recent years. There is no sexual predilection, and the tumor occurs bilaterally in 30%–40% of cases. The mean age at diagnosis depends on family history and the laterality of the disease:

- patients with a known family history of retinoblastoma: 4 months
- patients with bilateral disease: 14 months
- patients with unilateral disease: 24 months

About 90% of cases are diagnosed in patients under 3 years old.

> Augsburger JJ, Oehlschlager U, Manzitti JE. Multinational clinical and pathologic registry of retinoblastoma. Retinoblastoma International Collaborative Study report 2. *Graefes Arch Clin Exp Ophthalmol.* 1995;233:469–475.
> Rubenfeld M, Abramson DH, Ellsworth RM, Kitchin FD. Unilateral vs. bilateral retinoblastoma: correlations between age at diagnosis and stage of ocular disease. *Ophthalmology.* 1986;93:1016–1019.
> Sanders BM, Draper GJ, Kingston JE. Retinoblastoma in Great Britain 1969–1980: incidence, treatment, and survival. *Br J Ophthalmol.* 1988;72:576–583.
> Tamboli A, Podgor MJ, Horm JW. The incidence of retinoblastoma in the United States: 1974 through 1985. *Arch Ophthalmol.* 1990;108:128–132.

Genetic Counseling

Retinoblastoma is caused by a mutation in the *RB1* gene located on the long arm of chromosome 13 at locus 14 (13q14). Both copies of the *RB1* gene must be mutated in order for a tumor to form. If a patient has bilateral retinoblastoma, there is approximately a 98%

Table 19-1 **Epidemiology of Retinoblastoma**

Most common intraocular cancer of childhood
Third most common intraocular cancer overall after melanoma and metastasis
Incidence is 1/14,000–1/20,000 live births
90% of cases present before 3 years of age
Occurs equally in males and females
Occurs equally in right and left eyes
No racial predilection
60%–70% unilateral (mean age at diagnosis, 24 months)
30%–40% bilateral (mean age at diagnosis, 14 months)

chance that it represents a germline mutation. Only 6% of retinoblastoma patients have a family history of retinoblastoma. The children of a retinoblastoma survivor who has the hereditary form of retinoblastoma have a 45% chance of being affected (50% chance of inheriting and 90% chance of penetrance). In these cases, the child inherits an abnormal gene from the affected parent. This abnormal gene coupled with somatic mutations in the remaining normal RB1 allele leads to the development of multiple tumors in 1 or both eyes.

Sporadic cases constitute about 94% of all retinoblastomas. Of these, 60% of patients have unilateral disease with no germline mutations. The remaining patients have new germline mutations and will develop multiple tumors. It should be noted that approximately 15% of the sporadic unilateral patients are carriers of a germline RB1 mutation. Unless there are multiple tumors in the affected eye, these patients cannot be distinguished from children without a germline mutation. Children with unilateral retinoblastoma and a germline mutation, much like their counterparts with bilateral retinoblastoma, are more likely to present at an earlier age. Commercial laboratories are now available to test the blood of all retinoblastoma patients for germline mutations. There is approximately a 95% chance of finding a new mutation if one exists.

Genetic counseling for retinoblastoma can be very complex (Fig 19-1). A bilateral retinoblastoma survivor has a 45% chance of having an affected child, whereas a unilateral survivor has a 7% chance of having an affected child. Normal parents of a child with bilateral involvement have less than a 5% risk of having another child with retinoblastoma. If 2 or more siblings are affected, the chance that another child will be affected increases to 45%. See Chapter 11 for further discussion of the genetic origins of the retinoblastoma tumor as well as descriptions of histologic features. BCSC Section 6, *Pediatric Ophthalmology and Strabismus,* also discusses retinoblastoma in its chapter on ocular tumors in childhood.

Abramson DH, Mendelsohn ME, Servodidio CA, Tretter T, Gombos DS. Familial retinoblastoma: where and when? *Acta Ophthalmol Scand.* 1998;76:334–338.

Gallie BL, Dunn JM, Chan HS, Hamel PA, Phillips RA. The genetics of retinoblastoma: relevance to the patient. *Pediatr Clin North Am.* 1991;38:299–315.

Murphree, AL. Molecular genetics of retinoblastoma. *Ophthalmol Clin North Am.* 1995;8:155–166.

Scott IU, O'Brien JM, Murray TG. Retinoblastoma: a review emphasizing genetics and management strategies. *Semin Ophthalmol.* 1997;12:59–71.

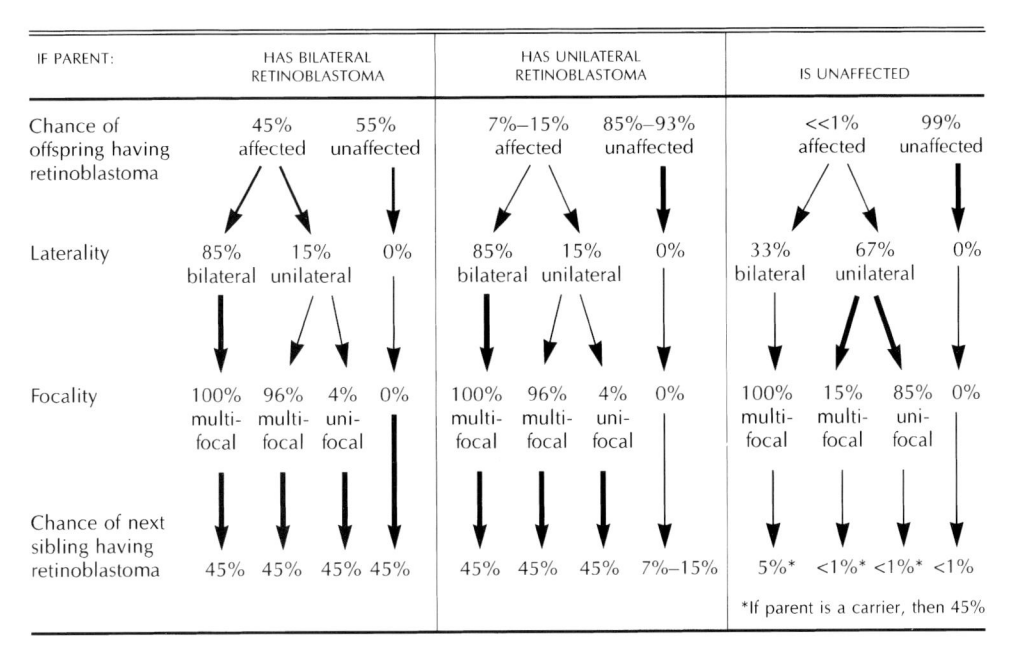

IF PARENT:	HAS BILATERAL RETINOBLASTOMA	HAS UNILATERAL RETINOBLASTOMA	IS UNAFFECTED
Chance of offspring having retinoblastoma	45% affected — 55% unaffected	7%–15% affected — 85%–93% unaffected	<<1% affected — 99% unaffected
Laterality	85% bilateral — 15% unilateral — 0%	85% bilateral — 15% unilateral — 0%	33% bilateral — 67% unilateral — 0%
Focality	100% multifocal — 96% multifocal — 4% unifocal — 0%	100% multifocal — 96% multifocal — 4% unifocal — 0%	100% multifocal — 15% multifocal — 85% unifocal — 0%
Chance of next sibling having retinoblastoma	45% 45% 45% 45%	45% 45% 45% 7%–15%	5%* <1%* <1%* <1%

*If parent is a carrier, then 45%

Figure 19-1 Genetic counseling for retinoblastoma. *(Chart created by David H. Abramson, MD.)*

Smith BJ, O'Brien JM. The genetics of retinoblastoma and current diagnostic testing. *J Pediatr Ophthalmol Strabismus.* 1996;33:120–123.

Diagnostic Evaluation

The presenting signs and symptoms of retinoblastoma are determined by the extent and location of tumor at the time of diagnosis. In the United States, the most common presenting signs of retinoblastoma are leukocoria (white pupillary reflex), strabismus, and ocular inflammation (Table 19-2; Fig 19-2). Other presenting features, such as heterochromia, spontaneous hyphema, and "cellulitis" are uncommon. In rare instances, a small lesion may be found on routine examination. Visual complaints are infrequent because most patients are preschool-age children.

The diagnosis of retinoblastoma can generally be suspected on the basis of a complete ocular examination in the office. The initial examination should include an assessment of visual function, slit-lamp biomicroscopy of the anterior segment and vitreous, and indirect ophthalmoscopy with scleral depression. Ultrasound may confirm the presence of intraocular calcifications.

Retinoblastoma begins as a translucent, gray to white intraretinal tumor, fed and drained by dilated, tortuous retinal vessels (Fig 19-3). As the tumor grows, foci of calcification develop, giving the characteristic chalky white appearance. Exophytic tumors grow beneath the retina and may have an associated serous retinal detachment (Fig 19-4). As the tumor grows, the retinal detachment may become extensive, obscuring visualization of the tumor (Fig 19-5). Endophytic tumors grow on the retinal surface into the vitreous

288 • Ophthalmic Pathology and Intraocular Tumors

Table 19-2 **Presenting Signs of Retinoblastoma**

Among Patients <5 Years of Age	Among Patients ≥5 Years of Age
Leukocoria (54%–62%)	Leukocoria (35%)
Strabismus (18%–22%)	Decreased vision (35%)
Inflammation (2%–10%)	Strabismus (15%)
Hypopyon	Floaters (4%)
Hyphema	Pain (4%)
Heterochromia	
Spontaneous globe perforation	
Proptosis	
Cataract	
Glaucoma	
Nystagmus	
Tearing	
Anisocoria	

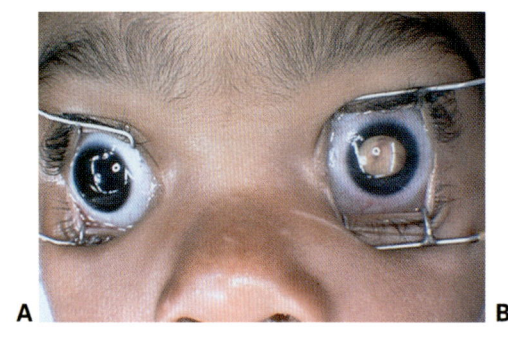

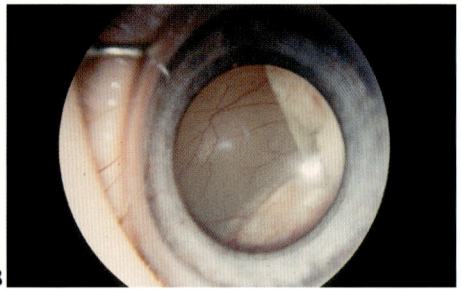

Figure 19-2 Retinoblastoma. **A,** Clinical appearance shows leukocoria and strabismus associated with advanced intraocular tumor. **B,** High magnification. Note large retrolental tumor and secondary total exudative retinal detachment. *(Courtesy of Timothy G. Murray, MD.)*

Figure 19-3 Retinoblastoma, clinical appearance. Small, discrete white tumor supplied by dilated retinal blood vessels. *(Courtesy of Timothy G. Murray, MD.)*

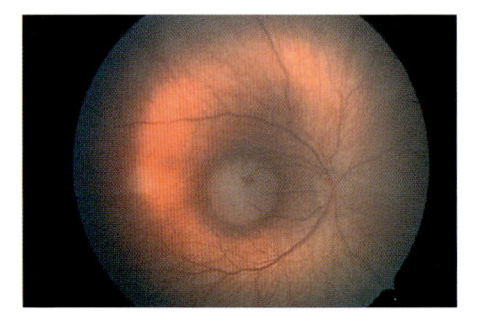

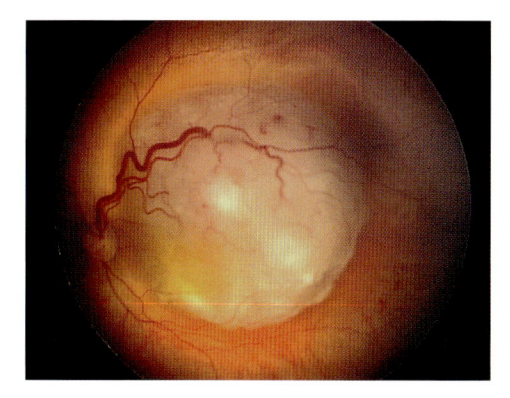

Figure 19-4 Retinoblastoma. Note the dilated retinal blood vessels, foci of calcification, cuff of subretinal fluid, and overlying luteal pigment. *(Courtesy of Matthew W. Wilson, MD.)*

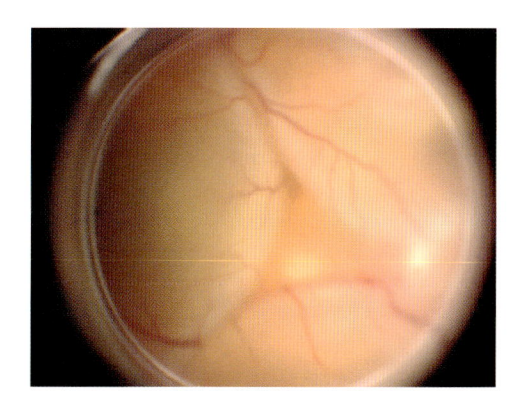

Figure 19-5 Retinoblastoma. Complete exudative detachment obscures tumor visualization. Note normal-appearing retinal vessels as opposed to those found in Coats disease. *(Courtesy of Matthew W. Wilson, MD.)*

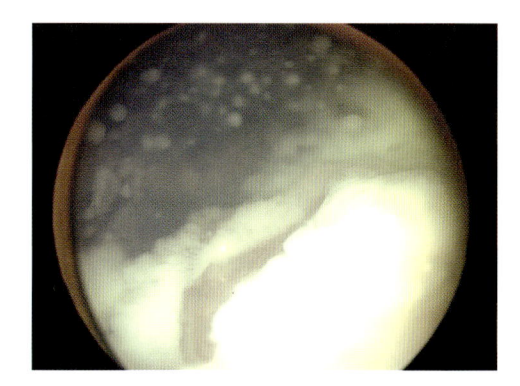

Figure 19-6 Retinoblastoma. Large endophytic tumor with extensive vitreous seeding. *(Courtesy of Matthew W. Wilson, MD.)*

cavity. Blood vessels may be difficult to discern in this tumor. Endophytic tumors are more apt to give rise to vitreous seeds (Fig 19-6). Cells shed from retinoblastoma remain viable in the vitreous and subretinal space and may eventually give rise to tumor implants throughout the eye. Vitreous seeds may also enter the anterior chamber, where they can aggregate on the iris to form nodules or settle inferiorly to form a pseudohypopyon (Fig 19-7). Secondary glaucoma and rubeosis iridis occur in about 50% of such cases. A rare variant of retinoblastoma is the *diffuse infiltrating retinoblastoma,* which is detected at a later age and is typically unilateral. Diffuse infiltrating retinoblastoma presents a diagnostic dilemma, as the retina may be difficult to see through the dense vitreous cells. It is often mistaken for an intermediate uveitis of unknown etiology.

Retinoblastoma cells most commonly escape the eye by invading the optic nerve and extending into the subarachnoid space. Figure 11-41 in Chapter 11 illustrates bulbous enlargement of the optic nerve following invasion by a retinoblastoma tumor. Tumor cells may also traverse emissary canals or erode through the sclera to enter the orbit. Extraocular extension may result in proptosis as the tumor grows in the orbit (Fig 19-8). In the anterior chamber, tumor cells may invade the trabecular meshwork, gaining access to the conjunctival lymphatics. The patient may subsequently develop palpable preauricular and cervical nodes. In the United States, patients rarely present with systemic metastasis and intracranial extension at the time of diagnosis. The most frequently identified sites of metastatic involvement in children with retinoblastoma include skull bones, distal bones, brain, spinal cord, lymph nodes, and abdominal viscera.

Abramson DH, Frank CM, Susman M, Whalen MR, Dunkel IJ, Boyd NW 3rd. Presenting signs of retinoblastoma. *J Pediatr.* 1998;132:505–508.

Albert DM. Historic review of retinoblastoma [review of 86 references]. *Ophthalmology.* 1987;94:654–662.

Figure 19-7 Retinoblastoma, clinical appearance. Pseudohypopyon resulting from migration of tumor cells into the anterior chamber (masquerade syndrome).

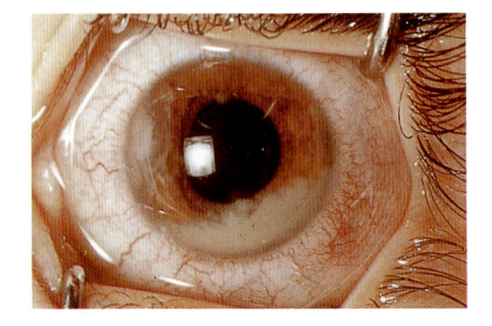

Figure 19-8 Retinoblastoma, clinical appearance. Proptosis caused by retinoblastoma with orbital invasion.

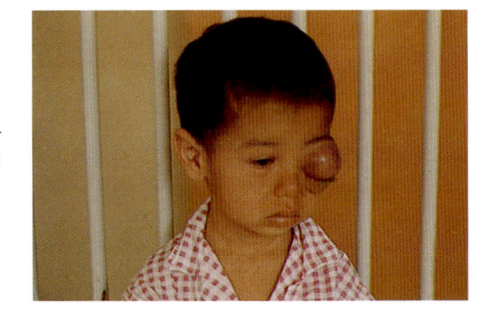

Clinical Examination

Children with retinoblastoma should have a complete history and physical examination by a pediatric oncologist. An examination under anesthesia (EUA) is needed in all patients to permit a complete assessment of the extent of ocular disease prior to treatment (Fig 19-9). The location of multiple tumors should be clearly documented. Intraocular pressure and corneal diameters should be measured intraoperatively. Ultrasonography can be helpful in the diagnosis of retinoblastoma by demonstrating characteristic calcifications within the tumor. Although these calcifications can also be seen on CT scan, MRI has become the preferred diagnostic modality for evaluating the optic nerve, orbits, and brain. Not only does MRI offer better soft tissue resolution, but it also avoids potentially harmful radiation exposure. Recent studies have suggested that systemic metastatic evaluation, typically bone marrow and lumbar puncture, is not indicated in children without neurologic abnormalities or evidence of extraocular extension. If optic extension is suspected, lumbar puncture may be performed. Parents and siblings should be examined for evidence of untreated retinoblastoma or retinoma, as this would provide evidence for a hereditary predisposition to the disease.

Differential Diagnosis

A number of lesions simulate retinoblastoma. Lesions that resemble small to medium-sized retinoblastomas include retinal astrocytic hamartomas commonly seen in tuberous sclerosis; exudative deposits, such as those that occur with Coats disease and retinal capillary hemangiomatosis; and peripheral or posterior pole granulomas, such as those associated with nematode endophthalmitis. The differential diagnoses for the patients with leukocoria and a retinal detachment include Coats disease, persistent fetal vasculature, ocular toxocariasis, and retinopathy of prematurity (Table 19-3). Most of these conditions can be differentiated from retinoblastoma on the basis of a comprehensive history, clinical examination, and appropriate ancillary diagnostic testing.

Coats disease

Coats disease is clinically evident within the first decade of life and is more common in boys. The lesion is typically characterized by unilateral retinal telangiectasia associated

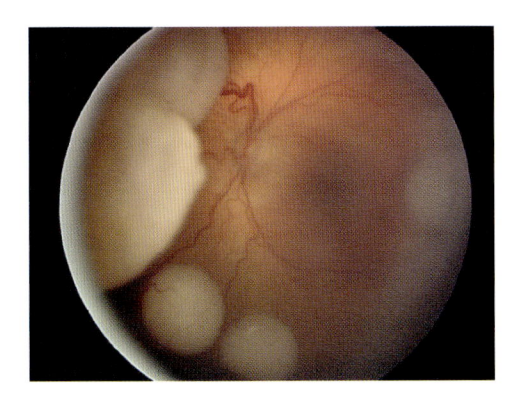

Figure 19-9 Retinoblastoma. Multiple tumor foci in an eye of a patient with a germline RB1 mutation. *(Courtesy of Matthew W. Wilson, MD.)*

Table 19-3 Differential Diagnosis of Retinoblastoma

Clinical Diagnosis in Pseudoretinoblastoma	265 Cases*	Percent	76 Cases†	Percent
Persistent fetal vasculature	51	19.0	15	20.0
Retinopathy of prematurity	36	13.5	3	4.0
Posterior cataract	36	13.5	5	7.0
Coloboma of choroid or optic disc	30	11.5	7	9.0
Uveitis	27	10.0	2	3.0
Larval granulomatosis	18	6.5	20	26.0
Congenital retinal fold	13	5.0		
Coats disease	10	4.0	12	16.0
Organizing vitreous hemorrhage	9	3.5	3	4.0
Retinal dysplasia	7	2.5		
Assorted other disorders	28	10.5	9	12.0

*From Howard GM, Ellsworth RM. Dfferential diagnosis of retinoblastoma. Am J Ophthalmol. 1965; 60: 610–618.

†From Shields JA, Stephens RT, Sarin LK. The differential diagnosis of retinoblastoma. In: Harley RD, ed. Pediatric Ophthalmology. 2nd ed. Philadelphia: Saunders; 1983:114.

with intraretinal yellow exudation without a distinct mass (Fig 19-10). The progressive leakage of fluid may lead to an extensive retinal detachment. Ultrasound documents the absence of a retinal tumor and shows the convection of cholesterol in the subretinal fluid. Fluorescein angiography shows classic telangiectatic vessels. Laser photocoagulation or cryoablation of the vascular anomalies eliminates the exudative component of the disease and may restore visual function. Subretinal fluid may be drained to facilitate these procedures. Serial evaluation and follow-up is critical for these patients.

Persistent fetal vasculature

Persistent fetal vasculature (PFV), previously known as persistent hyperplastic primary vitreous (PHPV), is typically recognized within days or weeks of birth. The condition is unilateral in two thirds of cases and is associated with microphthalmos, a shallow or flat anterior chamber, a hypoplastic iris with prominent vessels, and a retrolenticular fibrovascular mass that draws the ciliary body processes inward. On indirect ophthalmoscopy, a vascular stalk may be seen arising from the optic nerve head and attaching to the posterior lens capsule. Ultrasound confirms the diagnosis by showing persistent hyaloid remnants arising from the optic nerve head, usually in association with a closed funnel retinal detachment. No retinal tumor is seen, and the axial length of the eye is shortened. Calcification may be present. PFV may be managed with combined lensectomy and vitrectomy approaches in selected cases. See Chapter 10 in this volume and BCSC Section 6, *Pediatric Ophthalmology and Strabismus.*

Ocular toxocariasis

Ocular toxocariasis typically occurs in older childrven with a history of soil ingestion or exposure to puppies. Toxocara presents with posterior and peripheral granulomas, with an associated uveitis. Organized vitreoretinal traction and cataracts may be present. Ultrasound shows the vitritis, granulomas, retinal traction, and the absence of calcium. See BCSC Section 9, *Intraocular Inflammation and Uveitis.*

CHAPTER 19: Retinoblastoma • 293

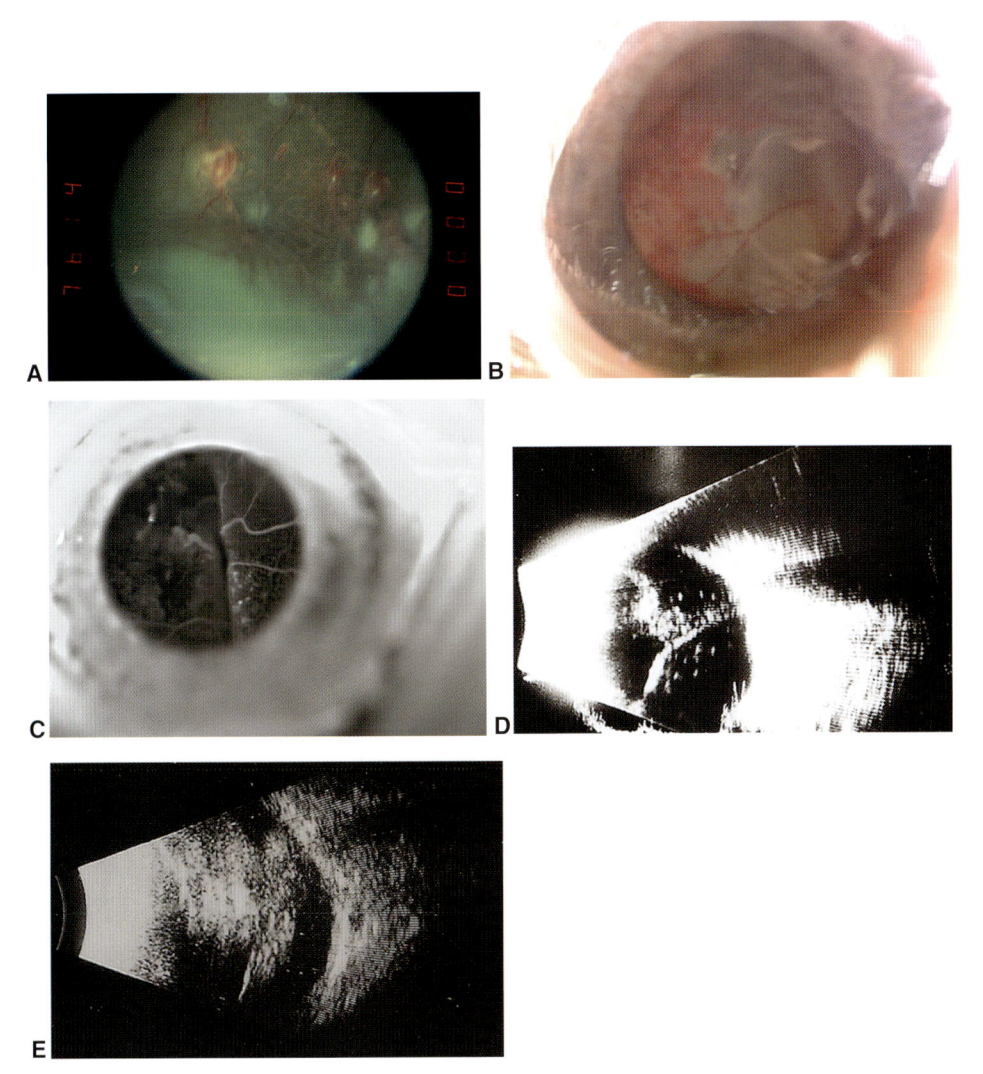

Figure 19-10 Coats disease. **A,** Clinical appearance of characteristic lightbulb aneurysms seen in a patient with Coats disease. There is an inferior exudative retinal detachment. **B,** In advanced cases, there can be a complete exudative retinal detachment. In this case, the retina is visible behind the lens. **C,** Fluorescein angiogram showing classic telangiectatic vessels. **D,** Patient with Coats disease shows an exudative retinal detachment on ultrasound. **E,** In contrast, this ultrasound scan of a patient with retinoblastoma shows a total retinal detachment, but in this case a large tumor mass is also present. *(Parts B and C courtesy of Matthew W. Wilson, MD.)*

Astrocytoma

Retinal astrocytoma, or astrocytic hamartoma, generally appears as a small, smooth, white, glistening tumor located in the nerve fiber layer of the retina (Fig 19-11). It may be single or multiple, unilateral or bilateral. In some cases, it may become larger and calcified, typically having a mulberry appearance. Astrocytomas occasionally arise from the optic disc; such tumors are often referred to as *giant drusen*. Astrocytomas of the retina

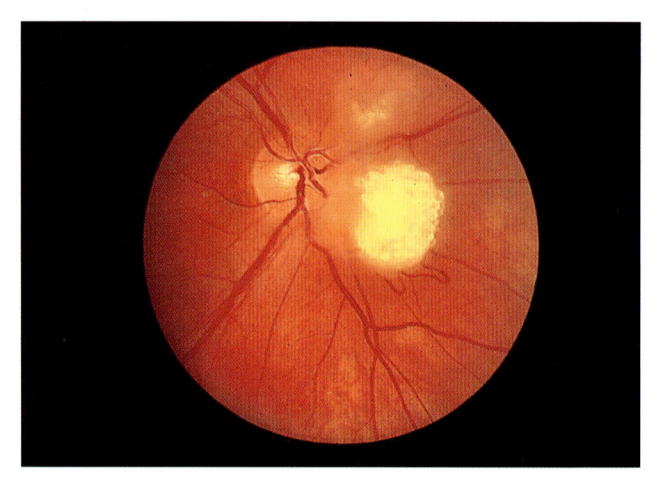

Figure 19-11 Retinal astrocytic hamartomas, clinical appearance. Note the more subtle opalescent lesion superonasal from the optic disc and the larger mulberry lesion inferonasal from the disc.

commonly occur in patients with tuberous sclerosis but may also be seen in patients with neurofibromatosis. Most retinal astrocytomas are not associated with a phakomatosis.

> Shields JA, Parsons HM, Shields CL, Shah P. Lesions simulating retinoblastoma. *J Pediatr Ophthalmol Strabismus.* 1991;28:338–340.
>
> Shields JA, Shields CL. *Intraocular Tumors: A Text and Atlas.* Philadelphia: Saunders; 1992: 341–362.
>
> Ulbright TM, Fulling KH, Helveston EM. Astrocytic tumors of the retina. Differentiation of sporadic tumors from phakomatosis-associated tumors. *Arch Pathol Lab Med.* 1984;108: 160–163.

Classification

The Reese-Ellsworth clinical classification is the most commonly used method of categorizing intraocular retinoblastoma (Table 19-4); it does not classify extraocular retinoblastoma. The classification takes into account the number, size, and location of tumors and the presence or absence of vitreous seeds. According to this classification, eye tumors are grouped from very favorable (group I) to very unfavorable (group V) by probability of eye preservation when treated with external-beam radiation alone. The Reese-Ellsworth classification does not provide prognostic information about patient survival or vision. The use of external-beam radiotherapy has given way to the use of primary systemic chemotherapy for the treatment of bilateral retinoblastoma. As a result, the Children's Oncology Group (COG) is currently evaluating a new International Classification System, which will be used in a series of upcoming clinical trials. The hope is to develop a schema that better predicts an eye's response to chemotherapy (Table 19-5). For American Joint Com-

Table 19-4 Reese-Ellsworth Classification of Retinoblastoma

Group	A	B
Group I (very favorable)	Solitary tumor 4 disc diameters (DD) at or behind equator	Multiple tumors 4 DD at or behind equator
Group II (favorable)	Solitary tumor 4–10 DD or behind equator	Multiple tumors 4–10 DD at or behind equator
Group III (doubtful)	Any lesion anterior to equator	Solitary tumor 10 DD posterior to equator
Group IV (unfavorable)	Multiple tumors, some larger than 10 DD	Any lesion anterior to ora serrata
Group V (very unfavorable)	Massive tumor occupying half or more of retina	Vitreous seeding

Table 19-5 International Classification System

Group A	Small tumors (≤3 mm) confined to the retina; >3 mm from the fovea; >1.5 mm from the optic disc
Group B	Tumors (>3 mm) confined to the retina in any location, with clear subretinal fluid ≤6 mm from the tumor margin
Group C	Localized vitreous and/or subretinal seeding (<6 mm in total from tumor margin). If there is more than 1 site of subretinal/vitreous seeding, then the total of these sites must be <6 mm.
Group D	Diffuse vitreous and/or subretinal seeding (≥6 mm in total from tumor margin). If there is more than 1 site of subretinal/vitreous seeding, then the total of these sites must be ≥6 mm. Subretinal fluid >6 mm from tumor margin.

Group E	• No visual potential; *or*
	• Presence of any 1 or more of the following:
	  ▪ tumor in the anterior segment
	  ▪ tumor in or on the ciliary body
	  ▪ neovascular glaucoma
	  ▪ vitreous hemorrhage obscuring the tumor of significant hyphema
	  ▪ phthisical or pre-phthisical eye
	  ▪ orbital cellulitis–like presentation

mittee on Cancer (AJCC) definitions and staging of retinoblastoma, see Table A-3 in the appendix.

>Gallie BL, Truong T, Heon E, et al. Retinoblastoma ABC classification survey. 11th International Retinoblastoma Symposium, Paris, France; 2003.
>
>Reese AB. *Tumors of the Eye*. 3rd ed. Hagerstown, MD: Harper & Row; 1976:90–132.
>
>Shields CL, Mashaykekhi A, Demirci H, Meadows AT, Shields JA. Practical approach to the management of retinoblastoma. *Arch Ophthalmol.* 2004;122:729–735.

Associated Conditions

Retinocytoma

Retinocytoma is clinically indistinguishable from retinoblastoma. Chapter 11 describes the histologic characteristics that distinguish retinocytoma from retinoblastoma (see Fig 11-43). The developmental biology of retinocytoma is subject to controversy. Some authorities consider retinocytoma to be retinoblastoma that has undergone differentiation, analogous to ganglioneuroma, the differentiated form of neuroblastoma. Many other authorities contend that retinocytoma is a benign counterpart of retinoblastoma.

Although histologically benign, retinocytoma carries the same genetic implications as retinoblastoma. A child harboring a retinoblastoma in 1 eye and a retinocytoma in the other should be considered capable of transmitting a faulty tumor suppressor gene to offspring.

Trilateral Retinoblastoma

The term *trilateral retinoblastoma* is reserved for cases of bilateral retinoblastoma associated with ectopic intracranial retinoblastoma. The ectopic focus is usually located in the pineal gland or the parasellar region and historically has been termed a *pinealoblastoma*. This tumor affects 2%–5% of children with a germline RB1 mutation. Rarely, a child may present with ectopic intracranial retinoblastoma prior to ocular involvement. More commonly, this independent malignancy presents months to years after treatment of the intraocular retinoblastoma.

Several different observations support the concept of primary intracranial retinoblastoma. CT helped to establish that intracranial tumors in some patients dying from retinoblastoma are anatomically separate from the primary tumors in the orbit. These intracranial tumors are not associated with metastatic disease elsewhere in the body, and, unlike metastatic retinoblastoma, they often demonstrate features of differentiation such as Flexner-Wintersteiner rosettes (see Fig 11-40 in Chapter 11). Embryologic, immunologic, and phylogenic evidence of photoreceptor differentiation in the pineal gland offers further support for the concept of trilateral retinoblastoma.

All patients with retinoblastoma should undergo baseline neuroimaging studies to exclude intracranial involvement. Patients with germline RB1 gene mutations (ie, bilateral retinoblastoma, unilateral multifocal retinoblastoma, or unilateral retinoblastoma with a positive family history) should undergo serial imaging of the CNS. Studies suggest that serial MRI with and without contrast is most sensitive for CNS involvement and does not expose the child to radiation. Median survival of patients with retinoblastoma with CNS involvement is approximately 8 months. Recent studies report a decrease in the incidence of trilateral retinoblastoma in patients treated with systemic chemotherapy, suggesting a possible prophylactic effect.

Holladay DA, Holladay A, Montebello JF, Redmond KP. Clinical presentation, treatment, and outcome of trilateral retinoblastoma. *Cancer.* 1991;67:710–715.

Jubran RF, Erdreich-Epstein A, Butturini A, Murphree AL, Villablanca JG. Approaches to treatment for extraocular retinoblastoma: Children's Hospital Los Angeles experience. *J Pediatr Hematol Oncol.* 2004;26:31–34.

Shields CL, Meadows AT, Shields JA, Carvalho C, Smith AF. Chemoreduction for retinoblastoma may prevent intracranial neuroblastic malignancy (trilateral retinoblastoma). *Arch Ophthalmol.* 2001;119:1269–1272.

Treatment

When treating retinoblastoma, it is first and foremost important to understand that it is a malignancy. When the disease is contained within the eye, survival rates exceed 95% in the Western world. However, with extraocular spread, survival rates decrease to under 50%. Therefore, in deciding on a treatment strategy, the first goal must be preservation of life, then preservation of the eye, and, finally, preservation of vision. The modern management of intraocular retinoblastoma currently incorporates a combination of different treatment modalities, including enucleation, chemotherapy, photocoagulation, cryotherapy, external-beam radiation therapy, and plaque radiotherapy. Metastatic disease is managed using intensive chemotherapy, radiation, and bone marrow transplantation. The treatment of children of children with retinoblastoma requires a team approach, including an ocular oncologist, pediatric ophthalmologist, pediatric oncologist, and radiation oncologist.

Abramson DH, Schefler AC. Update on retinoblastoma. *Retina.* 2004;24:828–848.

Shields CL, Meadows AT, Leahey AM, Shields JA. Continuing challenges in the management of retinoblastoma with chemotherapy. *Retina.* 2004;24:849–862.

Enucleation

Enucleation remains the definitive treatment for retinoblastoma, providing, in most cases, a complete surgical resection of the disease. Typically, enucleation is considered an appropriate intervention when

- the tumor involves more than 50% of the globe
- orbital or optic nerve involvement is suspected
- anterior segment involvement, with or without neovascular glaucoma, is noted

Enucleation techniques are aimed at minimizing the potential for inadvertent globe penetration while obtaining the greatest length of resected optic nerve that is feasible, typically longer than 10 mm. Porous integrated implants, such as hydroxyapatite or porous polyethylene, are currently used by most surgeons.

Attempts at globe-conserving therapy should be undertaken only by ophthalmologists well versed in the management of this rare childhood tumor and in conjunction with similarly experienced pediatric oncologists. Failed attempts at eye salvage may place a child at inadvertent risk of metastatic disease.

Chemotherapy

A significant advance in the management of bilateral intraocular retinoblastoma in the past decade has been the use of primary systemic chemotherapy. Systemic administration of chemotherapy reduces tumor volume, allowing for subsequent application of consolidative focal therapy with laser, cryotherapy, or radiotherapy (Fig 19-12). These changes have come about as a result of improvements in the treatment of both brain tumors and metastatic retinoblastoma. Current regimens incorporate varying combinations of carboplatin, vincristine, etoposide, and cyclosporine. Children receive drugs intravenously every 3–4 weeks for 4–9 cycles of chemotherapy. Meanwhile, serial EUAs are performed, during which tumor response is observed and focal therapies are administered. Drug regimens, routes of administration, and dose schedules should be determined by a pediatric oncologist experienced in the treatment of children with retinoblastoma. Newer transgenic mouse models of retinoblastoma may now facilitate the screening of newer chemotherapeutic agents (see the following section).

 Bechrakis NE, Bornfeld N, Schueler A, Coupland SE, Henze G, Foerster MH. Clinicopathologic features of retinoblastoma after primary chemoreduction. *Arch Ophthalmol.* 1998;116:887–893.

 Doz F, Khelfaoui F, Mosseri V, et al. The role of chemotherapy in orbital involvement of retinoblastoma: the experience of a single institution with 33 patients. *Cancer.* 1994;74:722–732.

 Dyer MA, Rodriguez-Galindo C, Wilson MW. Use of preclinical models to improve treatment of retinoblastoma. *PloS Med.* 2005;2:e332.

 Finger PT, Czechonska G, Demirci H, Rausen A. Chemotherapy for retinoblastoma: a current topic [review of 111 references]. *Drugs.* 1999;58:983–996.

 Gallie BL, Budning A, DeBoer G, et al. Chemotherapy with focal therapy can cure intraocular retinoblastoma without radiotherapy. *Arch Ophthalmol.* 1996;114:1321–1328. [Erratum: *Arch Ophthalmol.* 1997;115:525.]

 Murphree AL, Villablanca JG, Deegan WF III, et al. Chemotherapy plus local treatment in the management of intraocular retinoblastoma. *Arch Ophthalmol.* 1996;114:1348–1356.

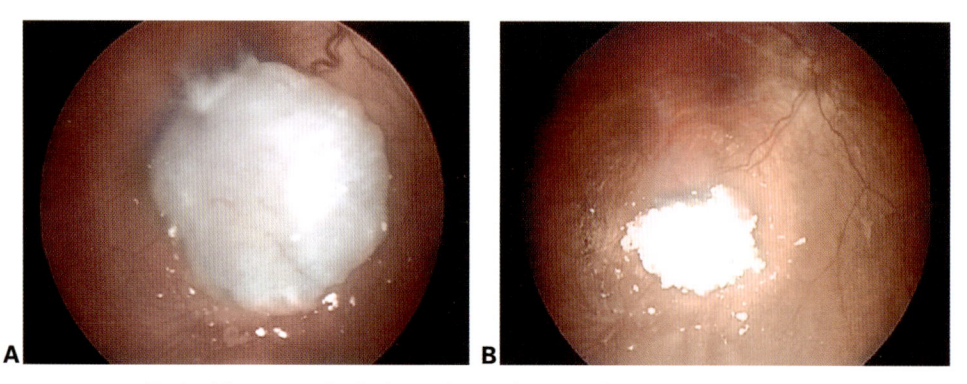

Figure 19-12 Retinoblastoma. **A,** Before chemotherapy. **B,** Reduced tumor volume after 2 cycles of chemotherapy alone.

Shields CL, De Potter P, Himelstein BP, Shields JA, Meadows AT, Maris JM. Chemoreduction in the initial management of intraocular retinoblastoma. *Arch Ophthalmol.* 1996;114: 1330–1338.

Wilson MW, Haik BG, Liu T, Merchant TE, Rodriguez-Galindo C. Effect on ocular survival of adding early intensive focal treatments to a two-drug chemotherapy regimen in patients with retinoblastoma. *Am J Ophthalmol.* 2005;140:397–406.

Periocular chemotherapy

Periocular chemotherapy is being included in upcoming COG trials based on recent data using subconjunctival carboplatin as treatment for retinoblastoma. In phase 1 and 2 clinical trials, both vitreous seeds and retinal tumors were found to be repsonsive to this treatment. Minor local toxicity in the form of orbit myositis has been seen after administration and responds to oral corticosteroids, and more severe reactions, including optic atrophy, have been reported.

Abramson DH, Frank CM, Dunkel IJ. A phase I/II study of subconjunctival carboplatin for intraocular retinoblastoma. *Ophthalmology.* 1999;106:1947–1950.

Harbour JW, Murray TG, Hamasaki D, et al. Local carboplatin therapy in transgenic murine retinoblastoma. *Invest Ophthalmol Vis Sci.* 1996;37:1892–1898.

Photocoagulation and Hyperthermia

Xenon arc and argon laser (532 nm) have traditionally been used to treat retinoblastomas smaller than 3 mm in apical height with basal dimensions less than 10 mm. Two to 3 rows of encircling retinal photocoagulation destroy the tumor's blood supply, with ensuing regression. Newer lasers now allow for direct confluent treatment of the tumor surface. The diode laser (810 nm) is used to provide hyperthermia. Direct application to the surface increases the tumor's temperature to the 45°–60° Celsius range and has a direct cytotoxic effect, which can be augmented by both chemotherapy and radiation (Fig 19-13).

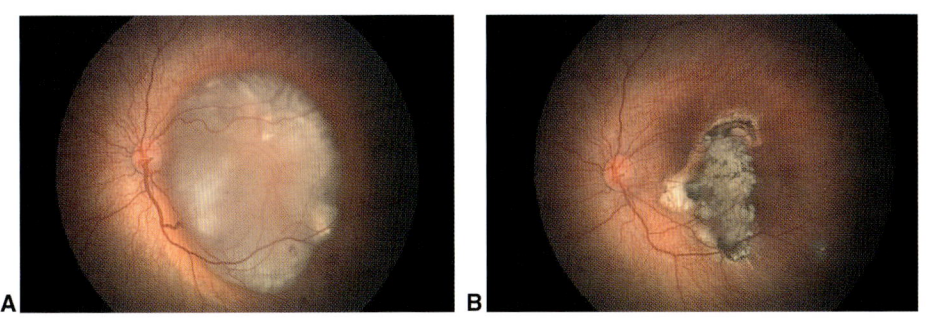

Figure 19-13 Retinoblastoma. **A,** Before treatment. **B,** Same eye 6 months later, after treatment with chemoreduction and laser therapy. *(Courtesy of Timothy G. Murray, MD.)*

Cryotherapy

Also effective for tumors in the size range of less than 10 mm in basal dimension and 3 mm in apical thickness, cryotherapy is applied under direct visualization with a triple freeze-thaw technique. Typically, laser photoablation is chosen for posteriorly located tumors and cryoablation for more anteriorly located tumors. Repetitive tumor treatments are often required for both techniques, along with close follow-up for tumor growth or treatment complications.

External-Beam Radiation Therapy

Retinoblastoma tumors are responsive to radiation. Current techniques use focused megavoltage radiation treatments, often employing lens-sparing techniques, to deliver 4000–4500 cGy over a 4–6 week treatment interval. Typically, those treated are children with bilateral disease not amenable to laser or cryotherapy. Globe salvage rates are excellent, with up to 85% of eyes being retained. Visual function is often excellent and limited only by tumor location or secondary complications.

Two major concerns have limited the application of external-beam radiotherapy using standard techniques:

1. the association of germline mutations of the *RB1* gene with a lifelong increase in the risk of second, independent primary malignancies (eg, osteosarcoma) that is exacerbated by exposure to external-beam radiotherapy
2. the potential for radiation-related sequelae, including midface hypoplasia, radiation-induced cataract, and radiation optic neuropathy and vasculopathy

Evidence suggests that combined-modality therapy that uses lower-dose external-beam radiotherapy coupled with chemotherapy may allow for increased globe conservation with decreased radiation morbidity. In addition, the use of systemic chemotherapy may delay the need for external-beam radiotherapy, allowing for greater orbital development and significantly decreasing the risk of second malignancies once the child is older than 1 year.

> Abramson DH, Frank CM. Second nonocular tumors in survivors of bilateral retinoblastoma: a possible age effect on radiation-related risk. *Ophthalmology.* 1998;105:573–574.
>
> Hungerford JL, Toma NM, Plowman PN, Doughty D, Kingston JE. Whole-eye versus lens-sparing megavoltage therapy for retinoblastoma. *Front Radiat Ther Oncol.* 1997;30:81–87.
>
> Murray T. Cancer incidence after retinoblastoma: radiation dose and sarcoma risk. *Surv Ophthalmol.* 1998;43:288–289.
>
> Tucker MA, D'Angio GJ, Boice JD Jr, et al. Bone sarcomas linked to radiotherapy and chemotherapy in children. *N Engl J Med.* 1987;317:588–593.

Plaque Radiotherapy (Brachytherapy)

Radioactive plaque therapy may be used both as salvage therapy for eyes in which globe-conserving therapies have failed to destroy all viable tumor and as a primary treatment for some children with relatively small to medium-sized tumors. This technique is generally applicable for tumors less than 16 mm in basal diameter and 8 mm in apical thickness. The most commonly used isotopes are iodine 125 and ruthenium 106. Intraoperative localization with ultrasound enhances local tumor control for plaque brachytherapy. A greater likelihood of radiation optic neuropathy or vasculopathy may be associated with this radiotherapy modality compared with external-beam radiotherapy. Limiting the radiation dose to periocular structures may lower the incidence of radiation-induced second malignancies.

> Freire JE, De Potter P, Brady LW, Longton WA. Brachytherapy in primary ocular tumors. *Semin Surg Oncol.* 1997;13:167–176.
>
> Shields CL, Shields JA, De Potter P, et al. Plaque radiotherapy in the management of retinoblastoma: use as a primary and secondary treatment. *Ophthalmology.* 1993;100:216–224.

Targeted Therapy

New frontiers in the treatment of retinoblastoma include the use of gene therapy for treating vitreous seeds. Adenoviral-mediated transfection of tumor cells with thymidine kinase renders the tumor susceptible to systemically administered ganciclovir. Phase 1 clinical trials have been completed, documenting both safety and efficacy. Although currently reserved as salvage therapy for remaining eyes failing all conventional modalities of treatment, there is hope that this new targeted therapy may become a mainstream treatment.

> Chévez-Barrios P, Chintagumpala M, Mieler W, et al. Response of retinoblastoma with vitreous tumor seeding to adenovirus-mediated delivery of thymidine kinase followed by ganciclovir. *J Clin Oncol.* 2005;23:7927–7935.

Spontaneous Regression

Retinoblastoma is one of the more common malignant tumors to undergo complete and spontaneous necrosis (although this is rarely recognized with active disease). Spontaneous regression is recognized clinically after involutional changes such as phthisis have occurred. The incidence of spontaneous regression is unknown, as no child with active retinoblastoma is observed in the hopes of spontaneous involution. Although the mechanism by which spontaneous regression occurs is not understood, its histologic appearance is diagnostic. The vitreous cavities of these phthisical eyes are filled with islands of calcified cells embedded in a mass of fibroconnective tissue. Close inspection of the peripheral portion of these calcified islands reveals the ghosted contours of fossilized tumor cells. The process is often accompanied by exuberant proliferation of retinal pigment and ciliary epithelia.

Prognosis

Children with intraocular retinoblastoma who have access to modern medical care have a very good prognosis for survival, with overall survival rates of over 95% for children in developed countries. The most important risk factor associated with death is extraocular extension of tumor, either directly through the sclera or, more commonly, by invasion of the optic nerve, especially to the surgically resected margin (see Fig 11-42 in Chapter 11). The importance of choroidal invasion is unclear. Although a multivariate analysis of a large case series has shown that choroidal invasion is not predictive of metastases, the significance of this pathologic finding remains the subject of debate. A current multicenter study by the COG is investigating this further. Some evidence suggests, however, that bilateral tumors may increase the risk of death because of their association with primary intracranial tumors (see the discussion of trilateral retinoblastoma earlier in the chapter).

Children who survive bilateral retinoblastoma have an increased incidence of nonocular malignancies later in life. The mean latency for second tumor development is approximately 9 years from management of the primary retinoblastoma. The RB1 mutation is associated with a 26.5% incidence of second tumor development within 50 years in patients treated without exposure to radiation therapy. External-beam radiation therapy decreases the latency period, in turn increasing the incidence of second tumors in the first 30 years of life, as well as increasing the proportion of tumors in the head and neck. The most common type of second cancer in these patients appears to be osteogenic sarcoma. Other relatively common second malignancies include pinealomas, brain tumors, cutaneous melanomas, soft-tissue sarcomas, and primitive unclassifiable tumors (Table 19-6). Estimates suggest that as many as 10%–20% of patients who have bilateral retinoblastoma will develop an apparently unrelated neoplasm within 20 years and that 20%–40% will develop a third malignancy within 30 years. The prognosis for survival in retinoblastoma patients who later develop sarcomas is less than 50%.

Table 19-6 Nonretinoblastoma Malignancies in Retinoblastoma Survivors

Tumors Arising in the Field of Radiation of the Eye

Pathologic Type	No. Cases	Percent
Osteosarcoma	25	40.3
Fibrosarcoma	6	9.7
Soft-tissue sarcoma	5	8.1
Anaplastic and unclassifiable	5	8.1
Squamous cell carcinoma	3	4.8
Rhabdomyosarcoma	3	4.8
Assorted other	15	24.2
Total	62	

Tumors Arising Outside the Field of Radiation

Pathologic Type	No. Cases	Percent
Osteosarcoma	12	36.4
Malignant melanoma	4	12.1
Pinealoma	3	9.1
Ewing sarcoma	2	6.1
Papillary thyroid carcinoma	2	6.1
Assorted other	10	30.3
Total	33	

From Abramson DH, Ellsworth RM, Kitchin FD, el al. Second nonocular tumors in retinoblastoma survivors. Are they radiation-induced? *Ophthalmology.* 1984;91:1351–1355.

Eng C, Li FP, Abramson DH, et al. Mortality from second tumors among long-term survivors of retinoblastoma. *J Natl Cancer Inst.* 1993;85:1121–1128.

Kopelman JE, McLean IW, Rosenberg SH. Multivariate analysis of risk factors for metastasis in retinoblastoma treated by enucleation. *Ophthalmology.* 1987;94:371–377.

Roarty JD, McLean IW, Zimmerman LE. Incidence of second neoplasms in patients with bilateral retinoblastoma. *Ophthalmology.* 1988;95:1583–1587.

Shields CL, Shields JA, Baez K, Cater JR, De Potter P. Optic nerve invasion of retinoblastoma: metastatic potential and clinical risk factors. *Cancer.* 1994;73:692–698.

CHAPTER 20

Secondary Tumors of the Eye

Metastatic Carcinoma

Since the first description in 1872 of a metastatic tumor in the eye of a patient with carcinoma, a large body of literature has indicated that the most common type of intraocular or orbital tumor in adults is metastatic. There are several comprehensive studies of ocular metastatic tumor: some have reported the incidence of tumor metastases in a consecutive series in autopsies, some have dealt with tumor incidence in patients with generalized malignancy, and others have used a clinicopathologic approach. As long-term survival from systemic primary malignancy continues to increase, the ophthalmologist will be confronted with a growing incidence of intraocular and orbital metastatic disease requiring prompt recognition and appropriate diagnostic and therapeutic management.

Metastases to the eye are being diagnosed with increasing frequency for various reasons:

- increasing incidence of certain tumor types that metastasize to the eye (eg, lung, breast)
- prolonged survival of patients with certain cancer types (eg, breast cancer)
- increasing awareness among medical oncologists and ophthalmologists of the pattern of metastatic disease

Bloch RS, Gartner S. The incidence of ocular metastatic carcinoma. *Arch Ophthalmol.* 1971;85: 673–675.

Ferry AP, Font RL. Carcinoma metastatic to the eye and orbit. I. A clinicopathologic study of 227 cases. *Arch Ophthalmol.* 1974;92:276–286.

Grossniklaus HE, Green WR. Uveal tumors. In: Garner A, Klintworth GK, eds. *Pathobiology of Ocular Disease: A Dynamic Approach.* 2nd ed. New York: Marcel Dekker; 1994:1455–1459.

Shields CL, Shields JA, Gross NE, Schwartz GP, Lally SE. Survey of 520 eyes with uveal metastases. *Ophthalmology.* 1997:104:1265–1276.

Volpe NJ, Albert DM. Metastases to the uvea. In: Albert DM, Jakobiec FA, eds. *Principles and Practice of Ophthalmology.* 2nd ed. Philadelphia: Saunders; 2000:5073–5084.

Primary Tumor Sites

The vast majority of metastatic solid tumors to the eye are carcinomas from various organs. Cutaneous melanoma rarely metastasizes to the eye. Table 20-1 shows the most common primary tumors that metastasize to the choroid.

Table 20-1 Primary Sites of Choroidal Metastasis

Males (N = 137)	Females (N = 287)
Lung (40%)	Breast (68%)
Unknown (29%)	Lung (12%)
Gastrointestinal (9%)	Unknown (12%)
Kidney (6%)	Others (4%)
Prostate (6%)	Gastrointestinal (2%)
Skin (4%)	Skin (1%)
Others (4%)	Kidney (<1%)
Breast (1%)	

Modified from Shields CL, Shields JA, Gross NE, et al. Survey of 520 eyes with uveal metastases. *Ophthalmology*. 1997;104:1265–1276.

Mechanisms of Metastasis to the Eye

The mechanism of intraocular metastasis depends on hematogenous dissemination of tumor cells. The anatomy of the arterial supply to the eye dictates the predilection of tumor cell deposits within the eye. The posterior choroid, with its rich vascular supply, is the most favored site of intraocular metastases, and it is affected 10–20 times more frequently than is the iris or ciliary body. The retina and optic disc, supplied by the single central retinal artery, are rarely the sole site of involvement. Bilateral ocular involvement has been reported in 20%–25% of cases, and multifocal deposits are frequently seen within the involved eye. Many patients with ocular metastases also have concurrent CNS metastases.

Clinical Evaluation

The clinical features of intraocular metastases depend on the site of involvement. Metastases to the iris and ciliary body usually appear as white or gray-white gelatinous nodules (Figs 20-1, 20-2, 20-3). The clinical features of anterior uveal metastases may include

- iridocyclitis
- secondary glaucoma
- rubeosis iridis
- hyphema
- irregular pupil

Anterior segment tumors are best evaluated with slit-lamp biomicroscopy coupled with gonioscopy. High-resolution ultrasound imaging may quantify tumor size and anatomical relationships.

Patients with tumor in the posterior pole commonly complain of loss of vision. Pain and photopsia may be concurrent symptoms. Indirect binocular ophthalmoscopy may reveal a nonrhegmatogenous retinal detachment associated with a placoid amelanotic tumor mass (Figs 20-4, 20-5, 20-6). Multiple or bilateral lesions may be present in approximately 25% of cases, highlighting the importance of close evaluation of the fellow eye. These lesions are usually relatively flat and ill defined, often gray-yellow or yellow-white, with secondary alterations at the level of the RPE presenting as clumps of brown pigment ("leopard spotting"; Fig 20-7).

CHAPTER 20: Secondary Tumors of the Eye • 307

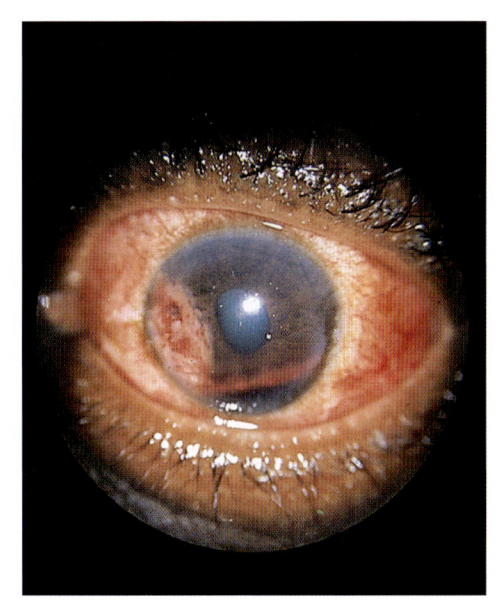

Figure 20-1 Metastasis to the iris associated with hyphema.

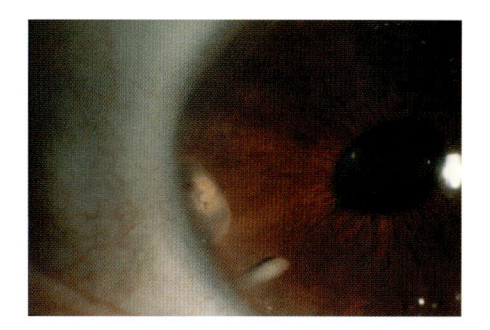

Figure 20-2 Metastasis from breast carcinoma to the iris. *(Courtesy of Timothy G. Murray, MD.)*

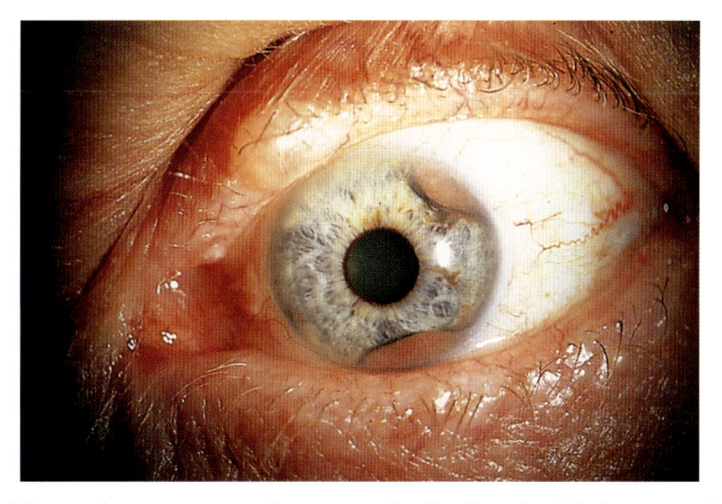

Figure 20-3 Metastatic cutaneous melanoma to the iris. Note both lesions at periphery.

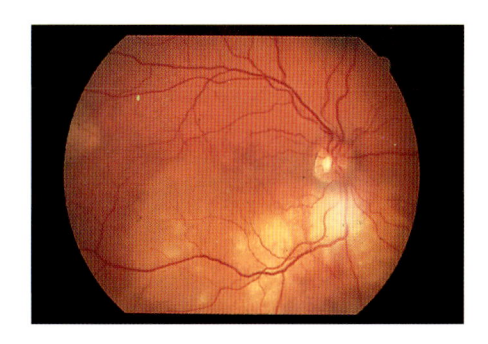

Figure 20-4 Multiple metastatic lesions to the choroid. Note the pale yellow color and relative flatness.

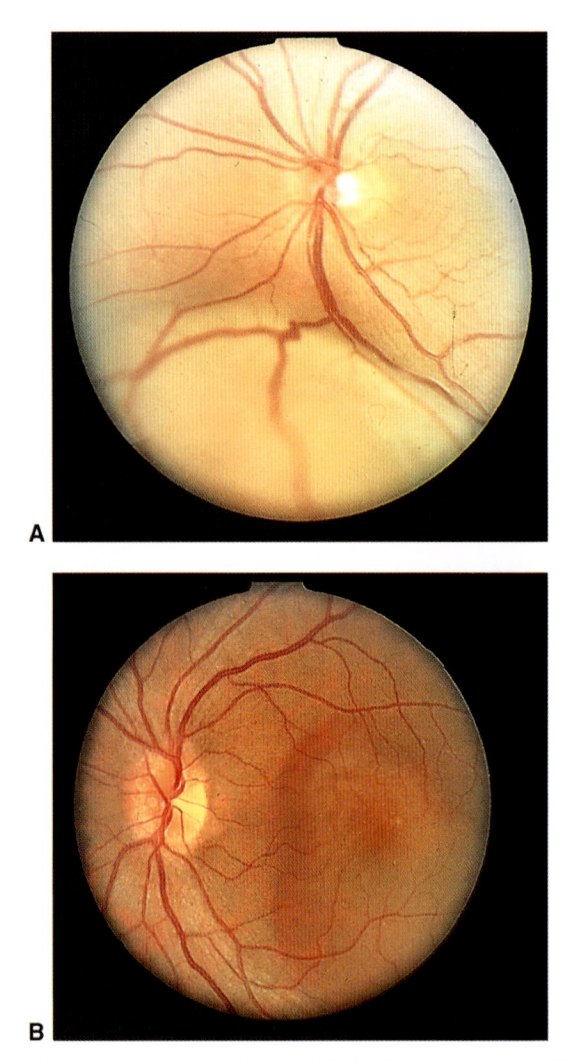

Figure 20-5 A, Metastatic lesion to the choroid inferiorly, associated with bullous retinal detachment. **B,** Subtle metastatic lesion to the choroid, near the fovea, associated with serous effusion.

The mushroom configuration frequently seen in primary choroidal melanoma from breakthrough of Bruch's membrane is rarely present in uveal metastases. The retina overlying the metastasis may appear opaque and become detached. Rapid tumor growth with necrosis and uveitis are occasionally seen. Dilated epibulbar vessels may be seen in the quadrant overlying the metastasis. For a differential diagnosis of choroidal metastasis, see Table 20-2.

Ancillary Tests

Although *fluorescein angiography* may be helpful in defining the margins of a metastatic tumor, it is typically less useful in differentiating a metastasis from a primary intraocular neoplasm. The double circulation pattern and prominent early choroidal filling often seen in choroidal melanomas are rarely found in metastatic tumors.

CHAPTER 20: Secondary Tumors of the Eye • 309

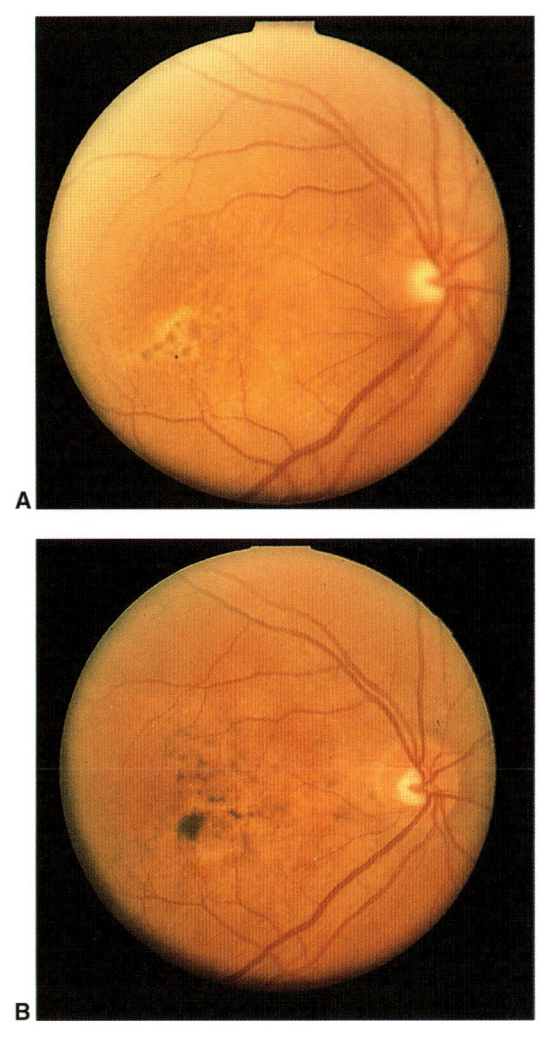

Figure 20-6 A, Metastatic carcinoma to the choroid. Vision was reduced to finger counting because of macular involvement. Note irregular pigmentation on surface. **B,** Same eye, 1 month after radiation therapy. Visual acuity has improved to 20/20. Note increased pigmentation, characteristic of irradiation effects.

Ultrasonography is diagnostically valuable in patients with metastatic tumor. B scan shows an echogenic choroidal mass with an ill-defined, sometimes lobulated, outline. Overlying secondary retinal detachment is commonly detected in these cases. A scan demonstrates moderate to high internal reflectivity.

Fine-needle aspiration biopsy may be helpful in rare cases when the diagnosis cannot be established by noninvasive procedures. Although metastatic tumors may recapitulate the histology of the primary tumor, they are often less differentiated. Special histochemical and immunohistochemical stains assist in the diagnosis of metastatic tumors, but they are usually not useful in determining the precise origin.

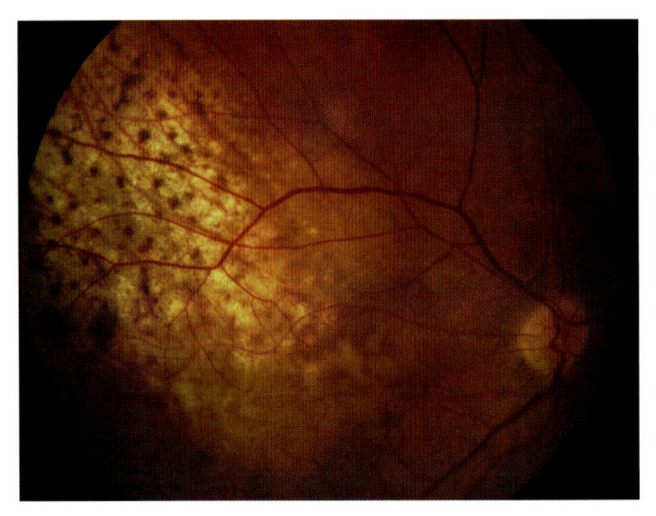

Figure 20-7 Breast metastases, clinical appearance. Note the amelanotic infiltrative choroidal mass with secondary overlying retinal pigment epithelial changes accounting for the characteristic "leopard spots." *(Courtesy of Matthew W. Wilson, MD.)*

Table 20-2 Differential Diagnosis of Choroidal Metastasis

Amelanotic nevus	VKH syndrome
Amelanotic melanoma	Central serous retinopathy
Choroidal hemangioma	Infectious lesions
Choroidal osteoma	Organized subretinal hemorrhage
Posterior uveal effusion syndrome	Extensive neovascular membranes
Posterior scleritis	Rhegmatogenous retinal detachment

Metastases to the optic nerve may produce disc edema, decreased visual acuity, and visual field defects. Because the metastases may involve the parenchyma or the optic nerve sheath, MRI as well as ultrasonography may be valuable in detecting the presence and location of the lesion(s).

Metastases to the retina, which are very rare, appear as white, noncohesive lesions, often distributed in a perivascular location suggestive of cotton-wool spots (Fig 20-8). Because of secondary vitreous seeding of tumor cells, these metastases sometimes resemble retinitis more than they do a true tumor. Vitreous aspirates for cytologic studies may confirm the diagnosis.

Other Diagnostic Factors

One of the most important diagnostic factors in the evaluation of suspected metastatic tumors is a history of systemic malignancy. More than 90% of patients with uveal metastasis from carcinoma of the breast, for example, have a history of treatment prior to the development of ocular involvement. In the remaining 10% of patients, the primary tumor can usually be diagnosed by breast examination at the time the suspicious ocular lesion is detected. For other patients, however, there is no prior history of malignancy.

CHAPTER 20: Secondary Tumors of the Eye • 311

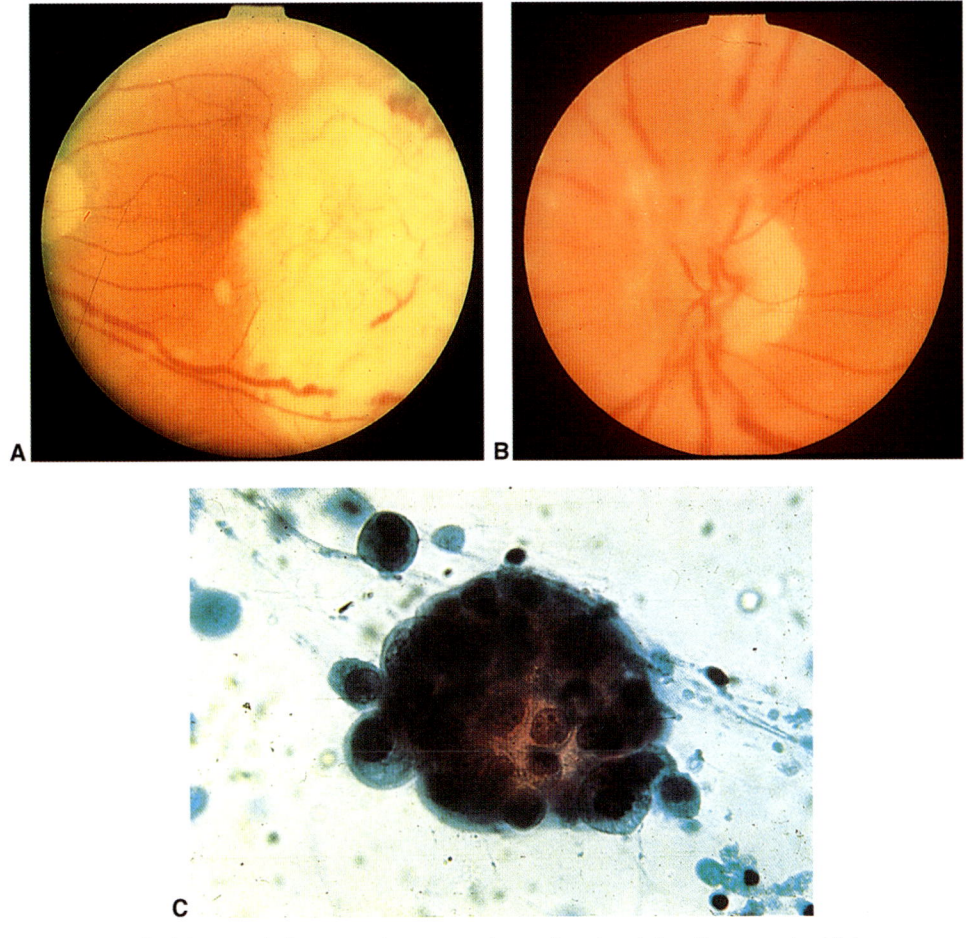

Figure 20-8 A, Metastatic lung carcinoma to the retina, involving the macula. Vision was reduced to finger counting. **B,** Same eye, showing characteristic perivascular distribution of metastases. **C,** Vitreous aspirate from same eye, showing a morula of cells, characteristic of adenocarcinoma of the lung.

This is especially true of patients with ocular metastasis from the lung. A complete review of systems, a family history, and a history of smoking may alert the ophthalmologist to the suspected site of an occult primary tumor. Any patient with an amelanotic fundus mass suspected of being a metastatic focus should have a thorough systemic evaluation, including imaging of the breast, chest, abdomen, and pelvis. CT-PET scanning may help direct a more targeted evaluation.

Prognosis

The diagnosis of tumor metastatic to the uvea implies a poor prognosis, because widespread dissemination of the primary tumor has usually occurred. In one report, the survival time following diagnosis of metastasis to the uvea ranged from 1 to 67 months, depending on the primary cancer type. Metastatic carcinoid is associated with long survival times. Patients with breast carcinoma metastatic to the uvea survive an average of 9–13 months after the metastasis is recognized, but cases with long-term survival have now been reported. Shorter survival time is typically seen in patients with lung carcinoma and carcinomas arising from the gastrointestinal or genitourinary tracts, in which metastases herald the presence of the primary tumor.

The goal in ophthalmic management of ocular metastases is preservation or restoration of vision and palliation of pain. Radical surgical procedures and treatments with risks greater than the desired benefits should be avoided.

Treatment

Indications for treatment include decreased vision, pain, diplopia, and severe proptosis. The patient's age and health status and the condition of the fellow eye are also critical in the decision-making process. The treatment modality in patients with metastatic ocular disease should be individually tailored. When ocular metastases are concurrent with widespread metastatic disease, systemic chemotherapy alone or in combination with local therapy is reasonable. In patients manifesting metastases in the eye alone, local therapy modalities may be safe, allowing conservation of visual functions with minimal systemic morbidity.

Chemotherapy or hormonal therapy for sensitive tumors (eg, breast cancer) may induce a prompt response. In such patients, no additional ocular treatment may be indicated. However, when vision is endangered by choroidal metastases in spite of chemotherapy, additional modalities of local therapy such as external irradiation, brachytherapy, and laser photocoagulation or transpupillary thermotherapy may be necessary. Radiotherapy is frequently associated with rapid improvement of the patient's symptoms, along with rapid resolution of exudative retinal detachment and, often, direct reduction in tumor size. Rarely, enucleation is performed because of severe, unrelenting pain.

> Amer R, Pe'er J, Chowers I, Anteby I. Treatment options in the management of choroidal metastases. *Ophthalmologica*. 2004;218:372–377.
>
> Shields JA, Shields CL, Brotman HK, Carvalho C, Perez N, Eagle RC Jr. Cancer metastatic to the orbit: the 2000 Robert M. Curts Lecture. *Ophthal Plast Reconstr Surg*. 2001;17:346–354.

Direct Intraocular Extension

Direct extension of extraocular tumors into the eye is rare. Intraocular extension occurs most commonly with conjunctival squamous cell carcinoma and less frequently with conjunctival melanoma and basal cell carcinoma of the eyelid. The sclera is usually an effective barrier against intraocular invasion. Only a small minority of carcinomas of the conjunctiva ever successfully penetrate the globe, but those that do are often variants of squamous cell carcinoma: mucoepidermoid carcinoma or spindle cell variant. These more aggressive neoplasms usually recur several times after local excision before they invade the eye.

CHAPTER 21

Lymphomatous Tumors

Intraocular Lymphoma

Intraocular lymphoma is almost always non-Hodgkin large cell lymphoma of the B-cell type. T-cell lymphoma involves the eye only rarely. Historically, the terminology for intraocular lymphoma was *histiocytic lymphoma* or *reticulum cell sarcoma*, but these terms are not used in the recent literature. Intraocular lymphoma can infiltrate any part of the eye, including the vitreous, retina, sub-RPE space, subretinal space, and uveal tract.

Two types of lymphoma may involve intraocular structures. The much more common one is *primary central nervous system lymphoma (PCNSL)*, in which approximately one quarter of the patients have intraocular involvement. In these cases, the vitreous and retina are involved. More rarely, the eye can be involved in *systemic/visceral/nodal lymphoma*. In these cases, the uveal tract is more commonly involved, usually in a pattern of metastatic disease. In advanced cases, the intraocular findings of the 2 types may overlap. In recent decades, the incidence of PCNSL has been increasing significantly in both immunocompetent and immunocompromised persons; thus, the incidence of intraocular lymphoma is more frequent than in the past.

Clinical Evaluation

Ocular signs and symptoms may occur before systemic or CNS findings. In such cases, the disease may manifest as a masquerade syndrome, simulating nonspecific uveitis. The onset of bilateral posterior uveitis in patients over the age of 50 years should be considered suggestive of large cell lymphoma, as should "chronic" uveitis in patients in their fifth to seventh decades. Although 30% of patients present with unilateral involvement, delayed involvement of the second eye occurs in approximately 85% of patients.

Diffuse vitreous cells may be associated with deep subretinal yellow-white infiltrates. Often, fine details of the retina are obscured by the density of the vitritis ("headlight in the fog"). Retinal vasculitis and/or vascular occlusion may be noted. The RPE may reveal characteristic clumping overlying the subretinal infiltrates (see Fig 10-16 in Chapter 10). Anterior chamber reaction may be minimal.

Photographic and fluorescein angiographic studies document baseline clinical findings but are rarely helpful in defining a differential diagnosis. Ultrasound examination may reveal discrete nodular or placoid infiltration of the subretinal space, associated retinal detachment, and vitreous syneresis with increased reflectivity. Clinical history and neurologic evaluation may reveal neurologic deficits in up to 10% of patients, and 60% of patients show concomitant CNS involvement at the time of presentation. If the diagnosis is suspected, neurologic consultation coupled with CT or MRI studies and lumbar puncture should be coordinated with diagnostic vitrectomy.

Pathologic Studies

Diagnostic confirmation of ocular involvement requires sampling of the vitreous and, when appropriate, the subretinal space. Coordinated planning with the surgical pathologist prior to surgery regarding sample handling is important. The surgical pathologist should be skilled in the handling of small-volume intraocular specimens and experienced in the evaluation of vitreous samples.

The best approach to pathologic evaluation of the specimen remains controversial. Complete diagnostic 3-port pars plana vitrectomy is indicated to obtain an undiluted vitreous specimen. If a subretinal nodule is accessible in a region of the retina unlikely to compromise visual function, subretinal aspiration of the lesion can be performed. A single-vitrectomy biopsy may not be adequate, and a repeat biopsy may be required. Evaluation of the vitreous and subretinal specimen may be performed using cytopathology (see Fig 10-16), including immunohistochemical studies for subclassification of the cells, flow cytometry, and PCR analysis for gene rearrangements (see Chapters 3, 4, and 10).

Preferably, a pathologist familiar with the diagnosis of intraocular large cell lymphoma should evaluate the specimen. If an adequate specimen is obtained, multiple pathologic approaches may be employed. Cytologic evaluation is essential in establishing the diagnosis, with flow cytometry and PCR serving as ancillary studies. Specimens that reveal malignant lymphocytic cells establish the diagnosis (Fig 21-1), and evaluation of cell surface markers may allow for subclassification of the tumor.

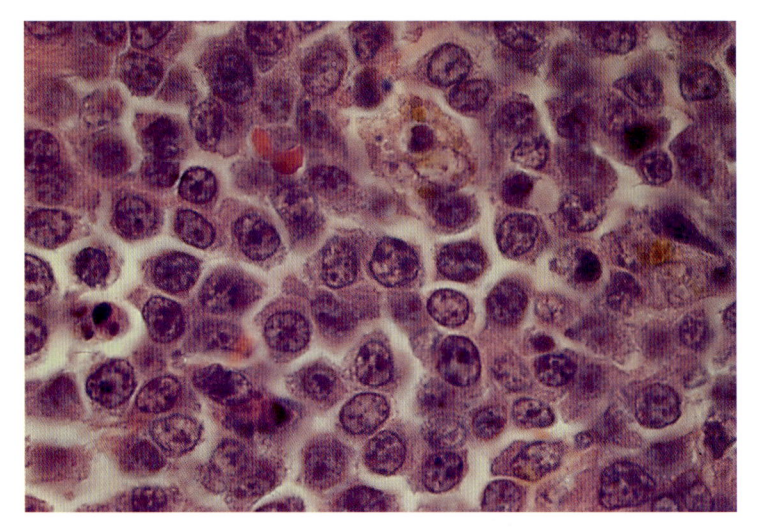

Figure 21-1 Large cell lymphoma, cytology. Note the unusual nuclei and prominent nucleoli of these neoplastic lymphoid cells obtained by fine-needle aspiration biopsy.

Treatment

Because the blood–ocular barriers may limit penetration of chemotherapeutic agents into the eye, irradiation of the affected eye using fractionated external-beam radiation has remained popular in many centers for treatment of intraocular lymphoma. However, although radiotherapy may induce an ocular remission, the tumor invariably recurs, and further irradiation places the patient at high risk for irreversible visual loss caused by radiation retinopathy. Concern regarding the disadvantages of ocular irradiation has led several groups to use intraocular chemotherapy, injecting high-dose methotrexate into the vitreous, with very good response and low recurrence rate. Parallel to the treatment of the intraocular disease is the treatment of the CNS and systemic lymphoma by a medical oncologist.

Prognosis

The prognosis for patients with large cell lymphoma is poor, although advances in early diagnosis have produced a cohort of long-term survivors. Serial follow-up with consultative management by an experienced medical oncologist is critical in the management of this disease. Patients with primary CNS lymphoma should be followed carefully by an ophthalmologist for possible ocular involvement, even after remission of the CNS disease.

Uveal Lymphoid Infiltration

Uveal lymphoid infiltration, formerly known as *reactive lymphoid hyperplasia,* typically presents in patients in the sixth decade; it can occur at any uveal site. Similar lymphoid proliferation can occur in the conjunctiva and orbit (see also Chapter 5 for conjunctival involvement, Chapter 12 for uveal involvement, and Chapter 14 for orbital involvement).

Clinical Evaluation

Patients typically notice painless, progressive visual loss. Ophthalmoscopically, a diffuse or, rarely, nodular amelanotic thickening of the choroid is noted. Exudative retinal detachment and secondary glaucoma may be present in up to 85% of eyes. Frequently, delay between the onset of symptoms and diagnostic intervention is significant.

This rare disorder is characterized pathologically by localized or diffuse infiltration of the uveal tract by lymphoid cells. The etiology is unknown. Clinically, this condition can simulate posterior uveal melanoma, metastatic carcinoma to the uvea, sympathetic ophthalmia, Vogt-Koyanagi-Harada syndrome, and posterior scleritis. Proptosis of the affected eye occurs in approximately 10%–15% of patients who develop simultaneous orbital infiltration with benign lymphoid cells. Ultrasound testing reveals a diffuse, homogeneous choroidal infiltrate with associated secondary retinal detachment. Extraocular extension or orbital involvement may be best demonstrated with echography.

Pathologic Studies

Biopsy confirmation should be targeted to the most accessible tissue. If extraocular involvement is present, biopsy of the involved conjunctiva or orbit may be considered.

FNAB or pars plana vitrectomy with biopsy may be indicated for isolated uveal involvement. Coordination with the surgical pathologist is crucial to achieve the greatest likelihood of appropriate confirmation and cell marker studies.

Treatment

Historically, eyes with this type of lymphoid infiltration were generally managed by enucleation because of presumed malignancy. Current management emphasizes globe-conserving therapy aimed at visual preservation. High-dose oral steroids may induce tumor regression and decrease exudative retinal detachment. Early intervention with low-dose ocular and orbital fractionated external-beam radiotherapy may definitively manage the disease.

Prognosis

The prognosis for survival is excellent for patients with uveal lymphoid infiltration, with the rare exception of patients with systemic lymphoma. Preservation of visual function appears related to primary tumor location and secondary sequelae, including exudative retinal detachment or glaucoma. Early intervention appears to enhance the likelihood for visual preservation.

Chan CC, Wallace DJ. Intraocular lymphoma: update on diagnosis and management. *Cancer Control.* 2004;11:285–295.

Coupland SE, Hummel M, Muller HH, Stein H. Molecular analysis of immunoglobulin genes in primary intraocular lymphoma. *Invest Ophthalmol Vis Sci.* 2005;46:3507–3514.

Grossniklaus HE, Martin DF, Avery R, et al. Uveal lymphoid infiltration: report of four cases and clinicopathologic review. *Ophthalmology.* 1998;105:1265–1273.

Read RW, Zamir E, Rao NA. Neoplastic masquerade syndromes. *Surv Ophthalmol.* 2002;47: 81–124.

Smith JR, Rosenbaum JT, Wilson DJ, et al. Role of intravitreal methotrexate in the management of primary central nervous system lymphoma with ocular involvement. *Ophthalmology.* 2002;109:1709–1716.

Specht CS, Laver NM. Benign and malignant lymphoid tumors, leukemia, and histiocytic lesions. In: Albert DM, Jakobiec FA, eds. *Principles and Practice of Ophthalmology.* 2nd ed. Philadelphia: Saunders; 2000:5146–5168.

CHAPTER 22

Ocular Manifestations of Leukemia

Ocular involvement with leukemia is common, occurring in as many as 80% of the eyes of patients examined at autopsy. Clinical studies have documented ophthalmic findings in as many as 40% of patients at diagnosis. Although retinal lesions are the most frequently observed clinical finding, histologic studies have shown that the choroid is affected more often. Furthermore, the uveal tract may serve as a "sanctuary site," predisposing the eye to be the first clinical manifestation of recurrent disease (Fig 22-1). Choroidal infiltrates may be difficult to detect with indirect ophthalmoscopy; they may be better detected on ultrasound as a thickening of the choroids. Serous retinal detachments may overlie these infiltrates. Leukemic involvement of the iris is also manifested as a diffuse thickening, and in some cases small nodules may be seen at the margin of the pupil (see Fig 17-4D). Tumor cells in the anterior chamber may layer to form a pseudohypopyon. Infiltration of the angle by these cells can give rise to a secondary glaucoma.

Retinal findings such as hard exudates, cotton-wool spots, and white-centered retinal hemorrhages (pseudo–Roth spots) are usually the result of associated anemia or thrombocytopenia. However, leukemic infiltrates can be seen as yellow deposits in the retina and the subretinal space. Gray-white nodules of various sizes have been seen in a case of chronic myelogenous leukemia. Occasionally, perivascular leukemic infiltrates can produce gray-white streaks in the retina.

Vitreous involvement by leukemias is rare; however, opacities may develop. If necessary, a diagnostic vitrectomy can be performed to establish a diagnosis. Leukemic infiltration of the optic nerve may present with severe visual loss and optic nerve edema. One or both eyes may be affected. This is an ophthalmic emergency and requires immediate treatment to preserve as much vision as possible. Systemic and intrathecal chemotherapy will be needed with or without radiation.

Leukemic infiltrates may also involve the orbital soft tissue, with resultant proptosis. These tumors, which are more common with myelogenous leukemias, are referred to as *granulocytic sarcomas* or *chloromas*. They have a predilection for the lateral and medial walls of the orbit.

Patients with leukemia and allied disorders may be immunocompromised and thus susceptible to opportunistic infections. Endogenous infections must be considered in the differential diagnosis of leukemic infiltration.

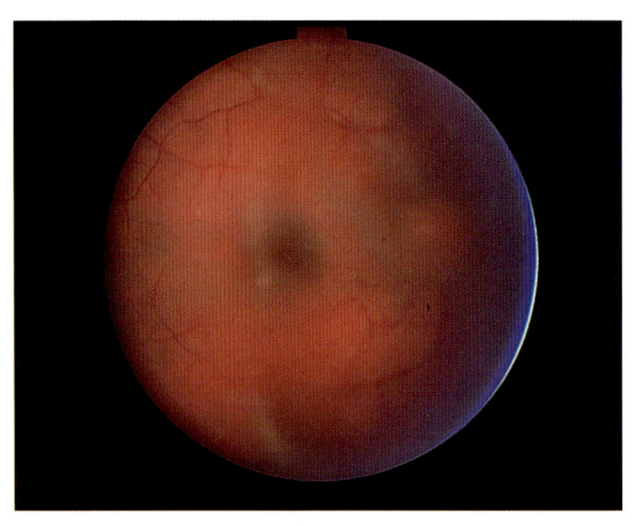

Figure 22-1 Leukemic infiltration of the vitreous, clinical appearance. View of the fundus is hazy because of dispersed tumor cells in the vitreous.

Treatment of leukemic involvement of the eye generally consists of low-dose radiation therapy to the eye and systemic chemotherapy. The prognosis for vision depends on the type of leukemia and the extent of ocular involvement.

> Guyer DR, Schachat AP, Vitale S, et al. Leukemic retinopathy: relationship between fundus lesions and hematologic parameters at diagnosis. *Ophthalmology.* 1989;96:860–864.
>
> Reddy SC, Jackson N. Retinopathy in acute leukaemia at initial diagnosis: correlation of fundus lesions and haematological parameters. *Acta Ophthalmol Scand.* 2004;82:81–85.
>
> Schachat AP, Jabs DA, Graham ML, Ambinder RF, Green WR, Saral R. Leukemic iris infiltration. *J Pediatr Ophthalmol Strabismus.* 1988;25:135–138.
>
> Schachat AP, Markowitz JA, Guyer DR, Burke PJ, Karp JE, Graham ML. Ophthalmic manifestations of leukemia. *Arch Ophthalmol.* 1989;107:697–700.
>
> Sharma T, Grewal J, Gupta S, Murray PI. Ophthalmic manifestations of acute leukaemias: the ophthalmologist's role. *Eye.* 2004;18:663–672.

CHAPTER 23

Rare Tumors

Medulloepithelioma

Medulloepithelioma, or diktyoma, is a tumor of the nonpigmented ciliary epithelium that occurs in both benign and malignant forms (see Fig 11-44). Medulloepitheliomas are congenital neuroepithelial tumors arising from primitive medullary epithelium. This type of tumor typically becomes clinically evident in children 4–12 years old, but it may also occur in adults. It usually appears as a variably pigmented mass arising from the ciliary body but has also been documented in the retina and optic nerve. The tumor may erode into the anterior chamber and become visible at the iris root. Large cysts may be seen on the surface of the tumor or within the lesion on diagnostic imaging (Fig 23-1). Chapter 11 discusses the histologic features of medulloepithelioma.

Management usually consists of enucleation or observation. Surgical resection is specifically avoided for the majority of these tumors because of late complications and documented metastases associated with this treatment. Fortunately, metastasis is rare with appropriate management, even if the tumor appears frankly malignant on histologic examination. Small lesions have been successfully treated with iodine 125 plaque brachytherapy.

> Davidorf FH, Craig E, Birnhaum L, Wakely P. Management of medulloepithelioma of the ciliary body with brachytherapy. *Am J Ophthalmol.* 2002;133:841–843.
> Garner A, Klintworth GK, eds. *Pathology of Ocular Disease: A Dynamic Approach.* 2nd ed. New York: Marcel Dekker; 1994:1405–1413.
> Lumbroso L, Desjardins L, Coue O, Ducourneau Y, Pechereau A. Presumed bilateral medulloepithelioma. *Arch Ophthalmol.* 2001;119:449–450.

Leiomyomas, Neurilemomas, and Neurofibromas

Leiomyomas, neurilemomas, and neurofibromas of the uveal tract are extremely rare tumors that are usually misdiagnosed clinically as amelanotic primary uveal melanomas. The role of ancillary diagnostic tests for such lesions is uncertain.

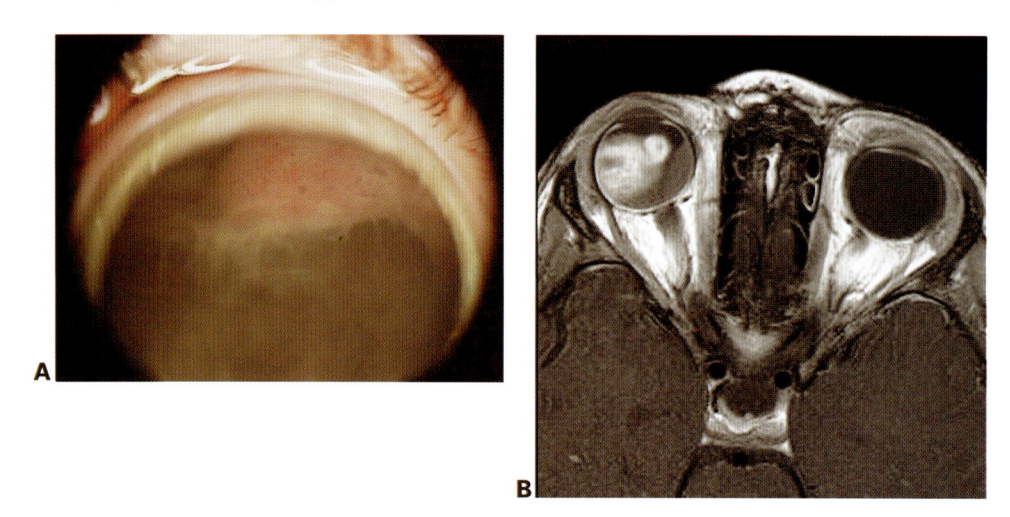

Figure 23-1 Medulloepithelioma. **A,** Pigmented lesion arising in ciliary body with amelanotic apex. **B,** T1-weighted MRI with gadolinium, showing diffuse enhancement and multiple cystic spaces. *(Courtesy of Matthew W. Wilson, MD.)*

APPENDIX

American Joint Committee on Cancer (AJCC) Definitions and Staging of Ocular Tumors, 2002

Table A-1 Carcinoma of the Conjunctiva

The following definitions apply to both clinical and pathologic staging

Primary Tumor (T)
- TX — Primary tumor cannot be assessed
- T0 — No evidence of primary tumor
- Tis — Carcinoma in situ
- T1 — Tumor ≤5 mm in greatest dimension
- T2 — Tumor >5 mm in greatest dimension, without invasion of adjacent structures
- T3 — Tumor invades adjacent structures, excluding the orbit
- T4 — Tumor invades the orbit with or without further extension
  - T4a Tumor invades orbital soft tissues without bone invasion
  - T4b Tumor invades bone
  - T4c Tumor invades adjacent paranasal sinuses
  - T4d Tumor invades brain

Regional Lymph Nodes (N)
- NX — Regional lymph nodes cannot be assessed
- N0 — No regional lymph node metastasis
- N1 — Regional lymph node metastasis

Distant Metastasis (M)
- MX — Distant metastasis cannot be assessed
- M0 — No distant metastasis
- M1 — Distant metastasis

Stage Grouping — No stage grouping is presently recommended

Histologic Grade (G)
- GX — Grade cannot be assessed
- G1 — Well differentiated
- G2 — Moderately differentiated
- G3 — Poorly differentiated
- G4 — Undifferentiated

Residual Tumor (R)
- RX — Presence of residual tumor cannot be assessed
- R0 — No residual tumor
- R1 — Microscopic residual tumor
- R2 — Macroscopic residual tumor

Table A-2 Malignant Melanoma of the Conjunctiva

Clinical Definitions (cTNM)

Primary Tumor (T)
- TX — Primary tumor cannot be assessed
- T0 — No evidence of primary tumor
- T1 — Tumor of the bulbar conjunctiva
- T2 — Tumor of the bulbar conjunctiva with corneal extension
- T3 — Tumor extending into the conjunctival fornix, palpebral conjunctiva, or caruncle
- T4 — Tumor invades the eyelid, globe, orbit, sinuses, or central nervous system

Pathologic Definitions (pTNM)

Primary Tumor (T)
- pTX — Primary tumor cannot be assessed
- pT0 — No evidence of primary tumor
- pT1 — Tumor of the bulbar conjunctiva confined to the epithelium
- pT2 — Tumor of the bulbar conjunctiva ≤0.8 mm in thickness with invasion of the substantia propria
- pT3 — Tumor of the bulbar conjunctiva >0.8 mm in thickness with invasion of the substantia propria or tumors involving palpebral or caruncular conjunctiva
- pT4 — Tumor invades the eyelid, globe, orbit, sinuses, or central nervous system

Regional Lymph Nodes (N)
- pNX — Regional lymph nodes cannot be assessed
- pN0 — No regional lymph node metastasis
- pN1 — Regional lymph node metastasis

Distant Metastasis (M)
- pMX — Distant metastasis cannot be assessed
- pM0 — No distant metastasis
- pM1 — Distant metastasis

Stage Grouping — No stage grouping is presently recommended

Histologic Grade (G)
(Histopathologic grade represents the origin of the primary tumor)
- GX — Origin cannot be assessed
- G0 — Primary acquired melanosis without cellular atypia
- G1 — Conjunctival nevus
- G2 — Primary acquired melanosis with cellular atypia (epithelial disease only)
- G3 — De novo malignant melanoma

Residual Tumor (R)
- RX — Presence of residual tumor cannot be assessed
- R0 — No residual tumor
- R1 — Microscopic residual tumor
- R2 — Macroscopic residual tumor

APPENDIX: American Joint Committee on Cancer (AJCC) Definitions • 323

Table A-3 **Retinoblastoma**

Clinical Definitions (cTNM)

Primary Tumor (T)

TX	Primary tumor cannot be assessed
T0	No evidence of primary tumor
T1	Tumor confined to the retina (no vitreous seeding or significant retinal detachment)
	T1a Any eye in which the largest tumor is ≤3 mm in height *and* no tumor is located closer than 1 DD (1.5 mm) to the optic nerve or fovea
	T1b All eyes in which the tumor(s) are confined to the retina regardless of location or size (up to half the volume of the eye). *No* vitreous seeding. *No* retinal detachment or subretinal fluid >5 mm from the base of the tumor.
T2	Tumor with contiguous spread to adjacent tissues or spaces (vitreous or subretinal space)
	T2a *Minimal tumor spread to vitreous and/or subretinal space.* Fine local or diffuse vitreous seeding and/or serous retinal detachment up to total detachment may be present, but *no* clumps, lumps, snowballs, or avascular masses are allowed in the vitreous or subretinal space. Calcium flecks in the vitreous or subretinal space are allowed. The tumor may fill up to 2/3 the volume of the eye.
	T2b *Massive tumor spread to the vitreous and/or subretinal space.* Vitreous seeding and/or subretinal implantation may consist of lumps, clumps, snowballs, or avascular tumor masses. Retinal detachment may be total. Tumor may fill up to 2/3 the volume of the eye.
	T2c Unsalvageable intraocular disease. Tumor fills more than 2/3 of the eye *or* there is no possibility of visual rehabilitation *or* one or more of the following are present: tumor-associated glaucoma, either neovascular or angle closure; anterior segment extension of tumor; ciliary body extension of tumor; hyphema (significant); massive vitreous hemorrhage; tumor in contact with lens; orbital cellulitis–like clinical presentation (massive tumor necrosis)
T3	Invasion of the optic nerve and/or optic coats
T4	Extraocular tumor

Regional Lymph Nodes (N)

NX	Regional lymph nodes cannot be assessed
N0	No regional lymph node involvement
N1	Regional lymph node involvement (preauricular, submandibular, or cervical)
N2	Distant lymph node involvement

Distant Metastasis (M)

MX	Distant metastasis cannot be assessed
M0	No distant metastasis
M1	Metastases to central nervous system and/or bone, bone marrow, or other sites

(Continued)

Table A-3 *(continued)*

Pathologic Definitions (pTNM)

Tumor (pT)
- pTX — Primary tumor cannot be assessed
- pT0 — No evidence of primary tumor
- pT1 — Tumor confined to the retina, vitreous, or subretinal space. No optic nerve or choroidal invasion
- pT2 — Minimal invasion of optic nerve and/or optic coats
  - pT2a Tumor invades optic nerve up to, but not through, the level of the lamina cribrosa
  - pT2b Tumor invades choroid focally
  - pT2c Tumor invades optic nerve up to but not through the level of the lamina cribrosa *and* invades the choroid focally
- pT3 — Significant invasion of the optic nerve and/or optic coats
  - pT3a Tumor invades optic nerve through the level of the lamina cribrosa but not to the line of resection
  - pT3b Tumor massively invades the choroid
  - pT3c Tumor invades the optic nerve through the lamina cribrosa but not to the line of resection *and* massively invades the choroid
- pT4 — Extraocular extension, which includes:
  - Tumor invades optic nerve to the line of resection
  - Tumor invades the orbit through the sclera
  - Tumor extends both anteriorly and posteriorly into orbit
  - Extension into the brain
  - Extension into the subarachnoid space of the optic nerve
  - Extension to the apex of the orbit
  - Extension to, but not through, the chiasm, or
  - Extension into the brain beyond the chiasm

Regional Lymph Nodes (N)
- pNX — Regional lymph nodes cannot be assessed
- pN0 — No regional lymph node metastasis
- pN1 — Regional lymph node metastasis

Distant Metastasis (M)
- pMX — Distant metastasis cannot be assessed
- pM0 — No distant metastasis
- pM1a — Bone marrow
- pM1b — Other sites

Stage Grouping — No applicable stage grouping for pathologic or clinical

Residual Tumor (R)
- RX — Presence of residual tumor cannot be assessed
- R0 — No residual tumor
- R1 — Microscopic residual tumor
- R2 — Macroscopic residual tumor

Table A-4 Malignant Melanoma of the Uvea

The following definitions apply to both clinical and pathologic staging

All Uveal Melanomas (T)
- TX — Primary tumor cannot be assessed
- T0 — No evidence of primary tumor

Iris (T)
- T1 — Tumor limited to the iris
  - T1a Tumor limited to the iris (≤3 clock-hours in size)
  - T1b Tumor limited to the iris (>3 clock-hours in size)
  - T1c Tumor limited to the iris with melanomalytic glaucoma
- T2 — Tumor confluent with or extending into the ciliary body and/or choroid
  - T2a Tumor confluent with or extending into the ciliary body and/or choroid with melanomalytic glaucoma
- T3 — Tumor confluent with or extending into the ciliary body and/or choroid with scleral extension
  - T3a Tumor confluent with or extending into the ciliary body with scleral extension and melanomalytic glaucoma
- T4 — Tumor with extraocular extension

Ciliary Body and Choroid (T)
- T1* — Tumor ≤10 mm in greatest diameter and ≤2.5 mm in greatest height (thickness)
  - T1a Tumor ≤10 mm in greatest diameter and ≤2.5 mm in greatest height (thickness) without microscopic extraocular extension
  - T1b Tumor ≤10 mm in greatest diameter and ≤2.5 mm in greatest height (thickness) with microscopic extraocular extension
  - T1c Tumor ≤10 mm in greatest diameter and ≤2.5 mm in greatest height (thickness) with macroscopic extraocular extension
- T2* — Tumor >10 mm but ≤16 mm in greatest basal diameter and between 2.5 and 10 mm in maximum height (thickness)
  - T2a Tumor 10–16 mm in greatest basal diameter and between 2.5 and 10 mm in maximum height (thickness) without microscopic extraocular extension
  - T2b Tumor 10–16 mm in greatest basal diameter and between 2.5 and 10 mm in maximum height (thickness) with microscopic extraocular extension
  - T2c Tumor 10–16 mm in greatest basal diameter and between 2.5 and 10 mm in maximum height (thickness) with macroscopic extraocular extension
- T3* — Tumor >16 mm in greatest diameter and/or >10 mm in maximum height (thickness) without extraocular extension
- T4* — Tumor >16 mm in greatest diameter and/or >10 mm in maximum height (thickness) with extraocular extension

(Continued)

Table A-4 *(continued)*

The following definitions apply to both clinical and pathologic staging

Regional Lymph Nodes (N)
- NX   Regional lymph nodes cannot be assessed
- N0   No regional lymph node metastasis
- N1   Regional lymph node metastasis

Distant Metastasis (M)
- MX   Distant metastasis cannot be assessed
- M0   No distant metastasis
- M1   Distant metastasis

Stage Grouping

Stage I	T1	N0	M0
	T1a	N0	M0
	T1b	N0	M0
	T1c	N0	M0
Stage II	T2	N0	M0
	T2a	N0	M0
	T2b	N0	M0
	T2c	N0	M0
Stage III	T3	N0	M0
	T4	N0	M0
Stage IV	Any T	N1	M0
	Any T	Any N	M1

Histologic Grade (G)
- GX   Grade cannot be assessed
- G1   Spindle cell melanoma
- G2   Mixed cell melanoma
- G3   Epithelioid cell melanoma

Residual Tumor (R)
- RX   Presence of residual tumor cannot be assessed
- R0   No residual tumor
- R1   Microscopic residual tumor
- R2   Macroscopic residual tumor

Venous Invasion (V)
- VX   Venous invasion cannot be assessed
- V0   Veins do not contain tumor
- V1   Microscopic venous invasion
- V2   Macroscopic venous invasion

* Note: When basal dimension and apical height do not fit this classification, the largest tumor diameter should be used for classification. In clinical practice, the tumor base may be estimated in optic disc diameters (DD) (average: 1 DD = 1.5 mm). The height may be estimated in diopters (average: 3 diopters = 1 mm). Techniques such as ultrasonography, visualization, and photography are frequently used to provide more accurate measurements.

APPENDIX: American Joint Committee on Cancer (AJCC) Definitions • 327

Table A-5 Carcinoma of the Eyelid

The following definitions apply to both clinical and pathologic staging

Primary Tumor (T)
- TX — Primary tumor cannot be assessed
- T0 — No evidence of primary tumor
- Tis — Carcinoma in situ
- T1 — Tumor of any size, not invading the tarsal plate, or, at the eyelid margin, ≤5 mm in greatest dimension
- T2 — Tumor invades tarsal plate or is at the eyelid margin, >5 mm but ≤10 mm in greatest dimension
- T3 — Tumor involves full eyelid thickness or is at the eyelid margin, >10 mm in greatest dimension
- T4 — Tumor invades adjacent structures, which include bulbar conjunctiva, sclera and globe, soft tissues of the orbit, perineural space, bone and periosteum of the orbit, nasal cavity and paranasal sinuses, and central nervous system

Regional Lymph Nodes (N)
- NX — Regional lymph nodes cannot be assessed
- N0 — No regional lymph node metastasis
- N1 — Regional lymph node metastasis

Distant Metastasis (M)
- MX — Distant metastasis cannot be assessed
- M0 — No distant metastasis
- M1 — Distant metastasis

Stage Grouping No stage grouping is presently recommended

Histologic Grade (G)
- GX — Grade cannot be assessed
- G1 — Well differentiated
- G2 — Moderately differentiated
- G3 — Poorly differentiated
- G4 — Undifferentiated or differentiation is not applicable

Residual Tumor (R)
- RX — Presence of residual tumor cannot be assessed
- R0 — No residual tumor
- R1 — Microscopic residual tumor
- R2 — Macroscopic residual tumor

Table A-6 Carcinoma of the Lacrimal Gland

The following definitions apply to both clinical and pathologic staging

Primary Tumor (T)
- TX — Primary tumor cannot be assessed
- T0 — No evidence of primary tumor
- T1 — Tumor ≤2.5 cm in greatest dimension, limited to the lacrimal gland
- T2 — Tumor >2.5 cm but ≤5 cm in greatest dimension limited to the lacrimal gland
- T3 — Tumor invades the periosteum
  - T3a Tumor ≤5 cm invades the periosteum of the lacrimal gland fossa
  - T3b Tumor >5 cm in greatest dimension with periosteal invasion
- T4 — Tumor invades the orbital soft tissues, optic nerve, or globe with or without bone invasion; tumor extends beyond the orbit to adjacent structures including the brain

Regional Lymph Nodes (N)
- NX — Regional lymph nodes cannot be assessed
- N0 — No regional lymph node metastasis
- N1 — Regional lymph node metastasis

Distant Metastasis (M)
- MX — Distant metastasis cannot be assessed
- M0 — No distant metastasis
- M1 — Distant metastasis

Stage Grouping   No stage grouping is presently recommended

Histologic Grade (G)
- GX — Grade cannot be assessed
- G1 — Well differentiated
- G2 — Moderately differentiated; includes adenoid cystic carcinoma without basaloid (solid) pattern
- G3 — Poorly differentiated; includes adenoid cystic carcinoma with basaloid (solid) pattern
- G4 — Undifferentiated

Residual Tumor (R)
- RX — Presence of residual tumor cannot be assessed
- R0 — No residual tumor
- R1 — Microscopic residual tumor
- R2 — Macroscopic residual tumor

APPENDIX: American Joint Committee on Cancer (AJCC) Definitions • 329

Table A-7 Sarcoma of the Orbit

The following definitions apply to both clinical and pathologic staging

Primary Tumor (T)
- TX — Primary tumor cannot be assessed
- T0 — No evidence of primary tumor
- T1 — Tumor ≤15 mm in greatest dimension
- T2 — Tumor >15 mm in greatest dimension without invasion of globe or bony wall
- T3 — Tumor of any size with invasion of orbital tissues and/or bony walls
- T4 — Tumor invasion of globe or periorbital structures, such as eyelids, temporal fossa, nasal cavity and paranasal sinuses, and/or central nervous system

Regional Lymph Nodes (N)
- NX — Regional lymph nodes cannot be assessed
- N0 — No regional lymph node metastasis
- N1 — Regional lymph node metastasis

Distant Metastasis (M)
- MX — Distant metastasis cannot be assessed
- M0 — No distant metastasis
- M1 — Distant metastasis

Stage Grouping — No stage grouping is presently recommended

Histologic Grade (G)
- GX — Grade cannot be assessed
- G1 — Well differentiated
- G2 — Moderately differentiated
- G3 — Poorly differentiated
- G4 — Undifferentiated

Residual Tumor (R)
- RX — Presence of residual tumor cannot be assessed
- R0 — No residual tumor
- R1 — Microscopic residual tumor
- R2 — Macroscopic residual tumor

Basic Texts

Ophthalmic Pathology and Intraocular Tumors

Albert DM, Jakobiec FA, eds. *Atlas of Clinical Ophthalmology.* Philadelphia: Saunders; 1996.

Albert DM, Jakobiec FA, eds. *Principles and Practice of Ophthalmology.* 6 vols. 2nd ed. Philadelphia: Saunders; 2000.

Apple DJ, Rabb MF. *Ocular Pathology: Clinical Applications and Self-Assessment.* 5th ed. St Louis: Mosby; 1998.

Bornfeld N, Gragoudas ES, Höpping W, et al, eds. *Tumors of the Eye.* New York: Kugler; 1991.

Char DH. *Clinical Ocular Oncology.* 2nd ed. Philadelphia: Lippincott Williams & Wilkins; 1998.

Cohen IK, Diegelmann RF, Lindblad WJ, eds. *Wound Healing: Biochemical and Clinical Aspects.* Philadelphia: Saunders; 1992.

Dutton JJ. *Atlas of Clinical and Surgical Orbital Anatomy.* Philadelphia: Saunders; 1994.

Garner A, Klintworth GK, eds. *Pathobiology of Ocular Disease: A Dynamic Approach.* 2nd ed. New York: Marcel Dekker; 1994.

Isenberg SJ, ed. *The Eye in Infancy.* 2nd ed. St Louis: Mosby; 1994.

Margo CE, Grossniklaus HE. *Ocular Histopathology: A Guide to Differential Diagnosis.* Philadelphia: Saunders; 1991.

McLean IW, Burnier MN, Zimmerman LE, Jakobiec FA. *Tumors of the Eye and Ocular Adnexa.* Washington: Armed Forces Institute of Pathology; 1994.

Nauman GOH, Apple DJ. *Pathology of the Eye.* New York: Springer-Verlag; 1986.

Rootman J, Stewart B, Goldberg RA. *Orbital Surgery. A Conceptual Approach.* Philadelphia: Lippincott; 1995.

Sanborn GE, Gonder JR, Shields JA. *Atlas of Intraocular Tumors.* Philadelphia: Saunders; 1994.

Sassani JW, ed. *Ophthalmic Pathology With Clinical Correlations.* Philadelphia: Lippincott Williams & Wilkins; 1997.

Shields JA, Shields CL. *Atlas of Eyelid and Conjunctival Tumors.* Philadelphia: Lippincott Williams & Wilkins; 1999.

Shields JA, Shields CL. *Atlas of Intraocular Tumors.* Philadelphia: Lippincott Williams & Wilkins; 1999.

Spencer WH, ed. *Ophthalmic Pathology: An Atlas and Textbook.* 4th ed. Philadelphia: Saunders; 1996.

Yanoff M, Fine BS. *Ocular Pathology.* 5th ed. St Louis: Mosby; 2002.

Related Academy Materials

Focal Points: Clinical Modules for Ophthalmologists

Galetta SL, Liu GT, Volpe NJ. Pseudotumor cerebri (Module 12, 2003).
Helm CJ. Melanoma and other pigmented lesions of the ocular surface (Module 11, 1996).
Lane Stevens JC. Retinoblastoma (Module 1, 1990).
Margo CE. Nonpigmented lesions of the ocular surface (Module 9, 1996).
Stefanyszyn MA. Orbital tumors in children (Module 9, 1990).

Publications

Berkow JW, Flower RW, Orth DH, Kelley JS. *Fluorescein and Indocyanine Green Angiography: Technique and Interpretation.* 2nd ed. (Ophthalmology Monograph 5, 1997).
Kline LB, ed. *Optic Nerve Disorders* (Ophthalmology Monograph 10, 1996).
Stewart WB, ed. *Surgery of the Eyelid, Orbit, and Lacrimal System* (Ophthalmology Monograph 8. Vol 1, 1993; reviewed for currency 2001. Vol 2, 1994; reviewed for currency 2003. Vol 3, 1995; reviewed for currency 2000).
Wilson FM II, ed. *Practical Ophthalmology: A Manual for Beginning Residents.* 5th ed. (2005).
Wirtschafter JD, Berman EL, McDonald CS. *Magnetic Resonance Imaging and Computed Tomography: Clinical Neuro-Orbital Anatomy* (Ophthalmology Monograph 6, 1992).

> **To order any of these materials, please call the Academy's Customer Service number at (415) 561-8540, or order online at www.aao.org.**

Study Questions

Although a concerted effort has been made to avoid ambiguity and redundancy in these questions, the authors recognize that differences of opinion may occur regarding the "best" answer. The discussions are provided to demonstrate the rationale used to derive the answer. They may also be helpful in confirming that your approach to the problem was correct or, if necessary, in fixing the principle in your memory.

1. Which of the following choices best describes the sequence of specific processes that occur during wound healing in clear cornea?
   a. epithelial wound repair, wound edge digestion, fibroblast activation, wound contraction
   b. wound edge digestion, epithelial wound repair, fibroblast activation, wound contraction
   c. fibroblast activation, wound contraction, wound edge digestion, epithelial wound repair
   d. wound edge digestion, fibroblast activation, epithelial wound repair, wound contraction

2. Which of the following special techniques in diagnostic pathology is quantitative in its standard form?
   a. immunohistochemistry
   b. electron microscopy
   c. flow cytometry
   d. PCR-based gene rearrangement studies

3. Which of the following best describes the differences between macular dystrophy of the cornea and granular and lattice dystrophies?
   a. deposited material and visual disability
   b. genetic transmission, deposited material, and visual disability
   c. genetic transmission, tissue distribution, visual disability, and deposited material
   d. genetic transmission and tissue distribution

4. Which of the following would *not* be detected by Prussian blue staining?
   a. Fleischer line
   b. Stocker line
   c. Ferry line
   d. Krukenberg spindle

5. The most important and helpful imaging tool in the diagnosis of choroidal and ciliary body melanoma is
   a. fluorescein angiography
   b. ultrasonography
   c. computed tomography (CT)
   d. magnetic resonance imaging (MRI)
   e. PET-CT

6. Which of the following about iris melanoma compared to choroidal melanoma is *true*?
   a. Iris melanoma is as common as choroidal melanoma.
   b. Iris melanoma metastasizes at a rate similar to that of choroidal melanoma.
   c. Histologically, iris melanoma may contain the same type of cells as choroidal melanoma.
   d. Like choroidal melanoma, iris melanoma is usually treated by brachytherapy.
   e. Iris melanoma is diagnosed, like choroidal melanoma, by both A-scan and B-scan modes of ultrasonography.

7. Two tumors commonly associated with so-called *masquerade syndromes* are
   a. conjunctival lymphoma, choroidal melanoma
   b. conjunctival lymphoma, intraocular lymphoma
   c. eyelid sebaceous carcinoma, intraocular lymphoma
   d. basal cell carcinoma, retinoblastoma

8. The most common secondary tumor in retinoblastoma patients is
   a. fibrosarcoma
   b. melanoma
   c. pinealoblastoma
   d. osteosarcoma

9. The primary treatment for a child with unilateral retinoblastoma filling more than 50% of the vitreous cavity with diffuse vitreous seeding is
   a. chemotherapy alone
   b. enucleation
   c. radiation alone
   d. chemotherapy and radiation

10. Which of the following statements about pleomorphic adenoma of the lacrimal gland is *false*?
    a. It can recur in a diffuse manner.
    b. It can transform to a malignant tumor if present long enough.
    c. Recurrences can transform to malignancy.
    d. It can resolve spontaneously.

11. Intraocular calcification in the eye of a child is most diagnostic of
    a. retinoblastoma
    b. toxocara
    c. persistent fetal vasculature
    d. Coats disease

12. Histopathologic characteristics of ciliochoroidal melanoma that correlate with patient prognosis include
    a. modified Callender classification, erosion through Bruch's membrane, intrinsic microvascular pattern
    b. tumor size, intrinsic microvascular patterns, immunohistochemical positivity for HMB-45
    c. modified Callender classification, tumor size, intrinsic microvascular patterns
    d. modified Callender classification, invasion of optic nerve, intrinsic microvascular patterns

13. Which of the following ocular histologic changes is not considered to be associated with diabetes mellitus?
    a. lacy vacuolization of the iris
    b. retinal hemorrhages
    c. iris hemorrhages
    d. thickened basement membranes

14. Histologic differentiation between primary and recurrent pterygia can be based on
    a. the degree of vascularity in the lesion
    b. the presence of more fibrous tissue in the recurrent lesion
    c. the absence of elastotic degeneration in recurrent pterygia
    d. the presence of Bowman's layer in recurrent but not primary pterygia

15. The most common primary sites and type of choroidal metastasis are
    a. lung carcinomas in males and females
    b. prostate carcinomas in males and breast carcinomas in females
    c. lung carcinomas in males and breast carcinomas in females
    d. gastrointestinal carcinomas in males and breast carcinomas in females
    e. carcinomas of unknown origin in males and breast carcinomas in females

16. Which of the following extraocular muscles inserts farthest from the limbus?
    a. superior rectus
    b. inferior rectus
    c. inferior oblique
    d. superior oblique

17. Which of the following antigens would allow identification of a spindle cell tumor as a melanoma?
    a. cytokeratin
    b. S-100
    c. HMB-45
    d. desmin

342 • Study Questions

18. Histologically, the term *angle recession* refers to which of the following conditions?
    a. a tear between the ciliary body and the sclera
    b. a tear between the iris and the ciliary body
    c. a tear between the longitudinal and circular portions of the ciliary muscle
    d. posterior displacement of the iris root without alteration of the ciliary body

19. The following entity results in synechial angle-closure glaucoma:
    a. melanomalytic glaucoma
    b. iridocorneal endothelial (ICE) syndrome
    c. ghost cell glaucoma
    d. hemosiderosis bulbi

20. The sclera shows what variation in thickness and is composed primarily of what type of collagen?
    a. tenfold thickness variation; type I collagen
    b. threefold thickness variation; type IV collagen
    c. twofold thickness variation; type IV collagen
    d. threefold thickness variation; type I collagen

21. Anterior scleritis is likely to
    a. be bilateral in 50% of cases
    b. be associated with pain on eye movement
    c. cause exophthalmos
    d. be painless

22. Mutations in the fibrillin gene on chromosome 15 lead to lens displacement
    a. down
    b. inferonasally
    c. superotemporally
    d. anteriorly

23. Which of the following is the most common primary malignancy of the eyelid?
    a. basal cell carcinoma
    b. squamous cell carcinoma
    c. sebaceous carcinoma
    d. melanoma

24. When a parent has bilateral retinoblastoma, each child
    a. has an 85% chance of developing retinoblastoma
    b. who develops retinoblastoma will have bilateral disease
    c. will be affected only if male
    d. has a 45% chance of developing retinoblastoma

25. In the final scar of the average wound,
    a. myofibroblasts and fibroblasts contract
    b. most of the vessels persist
    c. the recently laid collagen parallels the uninjured surrounding collagen
    d. macrophages remain, producing enzymes

26. At the time of enucleation, most blind, painful eyes have either
    a. absolute glaucoma or expulsive hemorrhage
    b. phthisis bulbi or absolute glaucoma
    c. fibrous ingrowth or absolute glaucoma
    d. epithelial downgrowth or absolute glaucoma

27. Conjunctival and corneal epithelial cells
    a. never grow inside the eye
    b. can invade the eye by burrowing through intact cornea
    c. produce free-floating solid masses of cells in the eye
    d. may grow down a tract or wound edge to the inside of the eye

28. Cotton-wool spots
    a. are diagnostic of collagen vascular disease
    b. contain swollen glial cells
    c. never disappear once they are formed
    d. are transudates from the superficial capillary plexus
    e. represent coagulative necrosis of the nerve fiber layer

29. The most commonly used fixative in ophthalmic pathology is
    a. gluteraldehyde
    b. formalin
    c. B5
    d. RPMI

30. An appropriate use of surgical frozen sections is to
    a. provide a rapid diagnosis for anxious family members
    b. freeze all of the excised tissue
    c. determine if representative tissue has been sampled
    d. determine the margins of resection of primary acquired melanosis (PAM) with atypia

31. A giant cell with an annulus of nuclei surrounded by a lipid-filled zone is classified as a
    a. Langhans giant cell
    b. foreign body giant cell
    c. tumor giant cell
    d. Touton giant cell

344 • Study Questions

32. Vitreous amyloidosis is associated with
    a. peripheral neuropathy
    b. cranial nerve paralysis
    c. lattice dystrophy
    d. peripheral vascular disease

33. Which of the following statements about Descemet's membrane is *false*?
    a. It is developmentally derived from the neural crest.
    b. It is elaborated by the corneal endothelial cells.
    c. It remains static throughout life.
    d. It is composed of type IV collagen.

34. Band keratopathy is characterized by
    a. randomly distributed deposits in the cornea
    b. calcium deposition within the deep corneal stroma
    c. occurrence only in patients with hypercalcemia
    d. involvement of the epithelial basement membrane and Bowman's layer
    e. association with other congenital malformations

35. All of the following may be associated with congenital cataracts *except*
    a. anterior lenticonus
    b. cerulean cataracts
    c. aniridia
    d. rubella
    e. siderosis

36. Which of the following sites for ocular adnexal lymphoid neoplasms has the strongest association with systemic lymphoma?
    a. eyelid
    b. palpebral conjunctiva
    c. bulbar conjunctiva
    d. orbit

37. The conjunctival melanocytic proliferation most commonly associated with subsequent development of conjunctival malignant melanoma is
    a. ephelis
    b. nevus
    c. ocular melanocytosis
    d. primary acquired melanosis (PAM)

38. Exfoliation syndrome (pseudoexfoliation) does not include
    a. systemic deposition of fibrillin
    b. a history of infrared exposure
    c. transillumination defects of the iris
    d. deposition of a flaky material on lens zonule fibers

39. Which method is not effective in treating posterior uveal melanoma?
    a. enucleation
    b. brachytherapy
    c. charged-particle radiation
    d. conventional external-beam radiation
    e. surgical excision

40. Which of the following statements about uveal melanoma is *true*?
    a. Uveal melanomas rarely metastasize.
    b. Melanomas of the ciliary body have the best prognosis.
    c. Metastases always occur within 2½ years of treatment.
    d. Survival is directly related to tumor volume.

41. Which of the following statements about persistent hyperplastic primary vitreous (PHPV) is *true*?
    a. Visual prognosis is excellent.
    b. Early angle-closure glaucoma is common.
    c. Retinal detachment is rare.
    d. The eye is usually normal in size.
    e. Cataract is uncommon.

42. Medulloepitheliomas
    a. are tumors arising from surface ectoderm-derived cells
    b. are congenital lesions often containing cartilage
    c. are usually malignant in nature
    d. can be caused by trauma to the ciliary body
    e. usually metastasize to the liver

43. Which of the following tumors develops in the absence of a normal tumor-suppressor gene?
    a. choroidal melanoma
    b. melanocytoma
    c. medulloepithelioma
    d. retinoblastoma

346 • Study Questions

44. The average volume of the adult vitreous cavity is
    a. 3 cc
    b. 4 cc
    c. 5 cc
    d. 6 cc

45. Which of the following statements about corneal dystrophies is *true*?
    a. They may occur unilaterally.
    b. They are inherited disorders.
    c. Their development often follows surgical or accidental trauma to the eye.
    d. They rarely cause visual symptoms or impairment.
    e. They are never associated with stromal thinning.

46. von Hippel–Lindau syndrome is distinguished from von Hippel disease by the association of
    a. intracranial calcifications, ash leaf spots, retinal astrocytomas
    b. café-au-lait spots, Lisch nodules, optic pathway gliomas
    c. pheochromocytomas, cerebellar hemangioblastomas, renal cell carcinoma
    d. limbal dermoids, upper eyelid colobomas, ear tags

47. Which of the following statements regarding the sclera is *true*?
    a. It consists of type I collagen fibers.
    b. It appears white due to a regular, periodic arrangement of collagen fibers.
    c. The thickest areas are in the region of rectus muscle insertions.
    d. It derives nutrition from its own capillary bed.

48. In intraocular lymphoma associated with CNS lymphoma,
    a. T-cell lymphoma is common
    b. the vitreous and retina are usually involved
    c. the diagnosis is made using routine histopathologic preparations
    d. systemic and intrathecal chemotherapy usually result in a good response

49. Which of the following choices best matches the following description: a lymphoid infiltrate with a vaguely follicular pattern that includes the proliferation of monocytoid B lymphocytes and a heterogeneous mix of small lymphocytes and plasma cells?
    a. reactive lymphoid hyperplasia
    b. mucosa-associated lymphoid tissue (MALT)
    c. small B-cell lymphoma
    d. orbital inflammatory syndrome

Answers

1. **b.** Although many of the processes overlap, this is the overall sequence of events. If this sequence is disrupted, the wound healing process may be altered.

2. **c.** Although immunohistochemistry and PCR can be performed to yield quantitative results, only flow cytometric analysis is inherently quantitative.

3. **c.** Macular dystrophy is autosomal recessive, involves the entire cornea to the limbus, may cause earlier visual disability, and represents deposition of mucopolysaccharide.

4. **d.** Prussian blue detects iron. A Krukenberg spindle is composed of melanin pigment in the endothelium.

5. **b.** B-scan ultrasonography provides information about the size, shape, and position of the tumor; A-scan ultrasonography provides an accurate assessment of the lesion's internal reflectivity, vascularity, and height.

6. **c.** In iris melanoma, as in choroidal melanoma, spindle A, spindle B, and epithelioid cell types can be identified histologically.

7. **c.** Primary intraocular lymphoma and sebaceous cell carcinoma represent 2 of the most common and feared tumors; their presentation can simulate uveitis or other conditions. Although retinoblastoma can masquerade, basal cell carcinoma rarely does this.

8. **d.** Osteosarcoma represents 40% of secondary tumors within, and 36% outside, the field of radiation in patients previously treated for retinoblastoma.

9. **b.** Enucleation remains the recommended treatment for a child with unilateral retinoblastoma filling 50% of the vitreous cavity with diffuse vitreous seeding.

10. **d.** The first 3 behaviors are well accepted for this tumor; however, it does not characteristically resolve.

11. **a.** Intraocular calcification is most diagnostic of retinoblastoma.

12. **c.** The major risk factors found on histopathology that correlate with prognosis include cell type, as defined by the modified Callender classification; tumor size; tumor location (anterior to equator or adjacent to optic nerve); and intrinsic microvascular patterns. Erosion through Bruch's membrane is not correlated with prognosis and occurs frequently. Melanomas rarely invade the optic nerve, more often escaping the eye by eroding through the sclera. Most melanomas are HMB-45–positive, as an indication of their melanocytic origin.

13. **c.** Although iris neovascularization is a typical feature of diabetic ocular disease, iris hemorrhages are not.

14. **c.** Recurrent pterygia represent exuberant healing responses and do not show the elastotic degeneration typical of primary pterygia, which are of long-standing duration.

15. **c.** Breast carcinomas in women are by far the most common source of metastasis to the choroid. Lung carcinomas are the most common source of metastasis to the choroid in men.

16. **c.** The location of the oblique muscles is a key feature in orienting a globe. The inferior oblique inserts most posteriorly, in close proximity to the optic nerve and over the macula.

17. **c.** Although S-100 is expressed in melanomas, it is also expressed in other tumors and tissues of neuroectodermal origin. HMB-45 is more specific for melanocytic lesions and can differentiate a melanoma from other neuroectodermal tumors.

18. **c.** Choice *a* is a cyclodialysis, *b* is an iridodialysis. Angle recession involves separation of the longitudinal portion from the remainder of the ciliary muscle, with corresponding displacement of the iris and a change in angle configuration.

19. **b.** ICE syndrome involves the proliferation of corneal endothelium over the trabecular meshwork and iris, sealing the angle closed. Melanomalytic and ghost cell glaucoma are due to an accumulation of material in the trabecular meshwork, or secondary open-angle glaucoma. Hemosiderosis results in iron deposition and toxicity in the meshwork without other visible changes in the meshwork.

20. **d.** The sclera varies from 0.3 mm behind the rectus muscle insertions to 1 mm posteriorly and is composed mainly of type I collagen.

21. **a.** Anterior scleritis is typically painful and is bilateral in half the cases. Posterior scleritis is associated with exophthalmos and pain with eye movement.

22. **c.** Fibrillin gene mutations are seen in Marfan syndrome, in which the lens is typically displaced superotemporally.

23. **a.** Basal cell carcinoma is by far the most common primary malignancy of the eyelid. It is probably more common than squamous cell carcinoma, sebaceous carcinoma, and melanoma of the eyelid combined.

24. **d.** If a parent has bilateral disease, there is a 98% chance that he or she has a germinal mutation. If the parent has a germinal mutation, the risk for each child is 45%.

25. **a.** The final scar shrinks because of the contraction of myofibroblasts and fibroblasts. The vessels decrease markedly as the scar matures, but a few remain. Part of the distortion of any scar occurs because the collagen laid down in the healing process is not in synchrony with that in the surrounding tissues. Macrophages, which produce many factors in the active healing stage, subside and are absent from the final scar.

26. **b.** Blind eyes may become painful after many years and are enucleated to relieve the pain. Most eyes develop either high intraocular pressure and absolute glaucoma or cease to produce aqueous in adequate amounts to sustain the eye. In the latter case, the eye shrinks and becomes phthisical. The other choices are serious conditions, and each may lead to either glaucoma or phthisis.

27. **d.** The epithelial cells gain access to the globe by migrating along a preexisting tract or wound edge; they are unable to invade normal tissues. Once inside the eye, the epithelium may extend as a sheet over available surfaces, such as posterior cornea or iris, or may form epithelial cysts. Free-floating masses of solid epithelium do not form.

28. **e.** Cotton-wool spots are characteristic of, but not diagnostic of, collagen vascular diseases; they occur in a variety of ischemic retinopathies. They contain swollen nerve fibers, not glial cells. They usually disappear with time. They represent infarcts, with resultant coagulative necrosis of the nerve fiber layer. They are not typically associated with transudates.

29. **b.** Formalin is the most commonly used tissue fixative. Gluteraldehyde is used to fix tissue for electron microscopy. B5 is a mercury-based fixative used for preservation of cytologic detail, primarily in lymphoid tissue. RPMI may be used for flow cytometry specimens.

30. **c.** Frozen sections are not used to satisfy the curiosity of the surgeon or to relieve the anxiety of a patient's family. One should never freeze all excised tissue, because adequate fixation and avoidance of freezing artifact are needed to properly evaluate surgical specimens for diagnostic purposes. One should not try to evaluate the margins of melanocytic proliferations, including melanoma, with frozen sections. Adequate specimen preservation and processing are needed for such evaluation. An appropriate use of frozen sections is to determine if representative tissue is being sampled; if so, more tissue should be submitted in fixative for processing.

31. **d.** A Langhans giant cell has a horseshoe-shaped ring of nuclei around the periphery of the cytoplasm. Langhans giant cells may be encountered in tuberculosis and sarcoidosis, among other diseases. Foreign body giant cells have haphazardly arranged nuclei. Some malignant neoplasms, including melanoma, may contain multinucleated tumor giant cells. Touton giant cells have central nuclei and a peripheral lipid-filled area. Touton giant cells may be seen in association with chalazion, xanthogranuloma, and xanthelasma, among other diseases. Langhans, foreign body, and Touton giant cells are not diagnostic for any single disease process.

32. **a.** Vitreous amyloidosis and peripheral neuropathy are associated with a transthyretin abnormality.

33. **c.** The production of Descemet's membrane by the endothelial cells begins during fetal development and continues throughout adulthood. Therefore, the thickness of Descemet's membrane slowly increases with age.

34. **d.** Band keratopathy involves the interpalpebral region of the cornea and consists of calcium deposition in the epithelial basement membrane and Bowman's layer. Although band keratopathy may occur in patients with hypercalcemia, it also occurs in chronically inflamed eyes of patients with normal serum calcium levels. Band keratopathy is an acquired lesion and is, therefore, not associated with congenital malformations.

35. **e.** Siderosis is caused by the retention of iron-containing metallic foreign bodies in the lens, resulting in lens epithelial degeneration and necrosis. As such, it is an acquired condition rather than a congenital one.

36. **a.** Lymphomas manifesting in the eyelid are associated with systemic lymphoma in approximately 80% of cases; conjunctival and orbital lymphomas are more often localized than disseminated.

37. **d.** PAM with atypia is associated with approximately two thirds of cases of conjunctival melanoma; preexisting nevi are seen in fewer than one fourth. Ocular melanocytosis is

associated with an increased risk of melanoma. Ephelis, or freckle, is not associated with melanoma.

38. **b.** Unlike true exfoliation, exfoliation syndrome (pseudoexfoliation) is not associated with a history of infrared exposure.

39. **d.** Conventional external-beam radiation is not effective in treating uveal melanoma and is not used. Special methods of external-beam radiation such as fractionated stereotactic radiotherapy and gamma knife radiosurgery have been used with good results.

40. **d.** Smaller uveal tumors have the best prognosis overall. Melanomas often metastasize, and 30%–40% of patients die within 5 years of metastatic disease. Ciliary body melanomas in a relatively hidden area often become large before symptoms develop and have a poorer prognosis. The mean duration from treatment to the onset of metastases of uveal melanoma is 7 years.

41. **b.** Because the ciliary processes are often displaced centripetally by a central fibrovascular plaque, early angle-closure glaucoma is common. PHPV commonly occurs in microphthalmic eyes and is associated with cataract and retinal detachment. Visual prognosis is poor.

42. **b.** Medulloepitheliomas are derived from neuroectoderm. They are usually benign choristomas and, even if they are malignant, follow a benign course if the eye is removed with the tumor confined to it. There are developmental lesions—so-called adult medulloepitheliomas—that are actually reactive hyperplasias of the ciliary epithelium and usually related to ocular trauma.

43. **d.** Choroidal melanoma, melanocytoma, and medulloepithelioma are not associated with a tumor-suppressor gene.

44. **b.** The adult vitreous occupies four fifths of the eye, measures 4 cc, and weighs 4 g.

45. **b.** The corneal dystrophies are primary, inherited, bilateral disorders. Patients may have symptoms of recurrent erosion or loss of visual acuity. Some of the dystrophies, such as macular dystrophy, may be associated with stromal thinning.

46. **c.** von Hippel disease consists of a solitary retinal angioma, whereas von Hippel–Lindau includes the spectrum of pheochromocytomas, cerebellar hemangioblastomas, and renal cell carcinomas.

47. **a.** The sclera appears white due to the random arrangement and variable thickness of its collagen fibers compared with the collagen fibers of the cornea, which are parallel, relatively uniform, and regularly arranged. The sclera is thinnest in the region just posterior the rectus muscle insertions, a common location for traumatic scleral rupture. The scleral has blood vessels that pass through it—emissary vessels—but it does not have its own capillary bed. It derives its nutrition from the choroid and episcleral vessels.

48. **b.** Whereas in systemic/visceral/nodal lymphomas the uvea is the most common site of metastasis, in up to 25% of CNS lymphomas the vitreous and retina are the site of involvement.

49. **b.** The best diagnosis in this example is mucosa-associated lymphoid tissue (MALT), also known as extranodal marginal zone lymphoma (EMZL).

Index

(*f* = figure; *t* = table)

A-scan ultrasonography
   in choroidal/ciliary body melanoma, 262, 262*f*
   in choroidal hemangioma, 277, 278*f*
   in metastatic eye disease, 309
ABCA4 gene, in Stargardt disease, 167
Abrasions, corneal, 21–22
Acanthamoeba keratitis, 79, 79*f*
   contact lens wear and, 79, 79*f*
Acantholysis, definition of, 201
Acanthosis, definition of, 201
Accessory lacrimal glands
   of Krause, 199, 201*t*
   of Wolfring, 199, 201*t*
Acral-lentiginous melanoma, 218
Actin, in immunohistochemistry, 41
Actinic (Labrador) keratopathy (spheroidal degeneration), 81, 81*f*
Actinic (solar) keratosis, 210, 210*f*, 211*f*
Acute retinal necrosis, 144, 144*f*
Adenocarcinoma, of retinal pigment epithelium, 178, 275
Adenoid cystic carcinoma, of lacrimal glands, 227–228, 228*f*
Adenoma
   Fuchs (pseudoadenomatous hyperplasia), 177, 275
   pleomorphic (benign mixed tumor), of lacrimal gland, 226, 227*f*
   of retinal pigment epithelium, 178, 275
   of uvea/retina, 275
Adenomatous polyposis, familial (Gardner syndrome), retinal manifestations of, 143–144
Adipose tumors, of orbit, 236
Adult-onset foveomacular vitelliform dystrophy, 168–170, 169*f*
AFMVD. *See* Adult-onset foveomacular vitelliform dystrophy
Age/aging
   of sclera, 105, 106*f*
   syneresis and, 126, 127*f*
Age-related macular degeneration/maculopathy (senile macular degeneration), 161–165, 162*f*, 163*f*, 164*f*
   drusen associated with, 161–163, 162*f*
   dry (nonexudative), 163
   melanoma differentiated from, 264–265
   wet (exudative), 163–164, 164*f*
AJCC (American Joint Committee on Cancer), definitions/staging of ocular tumors by, 321–329*t*
Albinism, 140–142, 141*f*
Albinoidism, 140
Alcian blue stain, 38, 39*t*
Alizarin red stain, 39*t*
Alveolar rhabdomyosarcoma, 233, 233*f*
AMD. *See* Age-related macular degeneration
Amelanotic choroidal masses, differential diagnosis of, 264*t*
American Joint Committee on Cancer (AJCC), definitions/staging of ocular tumors by, 321–329*t*
Amiodarone, keratopathy caused by, 83

Amyloidosis/amyloid deposits
   conjunctival, 61–62, 62*f*
   corneal
      in Avellino dystrophy, 87
      in lattice dystrophy, 86–87, 87*f*, 205
   in eyelid, 205–207, 206*f*, 206*t*
   orbital, 225, 225*f*
   vitreous involvement in, 128–129, 129*f*
Anesthesia, examination under, in retinoblastoma, 291, 291*f*
Aneurysms
   Leber miliary, 142
   retinal arterial, microaneurysms, ischemia causing, 155, 155*f*
Angiography, fluorescein. *See* Fluorescein angiography
Angiomas (angiomatosis)
   encephalofacial/cerebrofacial/encephalotrigeminal. *See* Sturge-Weber disease/syndrome
   racemose (Wyburn-Mason syndrome), 282*f*, 283
   retinae, 280–281, 280*f*
Angiomatous tumors, 277–283. *See also specific type*
Angle-closure glaucoma, nanophthalmos and, 103
Angle recession, posttraumatic, 27, 27*f*, 97, 98*f*
   glaucoma and, 96–97
Aniridia, 181–182
Anomalies, congenital. *See specific type and* Congenital anomalies
Anterior basement membrane dystrophy, 83, 85*f*
Anterior chamber
   congenital anomalies of, 91–94, 93*f*
   degenerations of, 94–100
   depth of, 91
   disorders of, 91–100. *See also specific type*
   neoplastic, 100
   pigment in, 98–100, 98*f*
   topography of, 91, 92*f*
Anterior chamber angle, 92*f*
   traumatic recession of, 27, 27*f*, 97, 98*f*
      glaucoma and, 96–97
Anterior lenticonus, 114
Anterior segment, metastatic disease of, 306
Anterior uveitis, granulomatous, iris nodules in, 256*t*
Antiangiogenic agents, for retinal capillary hemangioma, 281
Antioxidants, age-related macular degeneration and, 161
Antoni A pattern/Antoni B pattern, in schwannomas, 236, 236*f*
Appendage neoplasms, 213–215, 214*f*, 215*f*
Arachnoid mater, optic nerve, 237, 238*f*
Argon laser therapy
   for choroidal hemangioma, 196
   for diabetic retinopathy/macular edema, 160
ARN. *See* Acute retinal necrosis
Array (microarray-based) comparative genomic hybridization (array CGH), 49*t*
Arterial occlusive disease, retinal
   branch retinal artery occlusion, 156
   central retinal artery occlusion, 156, 157*f*

351

Arteriovenous malformations, congenital retinal, 282*f*, 283
Arteritis, giant cell, optic nerve affected in, 240
Ascending optic atrophy, 241
Aspergillus (aspergillosis), orbital infection caused by, 222, 222*f*
Asteroid bodies, 128, 128*f*
　in sarcoidosis, 185
Asteroid hyalosis, 128, 128*f*
Astrocytes, 237
　gliomas originating in, 243
Astrocytoma (astrocytic hamartoma)
　pilocytic, juvenile, of optic nerve, 243, 244*f*
　retinoblastoma differentiated from, 293–294, 294*f*
Atrophia bulbi
　with disorganization (phthisis bulbi), 30–31, 31*f*
　with shrinkage, 31
　without shrinkage, 30, 31*f*
Atypia, cellular
　dysplastic nevi and, 218
　primary acquired melanosis and, 68–70, 70*f*, 71*f*
Avellino dystrophy, 87
Axenfeld anomaly/syndrome, 92, 93*f*
Axenfeld loop, 101, 102*f*
Axenfeld-Rieger syndrome, 91–94, 93*f*
　glaucoma associated with, 91

B&B stain (Brown and Brenn stain), 39*t*
B&H stain (Brown and Hopps stain), 39*t*
B-cell lymphomas
　intraocular, 313–315, 314*f*. *See also* Lymphomas, intraocular
　　vitreous involvement in, 133–135, 134*f*, 135*f*
　orbital, 228–230, 229*f*
B cells (B lymphocytes), 15
B-scan ultrasonography
　in choroidal/ciliary body melanoma, 262–263, 262*f*
　in choroidal hemangioma, 277–278, 278*f*
　in metastatic eye disease, 309
Bacteria
　conjunctivitis caused by, 57, 59*f*
　corneal infections caused by, 77–78
　endophthalmitis caused by, vitreous affected in, 125–126, 126*f*
　eyelid infections caused by, 202–203, 203*f*
　keratitis caused by, 77–78
　optic nerve infections caused by, 239
　orbital infections caused by, 221
Band keratopathy, 80, 81*f*
Basal cell carcinoma, of eyelid, 208*t*, 212–213, 212*f*, 213*f*
Basal cell nevus syndrome (Gorlin syndrome), eyelid manifestations of, 208*t*
Basal lamina (basal cell layer), drusen of (cuticular drusen), 163
Basal laminar deposits, 161
Basal linear deposits, 161
Basement membrane dystrophies, corneal epithelial, 83, 85*f*
Basophils, 14, 14*f*
Bear tracks (grouped pigmentation of retina), 265, 266*f*
Benign hereditary intraepithelial dyskeratosis, 64
Benign melanosis, 69*t*

Benign mixed tumor (pleomorphic adenoma), of lacrimal gland, 226, 227*f*
Benign reactive lymphoid hyperplasia. *See* Lymphoid hyperplasia
Bergmeister papilla, 125
Berlin edema (commotio retinae), 30
Best disease (vitelliform macular dystrophy), 167–168
Bestrophin, mutations in, 167
Biomicroscopy, slit-lamp
　in choroidal/ciliary body melanoma, 262
　in iris nevus, 251
Birth defects. *See specific type and* Congenital anomalies
Bladder (Wedl) cells, 115, 116*f*
Blindness
　age-related macular degeneration causing, 161
　diabetic retinopathy causing, 159
Blood, cornea stained by, 88–89, 89*f*
Blunt trauma, glaucoma and, 96–97
Bony orbit. *See* Orbit
Bony tumors, of orbit, 234–235
Borderline neoplastic proliferations, 17
Botryoid rhabdomyosarcoma, 234
Bowman's layer/membrane, 73, 74*f*
BPD. *See* Butterfly pattern dystrophy
Brachytherapy
　for choroidal hemangioma, 278
　for melanoma, 271, 271*f*
　　of iris, 255
　for metastatic eye disease, 312
　for retinoblastoma, 300–301
Branch retinal artery occlusion, 156
Branch retinal vein occlusion, 159
　neovascularization in, 155
BRAO. *See* Branch retinal artery occlusion
Brawny scleritis, 104, 104*f*
Breast cancer, eye involvement and, 306*t*, 307*f*, 310*f*, 312
Brown and Brenn (B&B) stain, 39*t*
Brown and Hopps (B&H) stain, 39*t*
Bruch's membrane
　choroidal neovascularization and, in age-related macular degeneration, 163–164, 164*f*
　rupture of, 28
Brücke's muscle, 180
Brushfield spots, 256*t*, 258*f*
BRVO. *See* Branch retinal vein occlusion
Bulbar conjunctiva, 53, 54*f*
Bullous keratopathy, 82–83, 82*f*
Burkitt lymphoma, of orbit, 229–230
Busacca nodules
　in iridocyclitis, 256*t*
　in sarcoidosis, 185, 258*f*
Butterfly pattern dystrophy, 168

c-Kit, in immunohistochemistry, 42
Calcific drusen, 163
Calcific plaques, senile, 105, 106*f*
Callender classification, of uveal melanomas, 190
Candlewax drippings, in sarcoidosis, 147, 185
Capillary hemangiomas
　of eyelid, 213
　of orbit, 230, 232*f*
　of retina, 280–281, 280*f*

Carcinoma, 17f, 17t. *See also* Adenocarcinoma; Carcinoma in situ
  adenoid cystic, of lacrimal glands, 227–228, 228f
  basal cell, of eyelid, 208t, 212–213, 212f, 213f
  of conjunctiva, 64–66, 65f
    squamous cell, 64–66, 65f
    staging of, 321t
  of eyelid, 211–213, 211f, 212f, 213f
  metastatic, 305–312. *See also specific type and structure affected*
    ancillary tests in evaluation of, 308–310, 311f
    clinical features of, 306–308, 307f, 308f, 309f, 310f, 310t
    diagnostic factors in, 310–311
    mechanisms of spread and, 306
    primary sites and, 305, 306t
    prognosis for, 311–312
    treatment of, 312
  sebaceous, 213–215, 214f, 215f
  squamous cell
    of conjunctiva, 64–66, 65f
    of eyelid, 211–212, 211f
      actinic keratosis and, 210, 211
      retinoblastoma associated with, 302t
  thyroid, retinoblastoma associated with, 302t
Carcinoma in situ
  of conjunctiva, 63f, 65f
  of cornea, 90
Carney complex, eyelid manifestations of, 206t
Caruncle, 53
Caseating granulomas, 14, 15f
Cataract, 113–118
  cerulean, 114
  congenital and infantile, 111–112
  coronary, 114
  hypermature, phacolytic glaucoma and, 96, 113
  morgagnian, 117, 118f
  nuclear, 118, 119f
  persistent fetal vasculature (persistent hyperplastic primary vitreous) and, 112
  posterior polar, 112
    retinoblastoma differentiated from, 292t
  rubella, 112
  subcapsular
    anterior (subcapsular fibrous plaques), 115, 115f
    posterior (cupuliform), 115, 116f
  traumatic, 28
Cataract surgery, endophthalmitis after, 120
Cavernous hemangioma, 12
  of orbit, 12, 230, 232f
  of retina, 281–283, 282f
Cavernous optic atrophy of Schnabel, 241–242, 242f
Cellular atypia
  dysplastic nevi and, 218
  primary acquired melanosis and, 68–70, 70f, 71f
Cellulitis, 202–203, 203f
  preseptal, 203, 203f
Central areolar pigment epithelial atrophy, 163
Central retinal artery, occlusion of, 156, 157f
Central retinal vein, occlusion of, 157–158, 158f
  nonperfused, 157
Cerulean cataract, 114

CGH. *See* Comparative genomic hybridization
Chalazion, 203–205, 204f
Chandler syndrome, 94
Charged-particle radiation
  for choroidal hemangioma, 278
  for melanoma, 271–272
  for retinal capillary hemangioma, 281
CHED. *See* Congenital hereditary endothelial dystrophy
Chédiak-Higashi syndrome, 141
Chemotherapy (cancer)
  for lymphoma, 315
  for melanoma, 273
  for metastatic eye disease, 312
  for retinoblastoma, 298–299, 298f, 299f
Children, staphylomas in, 77, 106
Chlamydia trachomatis, conjunctivitis caused by, 57–58, 59f
Chloroma (granulocytic sarcoma), 317
Cholesterol emboli (Hollenhorst plaques), in branch retinal artery occlusion, 156
Choriocapillaris, 181, 182f
Chorioretinitis
  fungal, 145–146, 146f
  sclopetaria, 30, 197
Choristomas, 12
  complex, 54
  conjunctival, 53–54, 55f
  episcleral osseous, 103
  phakomatous (Zimmerman tumor), 202
  scleral, 102
Choroid
  amelanotic masses of, differential diagnosis of, 264t
  coloboma of, retinoblastoma differentiated from, 292t
  detachment of, 197
  focal posttraumatic granulomatous inflammation of, 30, 30f
  hemangiomas of, 195–196, 195f, 277–280, 278f, 279f
    in Sturge-Weber syndrome, 195, 277
  in leukemia, 317
  lymphoid proliferation in, 196–197
  melanocytoma of, 189, 254
  melanoma of, 189–193, 191f, 192f, 193f, 194f, 249, 259–275, 261f. *See also* Choroidal/ciliary body melanoma
    nevus differentiated from, 252, 264
    staging of, 325–326t
  neovascularization of, 30, 187, 187f
    in age-related macular degeneration, 163–164, 164f
  nevus of, 189, 189f, 251–254, 253f
    melanoma differentiated from, 252, 264
  osteoma of, 196
    melanoma differentiated from, 266–267, 267f
  rupture of, 30, 30f, 197
  topography of, 179f, 181, 182f
  tumors of, 189–193
    metastatic, 194, 194f, 306, 306t, 307f, 308f, 309f, 310t
  vasculature of, retina supplied by, 138
  wound healing and, 25

Choroidal/ciliary body melanoma (posterior uveal melanoma), 189–193, 191f, 192f, 193f, 194f, 249, 259–275, 260f, 261f
  classification of, 267, 268t
  diagnosis of, 260–264, 262f, 263f
    differential, 264–267, 264t, 265f, 266f
  epithelioid, 190, 191f
  incidence of, 189, 259
  metastatic, 194
    evaluation of, 268–269, 269t
  prognosis for, 190–191, 273–275
  spindle cell, 190, 191f
  spread of, 191–193, 192f, 193f, 194
  staging of, 325–326t
  treatment of, 270–273
Choroidal neovascularization, 30, 187, 187f
  in age-related macular degeneration, 163–164, 164f
Choroidal/suprachoroidal hemorrhage, expulsive, 27, 28f
Choroidal vasculopathy, polypoidal (posterior uveal bleeding syndrome), 165–167, 166f
Chromogens, in immunohistochemistry, 41, 43f
Chromogranin, in immunohistochemistry, 42, 43f
Chromosomal banding, 48t
Chronic lymphocytic leukemia (CLL) type lymphoma, of orbit, 229
CHRPE. See Congenital hypertrophy of retinal pigment epithelium
Ciliary body
  hyalinization of, 187
  melanocytoma of, 189, 254
  melanoma of, 189–193, 191f, 192f, 193f, 194f, 249, 259–275, 260f. See also Choroidal/ciliary body melanoma
    nevus differentiated from, 252, 264
    staging of, 325–326t
  metastatic disease of, 306
  neoplastic disorders of, 189–193
  nevus of, 189f, 198, 251–254
  tear in (angle recession), 27, 27f, 97, 98f
    glaucoma and, 96–97
  topography of, 179f, 180, 181f
  wound healing and, 25
Ciliary epithelium
  benign adenomas and cysts of, 275
  medulloepithelioma (diktyoma) of, 176–177, 177f, 319, 320f
  pigmented, acquired hyperplasia of, 276
CIN. See Conjunctival intraepithelial neoplasia
Circumscribed (localized) choroidal hemangioma, 195, 277, 278f
Circumscribed iris nevus, 251
CLL type lymphoma. See Chronic lymphocytic leukemia (CLL) type lymphoma
Clump cells, in iris, 180
CMV. See Cytomegaloviruses
Coats disease, 142, 143f
  retinoblastoma differentiated from, 291–292, 292t, 293f
Cobblestone (paving-stone) degeneration, 149, 150f
Coccidioides immitis (coccidioidomycosis), optic nerve infection caused by, 239
Cogan microcystic dystrophy, 83, 85f

Cogan-Reese (iris nevus) syndrome, 94, 256t
Coherence tomography, optical. See Optical coherence tomography
Collaborative Ocular Melanoma Study (COMS), 249, 268, 274–275
Colloidal iron stain, 38, 39t
Colobomas
  optic nerve/optic disc, 239
  retinoblastoma differentiated from, 292t
  uveal, 182
Combined hamartoma, of retina and retinal pigment epithelium, 177–178, 276, 276f
Commotio retinae (Berlin edema), 30
Communication, between clinician and pathologist, 33–34
Comparative genomic hybridization (CGH), 48–49t
  microarray-based (array CGH), 49t
Complex choristomas, 54
Compound nevi
  of conjunctiva, 68, 69f
  of eyelid, 216, 217f
Compromised host. See Immunocompromised host
Computed tomography (CT scan)
  in choroidal/ciliary body melanoma, 264
  in retinoblastoma, 291, 296
COMS (Collaborative Ocular Melanoma Study), 249, 268, 274–275
Cone inner segments, 138, 138f
Cone outer segments, 138, 138f
Cones, 138, 138f
  retinoblastoma and, 171
Congenital anomalies, 12, 13f. See also specific type
  of anterior chamber, 91–94, 93f
  of conjunctiva, 53–55, 54f, 55f
  of cornea, 74–77
  of eyelid, 201–202
  of lens, 110–112, 111f, 111t
  of optic disc and nerve, 239, 239f
  of orbit, 220, 221f
  of retina and retinal pigment epithelium, 139–144, 141f, 143f
  of sclera, 102–103
  of trabecular meshwork, 91–94, 93f
  of uveal tract, 181–182
  of vitreous, 124–125, 124f
Congenital cataract, 111
Congenital hereditary endothelial dystrophy, 74–75, 75f
Congenital hypertrophy of retinal pigment epithelium (CHRPE), 142–144, 143f
  melanoma differentiated from, 143, 265, 265f
Congenital rubella syndrome, cataracts and, 112
Congenital syphilis, corneal manifestations of/interstitial keratitis, 80
Congo red stain, 38, 39t
Conjunctiva
  amyloid deposits in, 61–62, 62f
  bulbar, 53, 54f
  carcinoma of, 64–66, 65f
    squamous cell, 64–66, 65f
    staging of, 321t
  congenital anomalies of, 53–55, 54f, 55f
  cysts of, 56, 56f
    nevi and, 68, 69f

degenerations of, 60–62, 60f, 61f, 62f
disorders of, 53–71. *See also specific type*
  neoplastic, 62–71
dysplasia of, 63f, 64, 65f
epithelium of
  cysts of, 56, 56f
    nevi and, 68, 69f
  dysplasia of, 63f, 64, 65f
  tumors of, 62–66, 63f, 65f
foreign body on, 60
forniceal, 53, 54f
goblet cells in, 53, 54f, 201t
infection/inflammation of, 55–60, 56f. *See also* Conjunctivitis
intraepithelial neoplasia of (CIN), 63f, 64, 65f
lymphoma of, 67, 67f, 68f
melanocytic lesions of, 68–71, 69f, 69t, 70f, 71f
melanoma of, 70–71, 71f
  primary acquired melanosis and, 70, 71f
  staging of, 322t
nevus of, 68, 69f, 69t
palpebral, 53, 54f, 199–201, 200f
papillomas of, 62–64, 63f
stroma of, 53
subepithelial lesions of, 66–67, 66f, 67f, 68f
topography of, 53, 54f
tumors of, 62–71
  human papillomaviruses causing, 62–64, 63f
  staging of, 321–322t
Conjunctival inclusion cysts, 56, 56f
  nevi and, 68, 69f
Conjunctival intraepithelial neoplasia (CIN), 63f, 64, 65f
Conjunctivitis, 55–60
  acute, 55
  bacterial, 57, 59f
  chronic, 55–56
  follicular, 56, 57f, 58f
  giant papillary (contact lens–induced), 56
  Haemophilus causing, 57
  infectious, 57–58, 59f
  noninfectious, 58–60
  papillary, 56, 57f
  in Parinaud oculoglandular syndrome, 60
  viral, 57, 59f
Contact inhibition, in corneal wound repair, 21
Contact lenses
  Acanthamoeba keratitis associated with, 79, 79f
  conjunctivitis caused by (giant papillary conjunctivitis), 56
Contraction, wound, 21
Copper, corneal deposition of, Kayser-Fleischer ring caused by, 89
Cornea
  abrasions of, 21–22
  amyloid deposits in
    in Avellino dystrophy, 87
    in lattice dystrophy, 86–87, 87f, 205
  blood staining of, 88–89, 89f
  Bowman's layer/membrane of, 73, 74f
  congenital/developmental anomalies of, 74–77
  degenerations/dystrophies of, 80–88. *See also specific type and* Corneal degenerations; Corneal dystrophies

diameter of, 73
disorders of, 73–90. *See also specific type and* Keratitis; Keratopathy
  intraocular lenses and, 121
  neoplastic, 89–90, 90f. *See also specific tumor type*
dysplasia of, 89–90, 90f
edema of, intraocular lenses and, 121
endothelium of, 73, 74f
  wound healing/repair of, 23f, 24
epithelium of, 73, 74f
  dysplasia of, 89–90, 90f
  wound healing/repair of, 21–22, 23–24, 23f
foreign body in, 80
guttae in, in Fuchs dystrophy, 88, 88f
infection/inflammation of, 77–80, 78f, 79f. *See also* Keratitis
intraepithelial neoplasia of, 89
pigmentation/pigment deposits in, 88–89, 89f
scleralization of, 76–77
staphyloma of, congenital, 77
stroma of, 73, 74f
  wound healing/repair of, 22–23
thickness of, 73
topography of, 73, 74f
tumors of, 89–90, 90f. *See also specific type*
wound healing/repair of, 21–24, 23f
Corneal buttons, 83, 88
Corneal degenerations, 80–83. *See also specific type and* Keratopathy
  drug-related, 83
Corneal dystrophies, 83–88, 87t. *See also specific type*
  endothelial, Fuchs, 88, 88f
  epithelial, basement membrane (map-dot-fingerprint/anterior membrane), 83, 85f
Corneal intraepithelial neoplasia, 89
Corneal nodules, Salzmann, 80
Corneoscleral meshwork, 91
Coronary cataract, 114
Cortex
  lens, 109
    degenerations of, 117, 117f, 118f
  vitreous, 123
Corticosteroids (steroids)
  for idiopathic orbital inflammation, 224
  for uveal lymphoid infiltration, 316
Cotton-wool spots, 151
  in leukemia, 317
Cowden disease, eyelid manifestations of, 208t
CRAO. *See* Central retinal artery, occlusion of
CRVO. *See* Central retinal vein, occlusion of
Cryotherapy
  for melanoma, 272
  for retinal angiomas/hemangiomas, 281
  for retinoblastoma, 300
Cryptococcus neoformans (cryptococcosis), optic nerve infection caused by, 239
Crystal violet stain, 39t
Cuticular (basal laminar) drusen, 163
Cyclodialysis, 27, 27f, 97
Cystic carcinoma, adenoid, of lacrimal glands, 227–228, 228f
Cystoid degeneration, peripheral, 147, 148f
Cystoid macular edema, intraocular lenses and, 121

Cytoid bodies, 151, 151f
Cytokeratins, in immunohistochemistry, 41
Cytomegaloviruses, retinitis caused by, 144, 145f

Dacryoadenitis, sclerosing, 224
Dalen-Fuchs nodules/spots, in sympathetic ophthalmia, 184, 184f
Decentration, of intraocular lenses, 119, 120f
Degenerations
  anterior chamber/trabecular meshwork, 94–100
  chorioretinal, generalized, 170f, 171
  conjunctival, 60–62, 60f, 61f, 62f
  corneal, 80–83
  definition of, 16
  elastotic/elastoid (elastosis), 60, 60f
    solar, of eyelid, 210, 211f
  eyelid, 205–207, 205f, 206f, 206t
  lens, 113–118. *See also* Cataract
  optic nerve, 241–243, 241f, 242f
  orbital, 225, 225f
  retinal, 147–171
  scleral, 105–106, 106f
  uveal tract, 186–187, 186t, 187f
  vitreous, 126–132
Degenerative retinoschisis, typical and reticular, 147–148
Dendrites, in herpes simplex virus keratitis, 78, 78f
Dermatan sulfate–proteoglycan, in cornea, macular dystrophy and, 84
Dermatomyositis, eyelid manifestations of, 206t
Dermis, eyelid, 199, 200f
  neoplasms of, 213
Dermoids (dermoid cysts/tumors), 12
  conjunctival, 53–54
  corneal, 75, 76f
  of eyelid, 202
  Goldenhar syndrome and, 54
  limbal, 53–54
  orbital, 220, 221f
Dermolipomas (lipodermoids), 54, 55f
  Goldenhar syndrome and, 54
Descemet's membrane/layer, 73, 74f
  guttae in, in Fuchs dystrophy, 88, 88f
  rupture of, 28, 28f, 29f
    in keratoconus, 28, 28f, 83, 84f
Descending optic atrophy, 241
Desmin, in immunohistochemistry, 41
Diabetic retinopathy, 159–160, 160f
Diagnostic electron microscopy, 42t, 47
Diathermy
  for retinal capillary hemangioma, 281
  transscleral, contraindications to, 272
Diffuse choroidal hemangioma, 195, 277, 279f
Diffuse drusen, 161, 162f
Diffuse iris nevus, 251
Diktyoma (medulloepithelioma), 176–177, 177f, 319, 320f
  teratoid, 177
Dilator muscle, 180, 180f
Diode laser, hyperthermia with
  for melanoma, 272
  for retinoblastoma, 299
Dislocated lens, 28, 110–111, 111f. *See also* Ectopia lentis

Dissection, gross, for pathologic examination, 35–37, 36f
Distichiasis, 202
Dot-and-blot hemorrhages, ischemia causing, 154f, 155
Down syndrome (trisomy 21/trisomy G syndrome), Brushfield spots in, 256t, 258f
Drugs, keratopathy caused by, 83
Drusen
  in age-related macular degeneration, 161–163, 162f
  calcific, 163
  cuticular (basal laminar), 163
  diffuse, 161, 162f
  giant, 243
    retinoblastoma differentiated from, 293–294
  hard, 161, 162f
  optic disc/nerve, 242–243, 242f
  soft, 162, 162f
Dura mater, optic nerve, 237, 238f
Dyskeratosis, 210, 210f, 211f
  benign hereditary intraepithelial, 64
  definition of, 201
Dysplasia
  of bony orbit, 234–235
  of conjunctival epithelium, 63f, 64, 65f
  of corneal epithelium, 89–90, 90f
  retinal, retinoblastoma differentiated from, 292t
Dysplastic nevus, 218
Dystrophies
  corneal, 83–88. *See also specific type*
  definition of, 16
  foveomacular, 168–170, 169f
  pattern, 168–170, 169f

Eccrine sweat glands, of eyelid, 201t
Ectopia lentis, 110–111, 111f, 111t
  simple, 110
  systemic conditions associated with, 111t
Ectropion uveae, 186
  iris nevus causing, 187
Edema
  macular. *See* Macular edema
  retinal, 152–154, 152f, 153f
Elastoid (elastotic) degeneration/elastosis, 60, 60f
  solar, of eyelid, 210, 211f
Electron microscopy, diagnostic, 42t, 47
Elevated intraocular pressure, lens epithelium affected by, 115
11p13 syndrome, in aniridia, 182
ELM. *See* External limiting membrane
ELOV4 gene, in Stargardt disease, 167
Elschnig pearls, 116, 116f
Emboli, cholesterol (Hollenhorst plaques), in branch retinal artery occlusion, 156
Embryonal rhabdomyosarcoma, 233, 233f, 234
Embryotoxon, posterior, 91, 93f
Emissaria/emissarial channels, 101, 102f
  melanoma spread via, 192, 193f
Encephalofacial angiomatosis. *See* Sturge-Weber disease/syndrome
Endophthalmitis
  bacterial, vitreous affected in, 125–126, 126f
  fungal
    iris nodule in, 256t
    vitreous affected in, 125

phacoantigenic (lens-induced granulomatous/
    phacoanaphylactic), 112, 112*f*, 113*f*
  postoperative, after cataract surgery, 120
  Propionibacterium acnes causing, 113, 114*f*
Endothelial dystrophies, congenital hereditary, 74–75, 75*f*
Endothelial meshwork, 91, 92*f*
Endothelium, corneal, 73, 74*f*
  wound healing/repair of, 23*f*, 24
Enucleation
  for melanoma, 270
  for retinoblastoma, 297
  rubeosis iridis and, 186
  for uveal lymphoid infiltration, 316
Eosinophils, 13–14, 13*f*
Ephelis, 216. *See also* Freckle
  conjunctival, 69*t*
Epidermal cysts, of orbit, 220
Epidermis, eyelid, 199, 200*f*
  neoplasms of, 207–213
Episclera, 101
  nodular fasciitis causing tumor of, 106–107
Episcleral osseous choristoma, 103
Episcleritis, 103
Epithelial cysts
  of ciliary epithelium, 275
  of orbit, 220, 221*f*
Epithelial dystrophies, 83, 85*f*
Epithelial hyperplasias
  of lens, 115–116, 115*f*
  of pigmented ciliary/retinal epithelium, 276
Epithelial inclusion cysts, conjunctival, 56, 56*f*
  nevi and, 68, 69*f*
Epithelial invasion of iris, 256*t*
Epithelial tumors, pigmented, of uvea and retina, 275–276, 276*f*
Epithelioid cell melanoma, 190, 191*f*
Epithelioid histiocytes, 14–15, 14*f*
Epithelium
  ciliary
    benign adenomas and cysts of, 275
    pigmented, acquired hyperplasia of, 276
  conjunctival, 53, 54*f*
    cysts of, 56, 56*f*
      nevi and, 68, 69*f*
    dysplasia of, 63*f*, 64, 65*f*
    lesions of, 62–66, 63*f*, 65*f*
  corneal, 73, 74*f*
    dysplasia of, 89–90, 90*f*
    wound healing/repair of, 21–22, 23–24, 23*f*
  lens, 109
    abnormalities of, 115–116, 115*f*, 116*f*
Erdheim-Chester disease, eyelid manifestations of, 206*t*
Essential iris atrophy, 94
Ethmoid bone, 219, 220*f*
Ewing sarcoma, retinoblastoma associated with, 302*t*
Examination, for retinoblastoma, 291, 291*f*
Exenteration, for melanoma, 273
Exfoliation, true, 95
Exfoliation syndrome (pseudoexfoliation), 95, 95*f*, 96*f*, 114, 114*f*
Exophthalmos. *See* Proptosis
Exorbitism. *See* Proptosis
Expulsive choroidal/suprachoroidal hemorrhage, 27, 28*f*

External-beam radiation
  for choroidal hemangioma, 278
  for lymphoma, 315
  for melanoma, 272
  for metastatic eye disease, 312
  for retinal capillary hemangioma, 281
  for retinoblastoma, 300
    secondary tumors and, 176, 302
  for uveal lymphoid infiltration, 316
External hordeolum (stye), 202
External limiting membrane, 138
Exudates, hard, 152, 152*f*, 153*f*
  in leukemia, 317
Eye
  congenital anomalies of, 12, 13*f*
  phthisical (phthisis bulbi), 30–31, 31*f*
  tumors of. *See* Intraocular tumors
Eyelids
  amyloid deposits in, 205–207, 206*f*, 206*t*
  basal cell carcinoma of, 208*t*, 212–213, 212*f*, 213*f*
  congenital anomalies of, 201–202
  degenerations of, 205–207, 205*f*, 206*f*, 206*t*
  disorders of, 199–218. *See also specific type*
    congenital, 201–202
    neoplastic, 207–218. *See also* Eyelids, tumors of
  dyskeratosis of, 210, 210*f*, 211*f*
  glands of, 199–201, 201*t*
  infection/inflammation of, 202–205, 203*f*, 204*f*
  keratosis of
    actinic (solar), 210, 210*f*, 211*f*
    seborrheic, 207–208, 207*f*, 208*f*
  papillomas of, 203
  retraction of, 199
  skin of, 199, 200*f*
  squamous cell carcinoma of, 211–212, 211*f*
    actinic keratosis and, 210, 211
  systemic diseases manifesting in, 205, 206*t*
  topography of, 199–201, 200*f*, 201*t*
  tumors of, 207–218
    appendage neoplasms, 213–215, 214*f*, 215*f*
    basal cell carcinoma, 208*t*, 212–213, 212*f*, 213*f*
    dermal, 213
    epidermal, 207–213
    malignant, staging of, 327*t*
    melanocytic, 215–218, 215*f*, 216*f*, 217*f*
      malignant (melanoma), 218
    papillomas, 203
    squamous cell carcinoma, 211–212, 211*f*
      actinic keratosis and, 210, 211
    systemic malignancies and, 208, 208*t*
  wound healing/repair and, 26

Familial adenomatous polyposis (Gardner syndrome), retinal manifestations of, 143–144
Familial amyloid polyneuropathy, 129, 129*f*, 205
FAP. *See* Familial amyloid polyneuropathy
Fasciitis, nodular, episcleral tumor caused by, 106–107
Ferry lines, 89
Fetal vasculature, persistent. *See* Persistent fetal vasculature
Fiber layer of Henle, 139. *See also* Nerve fiber layer
Fibrocellular proliferation, intraocular, 29–30
Fibroma, ossifying, of orbit, 235

Fibrosarcoma, retinoblastoma associated with, 302t
Fibrous dysplasia, of orbit, 234–235
Fibrous histiocytoma (fibroxanthoma)
    orbital, 234, 234f
    scleral, 106
Fibrovascular pannus, 82, 82f
Fibroxanthoma. See Fibrous histiocytoma
Fine-needle aspiration biopsy (FNAB), 42t, 47–50, 50f, 249
    in metastatic eye disease, 309
    in uveal lymphoid infiltration, 316
Fixatives, for tissue processing, 37, 37t
Flame hemorrhages, ischemia causing, 154f, 155
Fleischer ring/line, in keratoconus, 83, 84f, 89
Fleurettes, in retinoblastoma, 174, 174f
Flexner-Wintersteiner rosettes, in retinoblastoma, 173, 174f, 296
Flow cytometry, 44–45, 45f, 46f
Fluorescein angiography
    in choroidal/ciliary body melanoma, 263
    in choroidal hemangioma, 277
    of conjunctiva, 54–55
    in iris melanoma, 255
    in lymphoma, 313
    in metastatic eye disease, 308
    in retinal disease
        capillary hemangioma, 281
        cavernous hemangioma, 281
Fluorescence in situ hybridization (FISH), 48t
FNAB. See Fine-needle aspiration biopsy
Follicular center lymphoma, of orbit, 229
Follicular conjunctivitis, 56, 57f, 58f
Foreign bodies, intraocular
    conjunctival, 60
    corneal, 80
    of iris, 256t
    retained, siderosis and, 115
Foreign body giant cells, 15, 15f
Formalin, as tissue fixative, 37, 37t
Fornices, 53, 54f
Fovea (fovea centralis), 139
Foveola, 139, 140f
Foveomacular vitelliform dystrophy, adult-onset, 168–170, 169f
Fraser syndrome (cryptophthalmos-syndactyly), eyelid manifestations of, 206t
Freckle, 216
    conjunctival, 69t
    iris, 256t, 258f
Frontal bone, 219, 220f
Frozen section, for pathologic examination, 42t, 50–51
Fuchs adenoma (pseudoadenomatous hyperplasia), 177, 275
Fuchs dystrophy, 88, 88f
Fundus
    evaluation of, in choroidal/ciliary body melanoma, 262, 263
    flavimaculatus (Stargardt disease/juvenile macular degeneration), 167, 168f
    tomato catsup, 195, 277, 279f
Fundus photography, in choroidal/ciliary body melanoma, 263
Fungi
    chorioretinitis caused by, 145–146, 146f
    endophthalmitis caused by
        iris nodule in, 256t
        vitreous in, 125
    eyelid infections caused by, 202
    keratitis caused by, 78–79, 78f
    optic nerve infections caused by, 239
    orbital infections caused by, 221–222
    retinal infections caused by, 145–146, 146f

Ganglion cells, retinal, 137, 138f
Gardner syndrome (familial adenomatous polyposis), retinal manifestations of, 143–144
Gastrointestinal carcinoma, eye/orbital metastases of, 306t
Gelsolin gene, mutation in, amyloid deposits and, 205
Gene therapy, for retinoblastoma, 301
Genetic/hereditary factors, in retinoblastoma, 172, 249, 285–287, 287f
Genetic testing/counseling, in retinoblastoma, 285–287, 287f
Ghost cell glaucoma, 96, 97f, 126
Ghost cells, 96, 97f, 126, 127f
Giant cell arteritis, optic nerve affected in, 240
Giant cells
    foreign body, 15, 15f
    Langhans, 15, 15f
    multinucleated, 15, 15f
    Touton, 15, 15f
Giant congenital melanocytic nevi, 215
Giant drusen, 243
    retinoblastoma differentiated from, 293–294
Giant papillary (contact lens–induced) conjunctivitis, 56
Glands of Krause, 199, 201t
Glands of Moll, 201t
Glands of Wolfring, 199, 201t
Glaucoma
    angle-recession, 96–97
    Axenfeld-Rieger syndrome and, 91
    exfoliative, 95
    ghost cell, 96, 97f, 126
    hemolytic, 96
    hemorrhage-associated, 96–97, 97f
    hemosiderin in, 96
    lens-induced, 96, 97f, 113
    melanomalytic, 192
    nanophthalmos and, 103
    neovascular, rubeosis iridis and, 186
    phacolytic, 96, 97f, 113
    pigment dispersion syndrome and, 98–100, 99f
    secondary
        leukemia and, 317
        with material in trabecular meshwork, 95–100
        in uveal lymphoid infiltration, 315
    trauma and, 96–97, 97f
Glaukomflecken, 115
Glial cells, retinal, in retinal ischemia, 151
Glioblastomas, optic nerve (malignant optic gliomas), 244
Gliomas, optic nerve, 243–244, 244f
    malignant (glioblastomas), 244
Gliosis, of retina, 158, 178

Index • 359

Globe
 displacement of, 219
 gross dissection of, for pathologic examination, 35–37, 36f
 orientation of, pathologic examination and, 34, 34f
Goblet cells, 53, 54f, 201t
Goldenhar syndrome, dermoids/dermolipomas in, 54
Gomori methenamine silver stain, 38, 39t
Gonioscopy
 in choroidal/ciliary body melanoma, 262
 in iris nevus, 251
Gram stain, 38, 39t
Granular dystrophy, 86, 86f, 87t
Granulocytic sarcoma (chloroma), 317
Granulomas, 14, 14f, 15f
 in sarcoidosis, 58, 147
 zonal, 112
Granulomatosis
 larval, retinoblastoma differentiated from, 292t
 Wegener, eyelid manifestations of, 206t
Granulomatous inflammation, focal posttraumatic choroidal, 30, 30f
Graves disease. See Thyroid-associated orbitopathy
Gross dissection, for pathologic examination, 35–37, 36f
Grouped pigmentation of retina (bear tracks), 265, 266f

H&E (hematoxylin and eosin) stain, 38, 38f, 39t
Haab's striae, 83
Haemophilus/Haemophilus influenzae, conjunctivitis caused by, 57
Hamartomas, 12, 54–55
 astrocytic (astrocytomas)
  pilocytic, juvenile, 243, 244f
  retinoblastoma differentiated from, 293–294, 294f
 combined, of retina and retinal pigment epithelium, 177–178, 276, 276f
 conjunctival, 54–55
 of retinal pigment epithelium
  combined, 177–178, 276, 276f
  in Gardner syndrome, 143–144
Hard (hyaline) drusen, 161, 162f
Hard exudates, 152, 152f, 153f
 in leukemia, 317
"Hard" tubercles, 14, 14f
HBID. See Hereditary benign intraepithelial dyskeratosis
Healing, ophthalmic wound. See Wound healing/repair
Hemangioblastomas, retinal, 280–281, 280f
 with retinal angiomatosis (von Hippel–Lindau syndrome), 280–281
Hemangiomas (hemangiomatosis), 12, 277–283
 of choroid, 195–196, 195f, 277–280, 278f, 279f
  in Sturge-Weber disease/syndrome, 195, 277
 of eyelid, 213
 of orbit, 230, 232f
  capillary, 230, 232f
  cavernous, 12, 230, 232f
  racemose (Wyburn-Mason syndrome), 282f, 283
 of retina
  capillary, 280–281, 280f
  cavernous, 281–283, 282f
Hemangiopericytoma, of orbit, 230–231, 232f
Hematoxylin and eosin (H&E) stain, 38, 38f, 39t

Hemoglobin spherules, 126, 127f
Hemolytic glaucoma, 96
Hemorrhages
 choroidal, expulsive, 27, 28f
 glaucoma associated with, 96–97, 97f
 retinal
  ischemia causing, 154–155, 154f, 157
  in leukemia, 317
 vitreous, 126–128, 127f
  retinoblastoma differentiated from, 292t
Hemosiderin, in glaucoma, 96
Henle fiber layer, 139. See also Nerve fiber layer
Henle pseudoglands, 54f, 55
Her2Neu, in immunohistochemistry, 42
Hereditary benign intraepithelial dyskeratosis, 64
Hermansky-Pudlak syndrome, 141
Herpes simplex virus
 acute retinal necrosis caused by, 144, 144f
 keratitis caused by, 78, 78f
Herpes zoster, acute retinal necrosis caused by, 144, 144f
Histiocytes, 14
 epithelioid, 14–15, 14f
Histiocytic (large) cell lymphoma. See Lymphomas, intraocular
Histiocytoma, fibrous (fibroxanthoma)
 orbital, 234, 234f
 scleral, 106
HIV infection/AIDS, cytomegalovirus retinitis and, 144, 145f
HLA antigens. See Human leukocyte (HLA) antigens
HMB-45, in immunohistochemistry, 41
Hodgkin disease, in orbit, 228
Holes
 macular, 132, 133f
 optic (optic pits), 239, 239f
Hollenhorst plaques (cholesterol emboli), in branch retinal artery occlusion, 156
Homer-Wright rosettes, in retinoblastoma, 173–174, 174f
Homocystinuria, ectopia lentis in, 111
Hordeolum, external (stye), 202
Hormones, in cancer chemotherapy, for metastatic eye disease, 312
Horner-Trantas dots, 56
HPV. See Human papillomaviruses
Hudson-Stähli line, 89
Human leukocyte (HLA) antigens, in Vogt-Koyanagi-Harada syndrome, 185
Human papillomaviruses, 62–64
 eyelid infections caused by, 203
Hyaline deposits, corneal, in Avellino dystrophy, 87
Hyaline (hard) drusen, 161, 162f
Hyalocytes, 124
Hyaloid artery/system, persistence/remnants of, 125
Hyaloid face, of vitreous, 123
Hyaloideocapsular ligament, 123
Hyalosis, asteroid, 128, 128f
Hybridization
 comparative genomic (CGH), 48–49t
  microarray-based (array CGH), 49t
 fluorescence in situ (FISH), 48t
Hydrops, in keratoconus, 83
Hyperkeratosis, definition of, 201

Hyperlipoproteinemias, xanthelasma associated with, 205, 206t
Hypermature cataract, phacolytic glaucoma and, 96, 113
Hyperplasia
　epithelial
　　ciliary pigmented, 276
　　of lens, 115–116, 115f
　　pseudoadenomatous (Fuchs adenoma), 177, 275
　reactive/reactive lymphoid. *See* Lymphoid hyperplasia
Hyperthermia, diode laser
　for melanoma, 272
　for retinoblastoma, 299
Hyphema, glaucoma and, 96–97

ICE. *See* Iridocorneal endothelial (ICE) syndrome
Idiopathic orbital inflammation, 224, 224f, 225f
　orbital lymphoma differentiated from, 230
ILM. *See* Internal limiting membrane
Immunocompromised host, ocular infection in, cytomegalovirus retinitis, 144, 145f
Immunohistochemistry, 41–44, 43f, 44f
Immunotherapy/immunosuppression, for melanoma, 273
Implantation membrane, of iris, 256t
Inclusion cysts, epithelial, 56, 56f
　conjunctival, 56, 56f
　nevi and, 68, 69f
Index features, in diagnosis, 18
Indirect ophthalmoscopy, in choroidal/ciliary body melanoma, 261
Infantile cataract, 111
Infection (ocular), intraocular lenses and, 120
Inflammation (ocular), 13–16, 13f, 14f, 15f, 16f. *See also specific type or structure affected*
　acute, 13, 21
　chronic, 13
　conjunctival, 55–60, 56f
　corneal, 77–80, 78f, 79f
　eyelid, 202–205, 203f, 204f
　granulomatous, 13
　　focal posttraumatic choroidal, 30, 30f
　intraocular lenses and, 120
　lens-related, 112–113, 112f, 113f, 114f
　nongranulomatous, 13
　optic nerve, 239–240, 240f
　orbital, 221–224, 222f, 223f, 224, 225f
　retinal, 144–147, 144f, 145f, 146f, 147f
　in retinoblastoma, 287, 288t
　scleral, 103–105, 104f, 105f
　uveal tract, 183–187, 183f, 184f, 185f
　vitreal, 125–126, 126f
Inflammatory pannus (fibrovascular pannus), 82, 82f
Inner ischemic retinal atrophy, 150, 150f
　in branch retinal artery occlusion, 156
Inner nuclear layer, 137, 138f
Inner plexiform layer, 137, 138f
Internal limiting membrane, 137, 138f
Internal ulcer of von Hippel. *See* Keratoconus, posterior
International classification system, of retinoblastoma, 294–295, 295t
Interphotoreceptor retinoid-binding protein, 171
Intradermal nevus, 216, 217f
Intraepithelial dyskeratosis, benign hereditary, 64

Intraepithelial neoplasia
　conjunctival (CIN), 63f, 64, 65f
　corneal, 89
Intraocular chemotherapy. *See* Periocular chemotherapy
Intraocular lenses (IOLs), complications of, 119–121, 120f
Intraocular pressure, elevated/increased, lens epithelium affected by, 115
Intraocular tumors, 247–329. *See also specific type of tumor and structure affected*
　angiomatous, 277–283
　direct extension from extraocular tumors and, 312
　leukemia and, 317–318, 318f
　lymphoma (reticulum cell sarcoma/histiocytic [large] cell lymphoma/non-Hodgkin lymphoma of CNS), 313–315, 314f
　　vitreous involvement and, 133–135, 134f, 135f
　melanocytic, 251–276
　metastatic, 305–312. *See also* Metastatic eye disease
　rare, 319, 320f
　retinoblastoma, 285–303
　secondary, 305–312. *See also* Metastatic eye disease
　staging of, 321–329t
Intraretinal microvascular abnormalities (IRMAs), 155, 155f, 160
Intravitreal triamcinolone acetonide (IVTA), for macular edema, 153–154, 153f
Inverted follicular keratosis, 207, 208f
IOL. *See* Intraocular lenses
Iridocorneal endothelial (ICE) syndrome, 94–95, 94f
Iridocyclitis, iris nodules in, 256t
Iridodialysis, 27, 28f, 97, 98f
Iris
　absence of (aniridia), 181–182
　atrophy of, 94
　cysts of, 256t, 258f
　epithelial invasion of, 256t
　in leukemia, 256t, 258f, 317
　melanocytoma of, 254
　melanoma of, 188, 188f, 254–258, 255f, 257t, 259f
　metastatic disease of, 306, 307f
　neoplastic disorders of, 187–189, 188f
　neovascularization of (rubeosis iridis), 186, 186t
　topography of, 179–180, 179f, 180f
　transillumination of, in albinism, 141, 141f
　traumatic damage to
　　iridodialysis, 27, 28f, 97, 98f
　　repair of, 24–25
Iris freckle, 256t, 258f
Iris nevus, 187, 251, 252f, 256t
Iris nevus syndrome (Cogan-Reese syndrome), 94, 256t
Iris nodules, 256–257t, 258f
　differential diagnosis of, 256–257t
　in leukemia, 256t, 258f
　in metastatic disease, 306, 307f
　in retinoblastoma, 257t
　in sarcoidosis, 185
Iris pigment epithelium, 180, 180f
　cysts of, 256t, 258f
　proliferation of, 256t
Iritis, chronic, lens epithelium affected in, 115
IRMAs. *See* Intraretinal microvascular abnormalities

Iron
   corneal deposits of, in keratoconus, 83, 84f, 89
   foreign body of, siderosis caused by, 115
Iron lines, 89
Ischemia, retinal, 149–159. *See also* Retinal ischemia

Junctional nevus, of eyelid, 216, 216f
Juvenile pilocytic astrocytoma, of optic nerve, 243, 244f
Juvenile xanthogranuloma (nevoxanthoendothelioma), of iris, 256t
Juxtafoveal/parafoveal retinal telangiectasis, 142, 143f

Karyotype/karyotyping, 48t
Kayser-Fleischer ring, 89
Keratan sulfate, macular dystrophy and, 84
Keratic precipitates, mutton-fat, in sympathetic ophthalmia, 184
Keratinizing squamous cell carcinoma, well-differentiated (keratoacanthoma), eyelid, 208–209, 208t, 209f
Keratitis
   Acanthamoeba, 79, 79f
      contact lens wear and, 79, 79f
   bacterial, 77–78
   fungal, 78–79, 78f
   herpes simplex, 78, 78f
   noninfectious, 80
   syphilitic, 80
Keratoacanthoma, eyelid, 208–209, 208t, 209f
Keratoconus, 83, 84f
   Descemet's membrane rupture and, 28, 28f, 83, 84f
   posterior (internal ulcer of von Hippel), 76, 76f
Keratopathy
   actinic (Labrador keratopathy/spheroidal degeneration), 81, 81f
   band, 80, 81f
   bullous, 82–83, 82f
   drug-related, 83
   Labrador, 81, 81f
Keratosis
   actinic (solar), 210, 210f, 211f
   inverted follicular, 207, 208f
   seborrheic, 207–208, 207f, 208f
"Kissing" nevi, 215, 215f
c-Kit, in immunohistochemistry, 42
Koeppe nodules
   in iridocyclitis, 256t
   in sarcoidosis, 185, 258f
Koganei, clump cells of, 180
Krause, glands of, 199, 201t
Krukenberg spindles, 88, 89f, 99f, 100

Labrador (actinic) keratopathy, 81, 81f
Lacrimal bone, 219, 220f
Lacrimal glands, 219
   accessory, 199, 201t
   tumors of, 226–228, 227f, 228f
      staging of, 328t
Lacrimal system, wound healing/repair and, 26
Lamina cribrosa, 101, 237, 238f
Lamina fusca, 102, 181
Langhans giant cells, 15, 15f

Large (histiocytic) cell lymphoma. *See* Lymphomas, intraocular
Laser therapy (laser surgery). *See also* Photocoagulation
   for diabetic retinopathy, 160, 160f
   for retinoblastoma, 299, 299f
Lattice degeneration, 148, 149f
   radial perivascular, 148
Lattice dystrophy, 86–87, 87f, 87t, 205
Leber miliary aneurysm, 142
Leiomyoma, 319
   of ciliary body, 196
   of iris, 256t
   of orbit, 234
Leiomyosarcoma, of orbit, 234
Lens (crystalline)
   capsule of. *See* Lens capsule
   congenital anomalies and abnormalities of, 110–112, 111f, 111t
   cortex of, 109
      degenerations of, 117, 117f, 118f
   degenerations of, 113–118. *See also* Cataract
   dislocated, 28, 110–111, 111f
   disorders of, 109–121. *See also specific type*
      systemic disorders and, 118–119
   epithelium of, 109
      abnormalities of, 115–116, 115f, 116f
   glaucoma and, 96, 97f, 113
   infection/inflammation of, 112–113, 112f, 113f, 114f
   luxed/luxated, 28, 110
   nucleus of, 109
      degenerations of, 118, 119f
   subluxed/subluxated, 28, 110
   topography of, 109, 110f
   uveitis and, 112, 112f, 113f
   wound healing/repair and, 26
   zonular fibers/zonules of, 109, 110f
      tertiary vitreous, 124
Lens capsule, 109
   disorders of, 113–114, 114f
   rupture of, cataract formation and, 28
   wound healing/repair and, 26
Lens fibers
   degenerations of, 117, 117f, 118f
   zonular (zonules of Zinn), 109, 110f
      tertiary vitreous, 124
Lens-induced glaucoma, 96, 97f, 113
Lens-induced granulomatous endophthalmitis (phacoantigenic endophthalmitis), 112, 112f, 113f
Lens proteins
   in phacoantigenic endophthalmitis, 112
   in phacolytic glaucoma, 96, 113
Lenticonus
   anterior, 114
   posterior, 114, 114f
Lentigo maligna melanoma, 218
"Leopard spotting," 306, 310f
Leser-Trélat sign, 208
Leukemia, 17f, 17t
   ocular involvement in, 317–318, 318f
      choroid, 317
      iris, 256t, 258f, 317
      orbit, 229

retina, 317
vitreous, 317, 318*f*
Leukocoria
in Coats disease, 143*f*
in retinoblastoma, 287, 288*f*, 288*t*
differential diagnosis and, 291, 291*f*
Leukocyte common antigen, in immunohistochemistry, 42
Levator muscle (levator palpebrae superioris), 199
Limbal dermoids, 53–54
Limbal papillae, 56
Limbal papillomas, 62, 63*f*
Limbus, wound healing/repair and, 24, 25*f*
Limiting membrane
external, 138
internal, 137, 138*f*
Lipodermoids (dermolipomas), 54, 55*f*
Goldenhar syndrome and, 54
Lipomas, of orbit, 236
Liposarcomas, of orbit, 236
Lisch nodules, 257*t*, 258*f*
Localized (circumscribed) choroidal hemangioma, 195, 277, 278*f*
Lung cancer, eye involvement and, 306*t*, 311, 311*f*
Lupus erythematosus, systemic, eyelid manifestations of, 206*t*
Luxed/luxated lens, 28, 110. *See also* Ectopia lentis
Lymphangiomas, orbital, 230, 231*f*
Lymphocytes, 14–15, 14*f*
Lymphoid hyperplasia (lymphoid infiltration/reactive lymphoid hyperplasia/benign lymphoid pseudotumor/pseudolymphoma)
of conjunctiva, 66–67, 66*f*, 67*f*
of uveal tract (uveal lymphoid infiltration), 196–197, 315–316
Lymphoid proliferation, uveal tract involvement and, 196–197
Lymphoid tissues, mucosa-associated (MALT), lymphoma of, 229, 229*f*
Lymphomas, 17*f*, 17*t*, 313–315, 314*f*
Burkitt, of orbit, 229–230
conjunctival, 67, 67*f*, 68*f*
intraocular (reticulum cell sarcoma/histiocytic [large] cell lymphoma/non–Hodgkin lymphoma of CNS), 313–315, 314*f*
vitreous involvement and, 133–135, 134*f*, 135*f*
mucosa-associated (MALT), 229, 229*f*
orbital, 228–230, 229*f*
orbital inflammatory syndrome differentiated from, 230
of uveal tract, 197, 197*f*
vitreous, 133–135, 134*f*, 135*f*
Lymphoproliferative lesions/lymphomatous tumors, 313–316. *See also specific type* and Lymphoid hyperplasia; Lymphomas
of orbit, 228–230, 229*f*

Macrophages, 14
Macula, 139, 140*f*
lutea, 139
Macular degeneration, age-related. *See* Age-related macular degeneration
Macular dystrophy, 84, 85*f*, 87*t*, 167–171
vitelliform (Best disease), 167–168

Macular edema, 152–154, 152*f*, 153*f*
cystoid, intraocular lenses and, 121
Macular holes, 132, 133*f*
Magnetic resonance imaging (MRI)
in choroidal/ciliary body melanoma, 264
in retinoblastoma, 291, 296
Magnocellular nevus. *See* Melanocytoma
Malignant lymphoma. *See* Lymphomas
Malignant melanoma. *See* Melanomas
MALT lymphoma. *See* Mucosa-associated lymphoid tissue (MALT) lymphoma
Map-dot-fingerprint dystrophy (epithelial basement membrane/anterior membrane dystrophy), 83, 85*f*
Marfan syndrome, ectopia lentis in, 110–111
Masquerade syndromes, lymphoma and, 313
Masson trichrome stain, 38, 39*t*
Mast cells, 14
Maxilla, 219, 220*f*
Mean of the ten largest melanoma cell nuclei (MLN), 191
Medullated (myelinated) nerve fibers, 142
Medulloepithelioma (diktyoma), 176–177, 177*f*, 319, 320*f*
teratoid, 177
Meibomian glands, 199, 200*f*
Melan A, in immunohistochemistry, 41
Melanin, in retinal pigment epithelium, hypertrophy and, 143, 143*f*
Melanocytic nevus
of anterior chamber/trabecular meshwork, 100
congenital, 215–216, 215*f*
conjunctival, 68, 69*f*, 69*t*
of eyelid, 215–218, 216*f*, 217*f*
Melanocytic tumors, 251–276. *See also specific type and* Nevus
of anterior chamber/trabecular meshwork, 100, 100*f*
of conjunctiva, 68–71, 69*f*, 69*t*, 70*f*, 71*f*
of eyelid, 215–218, 215*f*, 216*f*, 217*f*
Melanocytoma
of iris/ciliary body/choroid, 189, 254
of optic disc/optic nerve, 243, 243*f*
melanoma differentiated from, 265–266, 266*f*
Melanocytosis, ocular/oculodermal, 69*t*
of iris, 257*t*
Melanomalytic glaucoma, 192
Melanomas
acral-lentiginous, 218
of anterior chamber/trabecular meshwork, 100, 100*f*
choroidal/ciliary body (uveal), 189–193, 191*f*, 192*f*, 193*f*, 194*f*, 249, 259–275. *See also* Choroidal/ciliary body melanoma
epithelioid cell, 190, 191*f*
nevus differentiated from, 252, 264
spindle cell, 190, 191*f*
spread of, 191–193, 192*f*, 193*f*, 194
staging of, 325–326*t*
conjunctival, 70–71, 71*f*
primary acquired melanosis and, 70, 71*f*
staging of, 322*t*
of eyelid, 218
of iris, 188, 188*f*, 254–258, 255*f*, 257*t*, 259*f*
lentigo maligna, 218
retinoblastoma associated with, 302, 302*t*
ring, 188, 190, 193, 194*f*

superficial spreading, 218
tapioca, 257t
uveal. *See* Melanomas, choroidal/ciliary body
Melanosis
 benign, 69t
 primary acquired, 68–70, 69f, 69t, 70f, 71f
  conjunctival melanoma and, 70, 71f
Membranes, implantation, of iris, 256t
Meningiomas, optic nerve, 244–245, 245f
Meretoja syndrome, 205
Mesectodermal leiomyoma, 196
Mesodermal dysgenesis. *See* Axenfeld-Rieger syndrome
Metastatic eye disease, 305–312. *See also specific type and structure affected*
 carcinoma, 305–312
  ancillary tests in evaluation of, 308–310, 311f
  clinical features of, 306–308, 307f, 308f, 309f, 310f, 310t
  diagnostic factors in, 310–311
  mechanisms of spread and, 306
  primary sites and, 305, 306t
  prognosis for, 311–312
  treatment of, 312
 of choroid, 306, 306t, 307f, 308f, 309f, 310t
 of iris, 306, 307f
 of optic nerve, 306, 310
 of orbit, 236
 of retina, 306, 310, 311f
 of uvea, 194–195, 194f, 311–312
Methenamine silver stain, Gomori, 38, 39t
Methotrexate, for intraocular lymphoma, 315
Microaneurysms, retinal, ischemia causing, 155, 155f
Microarray-based comparative genomic hybridization (array CGH), 49t
Microarrays, tissue, in immunohistochemistry, 44, 44f
Microglial cells, 237
 retinal, degeneration of in retinal ischemia, 151
Micrographic surgery, Mohs, for neoplastic disorders of eyelid
 basal cell carcinoma, 51, 213
 squamous cell carcinoma, 212
Microsporida (microsporidiosis), keratitis/keratoconjunctivitis caused by, 58
Mitomycin/mitomycin C
 for conjunctival intraepithelial neoplasia, 64
 for primary acquired melanosis, 70
Mittendorf dot, 112, 125
Mixed tumor, benign (pleomorphic adenoma), of lacrimal gland, 226, 227f
MLN. *See* Mean of the ten largest melanoma cell nuclei
Mohs micrographic surgery, for neoplastic disorders of eyelid
 basal cell carcinoma, 51, 213
 squamous cell carcinoma, 212
Molecular pathology techniques, 42t, 46–47, 48–49t
Moll, glands of, 201t
Molluscum contagiosum, of eyelid, 203, 204f
Monocytes, 14, 14f
Morgagnian cataract, 117, 118f
Morgagnian globules, 117, 117f
Mucoepidermoid carcinoma, 66
Mucor (mucormycosis)
 optic nerve involved in, 239
 orbit involved in, 221

Mucosa-associated lymphoid tissue (MALT) lymphoma, 229, 229f
Muir-Torre syndrome, eyelid manifestations of, 208t
Müller muscle (superior tarsal muscle), 180, 199
Multinucleated giant cells, 15, 15f
Multiple sclerosis, optic nerve involvement and, 240, 240f
Mutton-fat keratic precipitates, in sympathetic ophthalmia, 184
Mycotic (fungal) keratitis, 78–79, 78f
Myelinated (medullated) nerve fibers, 142
Myelitis, optic nerve involvement and, 240
Myoglobin, in immunohistochemistry, 41
Myositis, orbital, 224, 224f

Nanophthalmos, 103
Necrotizing retinitis, herpetic (acute retinal necrosis), 144, 144f
Necrotizing scleritis, 104–105, 104f, 105f
Neoplasia. *See also specific type and* Intraocular tumors; Tumors
 classification of, 16–17, 17f, 17t
 definition of, 16–17
Neovascular membrane, subretinal, in age-related macular degeneration, 164–165, 164f
Neovascularization
 choroidal, 30, 187, 187f
  in age-related macular degeneration, 163–164, 164f
 of iris (rubeosis iridis), 186, 186t
 retinal
  in age-related macular degeneration, 164–165, 164f
  ischemia causing, 155–156, 156f
  in retinopathy of prematurity, 161
Nerve fiber layer, 137, 138f, 139
Nerve fibers, medullated (myelinated), 142
Nerve (neural) sheath tumors
 of orbit, 235–236, 235f, 236f
 of uveal tract, 196
Neurilemoma (neurinoma, schwannoma)
 of orbit, 236, 236f
 of uveal tract, 196, 319
Neurofibromas
 of orbit, 235, 235f
 of uveal tract, 196, 319
Neurofibromatosis, von Recklinghausen (type 1)
 Lisch nodules associated with, 257t, 258f
 optic nerve gliomas and, 243–244
 optic nerve meningiomas and, 245
 orbital involvement in, 235, 235f
Neuroimaging, in retinoblastoma, 291, 296
Neurosensory retina, 137–138, 138f. *See also* Retina
Neutrophils (polymorphonuclear leukocytes), 13, 13f
Nevoxanthoendothelioma. *See* Juvenile xanthogranuloma
Nevus
 anterior chamber/trabecular meshwork affected by, 100
 of choroid, 189, 189f, 251–254, 253f
  melanoma differentiated from, 252, 264
 of ciliary body, 189f, 198, 251–254
 compound
  of conjunctiva, 68, 69f
  of eyelid, 217f
 congenital, 215–216, 215f

conjunctival, 68, 69f, 69t
dysplastic, 218
of eyelid, 215–218, 216f, 217f
intradermal, 216, 217f
iris, 187, 251, 252f, 256t
junctional, 216, 216f
"kissing," 215, 215f
macular, 216, 216f
magnocellular. *See* Melanocytoma
melanocytic
   of anterior chamber/trabecular meshwork, 100
   congenital, 215
   conjunctival, 68, 69f, 69t
   of eyelid, 215–218, 216f, 217f
nevocellular, 215–216, 216f
Spitz, 217
stromal, 68
subepithelial, 68
NFL. *See* Nerve fiber layer
Nodular episcleritis, 103
Nodular fasciitis, episcleral tumor caused by, 106–107
Non-Hodgkin lymphomas
of CNS (intraocular lymphoma/reticulum cell
   sarcoma/histiocytic [large cell] lymphoma),
   313–315, 314f
   vitreous involvement and, 133–135, 134f, 135f
orbital, 228–230, 229f
Nuclear cataracts, 118, 119f
Nuclear layer
inner, 137, 138f
outer, 138, 138f
Nucleus, lens, 109
degenerations of, 118, 119f

Occlusive retinal disease
arterial
   branch retinal artery occlusion, 156
   central retinal artery occlusion, 156, 157f
venous
   branch retinal vein occlusion, 159
   central retinal vein occlusion, 157–158, 158f
OCT. *See* Optical coherence tomography
Ocular albinism, 139–141
Ocular inflammation. *See* Inflammation
Ocular melanocytosis, 69t
of iris, 257t
Ocular (intraocular) surgery, for melanoma, 272
Oculocutaneous albinism, 139–141
Oculodermal melanocytosis, 69t
of iris, 257t
Oculoglandular syndrome, Parinaud, 60
Oil red O stain, 38
Oligodendrocytes, 237
Oncologist, ophthalmic, 49
Open-angle glaucoma
pigment dispersion syndrome and, 98–100, 99f
secondary, trauma causing, 96, 97f
Ophthalmia, sympathetic, 183–184, 183f, 184f
Ophthalmic artery, optic nerve supplied by, 237
Ophthalmic oncologist, 49
Ophthalmic pathology, 9–245
of anterior chamber and trabecular meshwork, 91–100
checklist for requesting, 42t

communication among health care team members
   and, 33–34
congenital anomalies and, 12, 13f
of conjunctiva, 53–71
of cornea, 73–90
degeneration and dystrophy and, 16
diagnostic electron microscopy in, 42t, 47
of eyelids, 199–218
fine-needle aspiration biopsy for, 42t, 47–50, 50f
flow cytometry in, 44–45, 45f, 46f
frozen section for, 42t, 50–51
history of, 5–8
immunohistochemistry in, 41–44, 43f, 44f
inflammation and, 13–16, 13f, 14f, 15f, 16f
of lens, 109–121
molecular pathologic techniques in, 42t, 46–47,
   48–49t
neoplasia and, 16–17, 17f, 17t
of optic nerve, 237–245
of orbit, 219–236
organizational paradigm for, 11–19, 18t
of retina, 137–178
of sclera, 101–107
special procedures in, 41–51, 42t
specimen handling for, 33–38, 39f
topography and, 12
of uveal tract, 179–197
of vitreous, 123–135
wound repair and, 21–31, 22f
Ophthalmic vein, 237
Ophthalmic wound healing/repair. *See* Wound healing/
   repair
Ophthalmopathy, thyroid. *See* Thyroid-associated
   orbitopathy
Ophthalmoscopy, in choroidal/ciliary body melanoma,
   261
Opportunistic infections, cytomegalovirus retinitis, 144,
   145f
Optic atrophy, 241–242, 241f
ascending, 241
cavernous, of Schnabel, 241–242, 242f
descending, 241
Optic disc (optic nerve head)
coloboma of, 239
   retinoblastoma differentiated from, 292t
drusen of, 242–243, 242f
melanocytoma (magnocellular nevus) of, 243, 243f
   melanoma differentiated from, 265–266, 266f
metastatic disease of, 306, 310
tumors of, 243–245, 243f, 244f, 245f
Optic nerve (cranial nerve II)
blood supply of, 237
coloboma of, 239
congenital abnormalities of, 239, 239f
degenerations of, 241–243, 241f, 242f
disorders of, 237–245. *See also specific type*
   neoplastic, 243–245, 243f, 244f, 245f
infection/inflammation of, 239–240, 240f
metastatic disease of, 306, 310
retinoblastoma involving, 174–175, 176f, 290
topography of, 237, 238f
Optic nerve glioblastoma (malignant optic glioma),
   244

Optic nerve (optic pathway) glioma (pilocytic
  astrocytoma), 243–244, 244f
 in children (juvenile), 243, 244f
 malignant (glioblastoma), 244
Optic pits (optic holes), 239, 239f
Optical coherence tomography (OCT), in idiopathic
  macular hole, 132
Orbicularis oculi muscle, 199, 200f
Orbit
 amyloid deposits in, 225, 225f
 bony, 219, 220f
 congenital disorders of, 220, 221f
 cysts of
  dermoid, 220, 221f
  epidermal, 220
 degenerations of, 225, 225f
 disorders of, 219–236. *See also specific type*
  neoplastic, 226–236. *See also* Orbit, tumors of
 infection/inflammation of, 221–224, 222f, 223f, 224,
  225f
  idiopathic (orbital inflammatory syndrome), 224,
   224f, 225f
   orbital lymphoma differentiated from, 230
 lacrimal gland neoplasia and, 226–228, 227f,
  228f
 leukemic infiltration of, 317
 lymphoproliferative lesions of, 228–230, 229f
 myositis affecting, idiopathic orbital inflammation
  presenting as, 224, 224f
 retinoblastoma affecting, 290, 290f
 soft tissues of, 219
 topography of, 219–220, 220f
 tumors of, 226–236
  adipose, 236
  bony, 234–235
  with fibrous differentiation, 234, 234f
  lymphoproliferative, 228–230, 229f
  metastatic, 236
  with muscle differentiation, 231–234, 233f
  nerve sheath, 235–236, 235f, 236f
  secondary, 236
  staging of, 329t
  vascular, 230–231, 231f, 232f
 wound healing/repair and, 26
Orbital inflammatory syndrome (idiopathic orbital
  inflammation/orbital pseudotumor/sclerosing
  orbitis), 224, 224f, 225f
 orbital lymphoma differentiated from, 230
Orbitis, sclerosing, 224, 224f, 225f
 orbital lymphoma differentiated from, 230
Orbitopathy, thyroid. *See* Thyroid-associated
  orbitopathy
Osseous choristoma, 103
Ossifying fibroma, of orbit, 235
Osteoma
 choroidal, 196
  melanoma differentiated from, 266–267, 267f
 orbital, 235
Osteosarcoma, retinoblastoma associated with, 176,
  302, 302t
Outer ischemic retinal atrophy, 150, 151f
Outer nuclear layer, 138, 138f
Outer plexiform layer, 137, 138f

Pagetoid spread
 of melanoma, 218
 in primary acquired melanosis, 68–70
 of sebaceous carcinoma, 214, 214f
Pain, in metastatic eye disease, 306
Palatine bone, 219, 220f
Palpebral conjunctiva, 53, 54f, 199–201, 200f
PAM. *See* Primary acquired melanosis
Pannus/micropannus, 82, 82f
 subepithelial fibrovascular, 82, 82f
Panuveitis, sympathetic ophthalmia and, 183–184, 183f,
  184f
Papillae
 Bergmeister, 125
 limbal, 56
Papillary conjunctivitis, 56, 57f
 giant (contact lens–induced), 56
Papillomas
 conjunctival, 62–64, 63f
 eyelid, 203
Papillomatosis, definition of, 201
Papillomaviruses. *See* Human papillomaviruses
Papillophlebitis, 157
Parafovea/parafoveal zone, 139
Parafoveal/juxtafoveal retinal telangiectasis, 142,
  143f
Parakeratosis, definition of, 201
Parasites, orbital infection caused by, 222
Parinaud oculoglandular syndrome, 60
Pars plana, 180, 181f
Pars plana vitrectomy
 for intraocular lymphoma diagnosis, 134, 314
 for uveal lymphoid infiltration diagnosis, 316
Pars plicata, 180, 181f
PAS (periodic acid–Schiff) stain, 38, 39t
Pathology, ophthalmic. *See* Ophthalmic pathology
Pattern dystrophies, 168–170, 169f
Paving-stone (cobblestone) degeneration, 149, 150f
PAX6 gene, mutation in, in aniridia, 182
PCNSL. *See* Primary intraocular/central nervous system
  lymphomas
PCR. *See* Polymerase chain reaction
PCV. *See* Polypoidal choroidal vasculopathy
PDT. *See* Photodynamic therapy
Pearl cyst, of iris, 256t
Periocular chemotherapy
 for intraocular lymphoma, 315
 for retinoblastoma, 299
Periodic acid–Schiff (PAS) stain, 38, 39t
Peripapillary vascular loops, 125
Peripheral cystoid degeneration, 147, 148f
Peripherin/RDS gene mutations
 in pattern dystrophies, 170
 in Stargardt disease, 167
Periphlebitis, in sarcoidosis, 185
Perls Prussian blue stain, 39t
Persistent fetal vasculature (persistent hyperplastic
  primary vitreous), 124, 125f
 cataract and, 112
 retinoblastoma differentiated from, 292, 292t
Persistent hyaloid artery/system, 125
PFV. *See* Persistent fetal vasculature

Phacoantigenic endophthalmitis (lens-induced granulomatous/phacoanaphylactic endophthalmitis/phacoanaphylaxis), 112, 112f, 113f
Phacolytic glaucoma, 96, 97f, 113
Phakomatous choristoma (Zimmerman tumor), 202
Photoablation, for melanoma, 272
Photocoagulation
 for choroidal hemangioma, 196, 278
 for diabetic retinopathy, 160, 160f
 for melanoma, 272
 for metastatic eye disease, 312
 for retinal capillary hemangioma, 281
 for retinoblastoma, 299, 299f
Photodynamic therapy, for choroidal hemangioma, 278
Photopsias, in metastatic eye disease, 306
Photoreceptors, 138, 138f
 atrophy of, in macular degeneration, 163
PHPV (persistent hyperplastic primary vitreous). See Persistent fetal vasculature
Phthisis bulbi (phthisical eye), 30–31, 31f
Pia mater, optic nerve, 237, 238f
Pigment dispersion syndrome
 anterior chamber and trabecular meshwork affected in, 98–100, 99f
 cornea affected in, 88, 89f
 glaucoma and, 98–100, 99f
Pigment epithelium. See Iris pigment epithelium; Retinal pigment epithelium
Pigmentations/pigment deposits
 corneal, 88–89, 89f
 trabecular meshwork, 98–100, 98f
Pinealoblastoma/pinealoma, retinoblastoma and, 296, 302t
Pinguecula, 60, 60f
PIOL. See Primary intraocular/central nervous system lymphomas
Pits, optic (optic holes), 239, 239f
PITX2 gene, in Axenfeld-Rieger syndrome, 92
Plaque radiotherapy. See Radioactive plaque therapy
Plaques
 Hollenhorst (cholesterol emboli), in branch retinal artery occlusion, 156
 optic nerve, 240
 senile scleral, 105, 106f
Plasma cells, 15–16, 16f
Pleomorphic adenoma (benign mixed tumor), of lacrimal gland, 226, 227f
Pleomorphic rhabdomyosarcoma, 233
Plexiform layer
 inner, 137, 138f
 outer, 137, 138f
Plexiform neurofibromas, of orbit, 235, 235f
Plica semilunaris, 53
Plus disease, 160–161
PMNs (polymorphonuclear leukocytes). See Neutrophils
PO (pupil–optic nerve) section, 35–36, 36f
Polyarteritis nodosa, eyelid manifestations of, 206t
Polychondritis, relapsing, eyelid manifestations of, 206t
Polymerase chain reaction (PCR), 46, 47f, 48t
Polymorphonuclear leukocytes. See Neutrophils
Polyneuropathy, familial amyloid, vitreous involvement in, 129, 129f

Polypoidal choroidal vasculopathy (posterior uveal bleeding syndrome), 165–167, 166f
Polyposis, familial adenomatous (Gardner syndrome), retinal manifestations of, 143–144
Posterior embryotoxon, 91, 93f
Posterior keratoconus. See Keratoconus, posterior
Posterior lenticonus, 114, 114f
Posterior polar cataract, 112
 retinoblastoma differentiated from, 292t
Posterior segment, metastatic tumors of, 306–308, 307f, 308f, 309f, 310f, 310t
Posterior subcapsular (cupuliform) cataract, 115, 116f
Posterior uveal bleeding syndrome (polypoidal choroidal vasculopathy), 165–167, 166f
Posterior uveal melanoma, 189–193, 191f, 192f, 193f, 194f, 249, 259–275. See also Choroidal/ciliary body melanoma
 nevus differentiated from, 252, 264
 staging of, 325–326t
Posterior vitreous detachment, 129–130, 130f
Postoperative endophthalmitis, after cataract surgery, 120
Posttraumatic angle recession, 27, 27f, 97, 98f
 glaucoma and, 96–97
Prealbumin. See Transthyretin
Pregnancy, rubella during, 112
Prematurity, retinopathy of, 160–161
 retinoblastoma differentiated from, 292t
Preseptal cellulitis, 203, 203f
Primary acquired melanosis (PAM), 68–70, 69f, 69t, 70f, 71f
 conjunctival melanoma and, 70, 71f
Primary intraocular/central nervous system lymphomas, 313–315, 314f
 vitreous involvement in, 133–135, 134f, 135f
Primary vitreous, 124
 persistent hyperplasia of. See Persistent fetal vasculature
Propionibacterium acnes, in endophthalmitis, 113, 114f
Proptosis (exophthalmos/exorbitism), 219
 in retinoblastoma, 290, 290f
 in rhabdomyosarcoma, 231
 in thyroid-associated orbitopathy, 222, 223f
 in uveal lymphoid infiltration, 315
Prostate cancer, eye/orbital metastases of, 306t
Prussian blue stain, Perls, 39t
Psammoma bodies, in optic nerve meningioma, 245
Pseudoadenomatous hyperplasia (Fuchs adenoma), 177, 275
Pseudoexfoliation (exfoliation syndrome), 95, 95f, 96f, 114, 114f
Pseudoglands of Henle, 54f, 55
Pseudogliomas, 171
Pseudohorn cysts, 207, 207f
Pseudohypopyon
 in leukemia, 317
 retinoblastoma causing, 290, 290f
Pseudomembrane, 55
Pseudoretinoblastoma, 292t
Pseudo-Roth spots, in leukemia, 317
Pseudotumor, orbital, 224, 224f, 225f
Pterygium, 61, 61f
Pupil–optic nerve (PO) section, 35–36, 36f

PVD. *See* Posterior vitreous detachment
PVR. *See* Vitreoretinopathies, proliferative

Racemose angioma/hemangioma (Wyburn-Mason syndrome), 282*f*, 283
Radial perivascular lattice degeneration, 148
Radiation therapy
　for choroidal hemangioma, 278
　for lymphoma, 315
　for melanoma, 271–272, 271*f*
　　of iris, 255
　for metastatic eye disease, 312
　for retinal capillary hemangioma, 281
　for retinoblastoma, 300–301
　　secondary tumors and, 176, 302
　for uveal lymphoid infiltration, 316
Radioactive plaque therapy (brachytherapy)
　for choroidal hemangioma, 278
　for melanoma, 271, 271*f*
　　of iris, 255
　for metastatic eye disease, 312
　for retinoblastoma, 300–301
RB1 (retinoblastoma) gene, 172, 249, 285–286
　secondary malignancies and, 176, 302–303, 302*t*
RDS/peripherin gene mutations
　in pattern dystrophies, 170
　in Stargardt disease, 167
Reactive lymphoid hyperplasia. *See* Lymphoid hyperplasia
REAL (Revised European-American) classification, for lymphomas, 228–229
"Real time" quantitative RT-PCR, 48*t*
Recurrent pterygia, 61
Reese-Ellsworth classification of retinoblastoma, 294, 295*t*
Regeneration, 21. *See also* Wound healing/repair
Relapsing polychondritis, eyelid manifestations of, 206*t*
Renal cell carcinoma, eye/orbital metastases of, 306*t*
Repair, 21. *See also* Wound healing/repair
Reticular degenerative retinoschisis, 147–148
Reticular peripheral cystoid degeneration, 147, 148*f*
Reticulum cell sarcoma, 133. *See also* Lymphomas, intraocular
Retina, 137–138, 137*f*. *See also under* Retinal
　atrophy of, ischemia causing. *See also* Retinal ischemia
　　in branch retinal artery occlusion, 156
　blood supply of. *See* Retinal blood vessels
　capillary hemangioma (hemangioblastoma) of, 280–281, 280*f*
　cavernous hemangioma of, 281–283, 282*f*
　congenital disorders of, 139–144, 141*f*, 143*f*
　degenerations of. *See* Retinal degenerations
　detachment of. *See* Retinal detachment
　disorders of. *See specific type and* Retinal disease
　dysplasia of, retinoblastoma differentiated from, 292*t*
　gliosis of, 158, 178
　hamartomas of, 177–178
　infection/inflammation of, 144–147, 144*f*, 145*f*, 146*f*, 147*f*. *See also* Retinitis
　in leukemia, 317
　necrosis of, acute (necrotizing herpetic retinitis), 144, 144*f*

　neovascularization of
　　disorders of in retinopathy of prematurity, 161
　　ischemia causing, 155–156, 156*f*
　neurosensory, 137–138, 138*f*
　topography of, 137–138, 138*f*
　tumors of, 171–178. *See also* Retinoblastoma
　　metastatic, 306, 310, 311*f*
　　pigmented, 275–276, 276*f*
　　in von Hippel–Lindau disease, 280–281
　wound healing/repair and, 26
Retinal angiomatosis (angiomatosis retinae), 280–281, 280*f*
　with hemangioblastomas (von Hippel–Lindau syndrome), 280–281
Retinal artery microaneurysms, ischemia causing, 155, 155*f*
Retinal artery occlusion
　branch, 156
　central, 156, 157*f*
Retinal blood vessels, 138
　anomalies of, 142, 143*f*
　ischemia and, 151–156, 152*f*, 153*f*, 154*f*, 155*f*, 156*f*
Retinal degenerations, 147–171
　lattice, 148, 149*f*
　　radial perivascular, 148
　paving-stone (cobblestone), 149, 150*f*
　peripheral cystoid, 147, 148*f*
Retinal detachment, 130–131, 131*f*, 132*f*
　choroidal hemangioma and, 196, 278
　in Coats disease, 142, 143*f*
　intraocular lenses and, 121
　lattice degeneration and, 148
　in leukemia, 317
　metastatic eye disease and, 306, 308, 308*f*
　in polypoidal choroidal vasculopathy, 167
　in retinoblastoma, 287, 289*f*
　rhegmatogenous, 131, 132*f*
　in uveal lymphoid infiltration, 315
　in von Hippel–Lindau disease, 280
Retinal dialyses, 29, 29*f*
Retinal disease, 137–178
　congenital, 139–144, 141*f*, 143*f*
　intraocular lenses and, 121
　neoplastic, 171–178
　　metastatic, 306, 310, 311*f*
　vascular
　　congenital, 142, 143*f*
　　parafoveal (juxtafoveal) telangiectasis, 142, 143*f*
Retinal edema, 152–154, 152*f*, 153*f*
Retinal fold, congenital, retinoblastoma differentiated from, 292*t*
Retinal hemorrhages
　ischemia causing, 154–155, 154*f*, 157
　in leukemia, 317
Retinal ischemia, 149–159
　cellular responses to, 150–151, 150*f*, 151*f*
　central and branch retinal artery and vein occlusions causing, 156–159, 157*f*, 158*f*
　inner ischemic retinal atrophy and, 150, 150*f*
　outer ischemic retinal atrophy and, 150, 151*f*
　retinopathy of prematurity and, 160–161
　vascular responses to, 151–156, 152*f*, 153*f*, 154*f*, 155*f*, 156*f*

Retinal neovascularization
　ischemia causing, 155–156, 156f
　in retinopathy of prematurity, 161
Retinal nerve fibers, myelinated (medullated), 142
Retinal pigment epithelium (RPE), 137, 139
　adenomas/adenocarcinomas of, 178, 275
　atrophy of, 163, 163f
　central areolar atrophy of, 163
　congenital abnormalities of, 139–144, 141f, 143f
　　hypertrophy, 142–144, 143f
　　　melanoma differentiated from, 143, 265, 265f
　detachment of, multiple recurrent serosanguineous (polypoidal choroidal vasculopathy), 165–167, 166f
　disorders of, 137–178
　geographic atrophy of, 163, 163f
　hamartoma of, 177–178
　　in Gardner syndrome, 143–144
　hypertrophy of, congenital, 142–144, 143f
　　melanoma differentiated from, 143, 265, 265f
　topography of, 139
Retinal scars, 26
Retinal tears, 130, 131f
Retinal telangiectasia/telangiectasis, parafoveal (juxtafoveal), 142, 143f
Retinal vein occlusion
　branch, 159
　　neovascularization in, 155
　central, 157–158, 158f
Retinitis
　cytomegalovirus, 144, 145f
　herpetic necrotizing (acute retinal necrosis), 144, 144f
　pigmentosa, 170f, 171
Retinoblastoma, 171–176, 285–303
　chemotherapy of, 298–299, 298f, 299f
　classification of, 294–295, 295t
　clinical evaluation/diagnosis of, 287–294, 288f, 288t, 289f, 290f, 291f
　　differential diagnosis and, 291–294, 292t, 293f, 294f
　conditions associated with, 296–297
　cryotherapy for, 300
　diffuse infiltrating, 290
　enucleation for, 297
　epidemiology of, 285, 285t
　fleurettes in, 174, 174f
　genetics of, 172, 249, 285–287, 287f
　　counseling and, 285–287, 287f
　histologic features of, 172–174, 172f, 173f, 174f
　intracranial, 296
　iris affected in, 257t
　metastatic, 290, 291
　optic nerve affected in, 174–175, 176f, 290
　orbit affected in, 290, 290f
　pathogenesis of, 171–172
　photocoagulation/hyperthermia for, 299, 299f
　presenting signs and symptoms of, 287–290, 288f, 288t, 289f
　prognosis for, 175, 301–303, 302t
　progression of, 174–175, 175f, 176f
　radiation therapy of, 300–301
　　secondary tumors and, 176, 302
　rosettes in, 173–174, 174f, 296
　secondary malignancies and, 176, 302–303, 302t
　spontaneous regression of, 301
　staging of, 323–324t
　targeted therapy of, 301
　treatment of, 297–301
　trilateral, 296
　vitreous seeding and, 289–290, 289f, 290
　　targeted therapy for, 301
Retinoblastoma *(RB1)* gene, 172, 249, 285–286
　secondary malignancies and, 176, 302–303, 302t
Retinocytoma (retinoma), 176, 176f, 296
Retinoid-binding proteins, interphotoreceptor, 171
Retinoma (retinocytoma), 176, 176f, 296
Retinopathy
　diabetic, 159–160, 160f
　of prematurity, 160–161
　　retinoblastoma differentiated from, 292t
Retinoschisis, 147–148
Retraction, eyelid, 199
Reverse transcriptase-polymerase chain reaction (RT-PCR), 48t
Revised European-American (REAL) classification, for lymphomas, 228–229
Rhabdomyosarcoma
　of orbit, 231–234, 233f
　retinoblastoma associated with, 302t
Rhegmatogenous retinal detachment. *See* Retinal detachment
Rhinosporidium seeberi, conjunctivitis caused by, 57
RHO (rhodopsin) gene, in retinitis pigmentosa, 171
Rieger anomaly/syndrome, 94
RIM proteins, mutations in, 167
Ring melanoma, 188, 190, 193, 194f
Rod inner segments, 138, 138f
Rod outer segments, 138, 138f
"Rodent" ulcer, 212, 212f
Rods, 138, 138f
ROP. *See* Retinopathy, of prematurity
Rosenthal fibers, in optic nerve gliomas, 244, 244f
Rosettes, in retinoblastoma, 173–174, 174f, 296
Roth spots, 155
RP. *See* Retinitis, pigmentosa
RP1 gene, in retinitis pigmentosa, 171
RPCD. *See* Reticular peripheral cystoid degeneration
RPE. *See* Retinal pigment epithelium
RPGR gene, in retinitis pigmentosa, 171
RT-PCR. *See* Reverse transcriptase-polymerase chain reaction
Rubella, congenital, cataracts and, 112
Rubeosis iridis (iris neovascularization), 186, 186t
Rush (plus) disease, 160–161
Russell bodies, 16, 16f, 66–67

S-100 protein, in immunohistochemistry, 41
Salzmann nodular degeneration, 80
Sarcoidosis
　conjunctivitis and, 58–60
　eyelid manifestations of, 206t
　optic nerve affected in, 240, 240f
　retina affected in, 147
　uveal tract affected in, 185, 185f, 258f
Sarcoma, 17f, 17t
　Ewing, retinoblastoma associated with, 302t
　granulocytic (chloroma), 317
　orbital, staging of, 329t

reticulum cell, 133. *See also* Lymphomas, intraocular
soft-tissue, retinoblastoma associated with, 302*t*
Scars
   retinal, 26
   wound repair and, 21
Schaumann bodies, in sarcoidosis, 185
Schlemm's canal, 91, 92*f*
Schnabel, cavernous optic atrophy of, 241–242, 242*f*
Schwalbe's line/ring, 91, 92*f*
Schwannoma (neurilemoma/neurinoma)
   of orbit, 236, 236*f*
   of uveal tract, 196, 319
Sclera
   aging of, 105, 106*f*
   congenital anomalies of, 102–103
   degenerations of, 105–106, 106*f*
   disorders of, 101–107. *See also specific type*
      neoplastic, 106–107
   infection/inflammation of, 103–105, 104*f*, 105*f*. *See also* Episcleritis; Scleritis
   stroma of, 101, 102*f*
   topography of, 101–102, 102*f*
   wound healing/repair of, 24
Scleral buckle, for retinal capillary hemangioma, 281
Scleral plaques, senile, 105, 106*f*
Scleritis, 103–105, 104*f*, 105*f*
   anterior, 104, 104*f*
   brawny, 104, 104*f*
   necrotizing, 104–105, 104*f*, 105*f*
   nonnecrotizing, 105
   posterior, 104, 104*f*
Sclerocornea, 76–77
Scleroderma, eyelid manifestations of, 206*t*
Scleromalacia perforans, 105
Sclerosing dacryoadenitis, 224
Sclerosing inflammation of orbit/sclerosing orbitis, 224, 224*f*, 225*f*
   orbital lymphoma differentiated from, 230
Sclopetaria, 30, 197
Sebaceous carcinoma/adenocarcinoma, 213–215, 214*f*, 215*f*
Sebaceous glands, of eyelid, 201*t*
Seborrheic keratosis, 207–208, 207*f*, 208*f*
Senile calcific plaques, 105, 106*f*
Sentinel vessels, 190
Siderosis, 115
Simple episcleritis, 103
Skin, eyelid, 199, 200*f*
Skin cancer, eye/orbital metastases of, 306*t*
Slit-lamp biomicroscopy. *See* Biomicroscopy, slit-lamp
Soemmering ring, 116, 116*f*
Soft drusen, 162, 162*f*
Soft-tissue sarcoma, retinoblastoma associated with, 302, 302*t*
Solar elastosis, of eyelid, 210, 211*f*
Solar (actinic) keratosis, 210, 210*f*, 211*f*
Specimen collection/handling, 33–38, 39*f*
   communication with health care team and, 33–34
   gross dissection and, 35–37, 36*f*
   orientation of globe and, 34, 34*f*
   processing/staining tissues and, 37–38, 37*t*, 38*f*, 39*t*
   special techniques and, 41–51, 42*t*
   transillumination and, 35, 35*f*

Sphenoid bone, 219, 220*f*
Spheroidal degeneration (actinic/Labrador keratopathy), 81, 81*f*
Sphincter muscle, 180, 180*f*
Spindle cell carcinoma, 66
Spindle cell melanoma, 190, 191*f*
Spitz nevus, 217
Spongiosis, definition of, 201
Squamous cell carcinoma
   of conjunctiva, 64–66, 65*f*
   of eyelid, 211–212, 211*f*
      actinic keratosis and, 210, 211
      well-differentiated keratinizing (keratoacanthoma), 208–209, 208*t*, 209*f*
   retinoblastoma associated with, 302*t*
Squamous cell papillomas, conjunctival, 62–64, 63*f*
Stains/staining techniques, 38, 38*f*, 39*t*
Staphylomas
   in children, 77, 106
   congenital, 77
   corneal, 77
   scleral, 104, 105*f*, 106
Stargardt disease (juvenile macular degeneration/fundus flavimaculatus), 167, 168*f*
STGD4 gene, in Stargardt disease, 167
Stickler syndrome, radial perivascular lattice degeneration in, 148
Stocker lines, 89
Storiform pattern, in fibrous histiocytoma, 106
Strabismus, in retinoblastoma, 287, 288*t*
Streptococcus, pneumoniae (pneumococcus), preseptal cellulitis caused by, 203
Stroma
   choroidal, 181
   conjunctival, 53
   corneal, 73, 74*f*
      wound healing/repair of, 22–23
   iris, 180
      wound healing and, 24–25
   scleral, 101, 102*f*
Stromal nevi, 68
Sturge-Weber disease/syndrome (encephalofacial angiomatosis), choroidal hemangioma in, 195, 277
Stye (external hordeolum), 202
Subcapsular cataract
   anterior (subcapsular fibrous plaques), 115, 115*f*
   posterior (cupuliform cataract), 115, 116*f*
Subepithelial fibrovascular pannus, 82, 82*f*
Subepithelial nevi, 68
Subluxed/subluxated lens, 28, 110. *See also* Ectopia lentis
Subretinal neovascular membranes, in age-related macular degeneration, 164–165, 164*f*
Substantia propria (conjunctival stroma), 53
Sunlight. *See* Ultraviolet light
Superior tarsal muscle of Müller, 199
Suprachoroidal detachment, melanoma differentiated from, 266
Surgery, for melanoma, 272
Sweat glands, of eyelid, 201*t*
Sympathetic ophthalmia, 183–184, 183*f*, 184*f*
Synaptophysin, in immunohistochemistry, 42
Syneresis, 126, 127*f*

Syphilis, congenital/intrauterine, corneal manifestations of, 80
Systemic lupus erythematosus, eyelid manifestations of, 206t
Systemic/visceral/nodal lymphoma, 313. *See also* Lymphomas, intraocular

T cells (T lymphocytes), 15
Taches de bougie, in sarcoidosis, 147
Tapioca melanoma, 257t
Tarsal plates/tarsus, 199, 200f
Telangiectasias, retinal, parafoveal (juxtafoveal), 142, 143f
Teratoid medulloepitheliomas, 177
Teratomas, 12, 13f
Theques, 68, 216
Thermotherapy, transpupillary
 for melanoma, 272
 for metastatic eye disease, 312
Thioflavin t (ThT) stain, 39t
Thyroid-associated orbitopathy (Graves disease/thyroid ophthalmopathy), 222, 223f
Thyroid carcinoma, retinoblastoma associated with, 302t
Thyroid ophthalmopathy. *See* Thyroid-associated orbitopathy
Tissue microarrays, in immunohistochemistry, 44, 44f
Tissue preparation, for pathologic examination, 37–38, 37t, 38f, 39t
 fixatives for, 37, 37t
 processing and, 37–38
 special techniques and, 41–51, 42t
 staining and, 38, 38f, 39t
TMAs. *See* Tissue microarrays
TNM staging system
 for conjunctival carcinoma, 321t
 for conjunctival melanoma, 322t
 for eyelid cancer, 327t
 for lacrimal gland carcinoma, 328t
 for orbital sarcoma, 329t
 for retinoblastoma, 323–324t
 for uveal melanoma, 325–326t
Tomato catsup fundus, 195, 277, 279f
Tomography, optical coherence. *See* Optical coherence tomography
Topography, 12
 anterior chamber, 91, 92f
 choroidal, 179f, 181, 182f
 ciliary body, 179f, 180, 181f
 conjunctival, 53, 54f
 corneal, 73, 74f
 eyelid, 199–201, 200f, 201t
 iris, 179–180, 179f
 lens, 109, 110f
 macular, 139, 140f
 optic nerve, 237, 238f
 orbital, 219–220, 220f
 retinal, 137–138, 138f
 retinal pigment epithelium, 139
 scleral, 101–102, 102f
 trabecular meshwork, 91, 92f
 uveal tract, 179–181, 179f, 180f, 181f, 182f
 vitreous, 123–124

Touton giant cells, 15, 15f
Toxocara (toxocariasis), retinoblastoma differentiated from, 292
Toxoplasma (toxoplasmosis), retinal, 146, 147f
TPCD. *See* Typical peripheral cystoid degeneration
Trabecular beams, 91
Trabecular meshwork
 congenital anomalies of, 91–94, 93f
 degenerations of, 94–100
 disorders of, 91–100. *See also specific type*
  neoplastic, 100
 endothelial, 91, 92f
 material in, secondary glaucoma and, 95–100
 pigment in, 98–100, 98f
 in pseudoexfoliation, 95
 topography of, 91, 92f
Transillumination, 35, 35f
 in choroidal/ciliary body melanoma diagnosis, 263, 263f
 iris, in albinism, 141, 141f
 in pathologic examination, 35, 35f
Transpupillary thermotherapy
 for melanoma, 272
 for metastatic eye disease, 312
Transscleral diathermy, contraindications to, 272
Transthyretin (prealbumin), amyloid deposits and, 129, 205
Trauma. *See also* Wound healing/repair
 corneal blood staining and, 88–89, 89f
 glaucoma and, 96–97, 97f
 histologic sequelae of, 27–31, 27f, 28f, 29f, 30f, 31f
 uveal tract, 197
Traumatic recession of anterior chamber angle, 27, 27f, 97, 98f
 glaucoma and, 96–97
Treacher Collins syndrome, eyelid manifestations of, 206t
Triamcinolone, intravitreal (IVTA), for macular edema, 153–154, 153f
Trichilemmomas, eyelid, 208t
Trilateral retinoblastoma, 296
Trisomy 21 (Down syndrome/trisomy G syndrome), Brushfield spots in, 256t, 258f
TTT. *See* Transpupillary thermotherapy
Tubercles, "hard," 14, 14f
Tumors. *See also specific type of tumor and structure affected and* Intraocular tumors
 of anterior chamber and trabecular meshwork, 100
 of choroid and ciliary body, 189–193
 conjunctival, 62–71
 corneal, 89–90, 90f
 eyelid, 207–218
 iris, 187–189, 188f
 optic disc/nerve, 243–245, 243f, 244f, 245f
 of orbit, 226–236
 scleral, 106–107
 secondary, 305–312. *See also* Metastatic eye disease
  retinoblastoma and, 176, 302–303, 302t
 uveal tract, 187–197
 of vitreous, 133–135, 134f, 135f
Tunica vasculosa lentis, remnant of, Mittendorf dot, 125
Typical degenerative retinoschisis, 147
Typical peripheral cystoid degeneration, 147, 148f

Ulcus rodens, 212, 212f
Ultrasonography/ultrasound
  in choroidal/ciliary body melanoma, 262–263, 262f
  in choroidal hemangioma, 277–278, 278f
  in iris melanoma, 255, 259f
  in lymphoma, 313
  in metastatic eye disease, 309
  in retinoblastoma, 291
  in uveal lymphoid infiltration, 315
Ultraviolet light (ultraviolet radiation), eye disorders/ injury associated with
  eyelid tumors, 210, 211, 212
  spheroidal degeneration (Labrador/actinic keratopathy), 81, 81f
Uvea (uveal tract). *See also specific structure*
  congenital anomalies of, 181–182
  degenerations of, 186–187, 186t, 187f
  disorders of, 179–197. *See also specific type*
    neoplastic, 187–197
  infection/inflammation of, 183–185, 183f, 184f, 185f. *See also* Uveitis
  lymphoid infiltration and, 196–197, 315–316
  lymphoid proliferation and, 196–197
  lymphoma of, 197, 197f
  melanocytoma of, 189, 254
  melanomas of, 189–193, 191f, 192f, 193f, 194f, 249, 259–275. *See also* Choroidal/ciliary body melanoma
    nevus differentiated from, 252, 264
    staging of, 325–326t
  metastatic disease of, 194–195, 194f, 311–312
  retinoblastoma involving, 175
  topography of, 179–181, 179f, 180f, 181f, 182f
  traumatic injury of, 197
  tumors of, 187–197
    miscellaneous, 195–197
    pigmented, 275–276, 276f
  wound healing/repair and, 24–25
Uveal (posterior) bleeding syndrome (polypoidal choroidal vasculopathy), 165–167, 166f
Uveal lymphoid infiltration, 196–197, 315–316
Uveal meshwork, 91
Uveal prolapse, 197
Uveitis, 183–185
  intraocular lymphoma and, 313
  lens-induced/phacoantigenic/phacoanaphylactic, 112, 112f, 113f
  retinoblastoma differentiated from, 292t
  sarcoidosis and, 185, 185f
  sympathetic ophthalmia and, 183–184, 183f, 184f
  Vogt-Koyanagi-Harada syndrome and, 184–185

Vascular endothelial growth factor (VEGF), in retinal ischemia, 151–152
Vascular loops, peripapillary, 125
Vascular system, of retina, 138
  anomalies of, 142, 143f
  ischemia and, 151–156, 152f, 153f, 154f, 155f, 156f
Vascular tumors, of orbit, 230–231, 231f, 232f
Vasculopathy, polypoidal choroidal (posterior uveal bleeding syndrome), 165–167, 166f
Venous occlusive disease, retinal
  branch retinal vein occlusion, 159
  central retinal vein occlusion, 157–158, 158f

Verhoeff–van Gieson stain, 39t
Verocay bodies, 236, 236f
Viruses
  conjunctivitis caused by, 57, 59f
  eyelid infections caused by, 203
  optic nerve infections caused by, 240
  retinal infections caused by, 144, 144f, 145f
Visual loss/impairment
  metastatic eye disease and, 306
  in uveal lymphoid infiltration, 315
Vitelliform macular dystrophy (Best disease), 167–168
Vitelliform macular dystrophy gene *(VMD2)*, 167
Vitrectomy
  for intraocular lymphoma diagnosis, 134, 314
  for uveal lymphoid infiltration diagnosis, 316
Vitreoretinopathies, proliferative, 131, 132f
Vitreous
  amyloidosis involving, 128–129, 129f
  congenital anomalies of, 124–125, 124f
  cortex of, 123
  cysts of, 125
  degenerations of, 126–132
  development of, 123–124
    abnormalities of, 124–125, 124f
  disorders of, 123–135. *See also specific type*
    neoplastic, 133–135, 134f, 135f
  inflammatory processes affecting, 125–126, 126f
  in leukemia, 317, 318f
  primary, 124
    persistent hyperplasia of. *See* Persistent fetal vasculature
  secondary, 124
  tertiary, 124
  topography of, 123–124
  wound healing/repair and, 26
Vitreous biopsy, in intraocular lymphoma, 134, 314, 314f
Vitreous detachment, posterior, 129–130, 130f
Vitreous hemorrhage, 126–128, 127f
  retinoblastoma differentiated from, 292t
Vitreous seeds, in retinoblastoma, 289–290, 289f, 290f
  targeted therapy for, 301
Vitritis, in intraocular lymphoma, 313
VKH. *See* Vogt-Koyanagi-Harada (VKH) syndrome
VMD2 (vitelliform macular dystrophy) gene, 167
Vogt-Koyanagi-Harada (VKH) syndrome, 184–185
von Hippel, internal ulcer of. *See* Keratoconus, posterior
von Hippel disease (retinal angiomatosis), 280–281, 280f
von Hippel–Lindau syndrome, 280–281
von Kossa stain, 39t
Vossius ring, 28

Wedl (bladder) cells, 115, 116f
Wegener granulomatosis, eyelid manifestations of, 206t
Wilms tumor, aniridia and, 182
Wilson disease, 89
Wolfring, glands of, 199, 201t
Wound contraction, 21
Wound healing/repair, 21–31, 22f. *See also specific tissue*
  of cornea, 21–24, 23f
  general aspects of, 21, 22f

histologic sequelae of trauma and, 27–31, 27f, 28f, 29f, 30f, 31f
  of sclera, 24
Wyburn-Mason syndrome (racemose angioma), 282f, 283

Xanthelasma. *See also* Xanthomas
  of eyelid, 205, 205f, 206t
Xanthogranuloma, juvenile (nevoxanthoendothelioma), of iris, 256t
Xanthomas, fibrous (fibrous histiocytoma)
  orbital, 234, 234f
  scleral, 106
Xanthophyll, in macula, 139

Zeis, glands of, 201t
Ziehl-Neelsen stain, 39t
Zimmerman tumor (phakomatous choristoma), 202
Zinn, zonules of (zonular fibers), 109, 110f
  tertiary vitreous, 124
Zonal granuloma, 112
Zonular fibers
  lens (zonules of Zinn), 109, 110f
  tertiary vitreous, 124
Zonules of Zinn (zonular fibers), 109, 110f
  tertiary vitreous, 124
Zygoma, 219, 220f
Zygomycetes (zygomycosis). *See Mucor* (mucormycosis)